CANINE AND FELINE CARDIAC ARRHYTHMIAS

SELF-ASSESSMENT

Larry Patrick Tilley, D.V.M.

Diplomate, American College of Veterinary Internal Medicine
(Internal Medicine)
President
Chief Medical Officer
Department of Cardiology
Cardiopet, Inc.
Floral Park, New York

Michael S. Miller, M.S., V.M.D.

Diplomate, American Board of Veterinary Practitioners
Staff Consultant
Cardiopet, Inc.
Staff Clinician
A & A Veterinary Hospital
Long Island, New York
Cardiology Ultrasound Referral Service
Wynnewood, Pennsylvania

Francis W. K. Smith, Jr., D.V.M.

Diplomate, American College of Veterinary Internal Medicine
(Internal Medicine)
Director of OnCall Services
Chief of Medicine
Cardiopet, Inc.
Floral Park, New York

CANINE AND FELINE CARDIAC ARRHYTHMIAS

SELF-ASSESSMENT

Lea & Febiger

1993

PHILADELPHIA LONDON

Lea & Febiger
200 Chester Field Parkway
Box 3024
Malvern, Pennsylvania 19355-9725
U.S.A.
(215) 251-2230

Executive Editor—Carroll C. Cann
Project Editor—Frances M. Klass
Production Manager—Samuel A. Rondinelli

Library of Congress Cataloging-in-Publication Data

Tilley, Lawrence P.
Canine and feline cardiac arrhythmias : self assessment / Larry Patrick Tilley. Michael S. Miller, Francis W.K. Smith, Jr.
p. cm.
Includes index.
ISBN 0-8121-1517-1
1. Dogs—Diseases. 2. Cats—Diseases. 2. Arrhythmia. 4. Veterinary cardiology. I. Miller, Michael S. (Michael Steven), 1950- . II. Smith, Francis W. K. III. Title.
SF992 C37T54 1992
636.7 0896128—dc20 92–18137
CIP

NOTE: Although the author(s) and the publisher have taken resonable steps to ensure the accuracy of the drug information included in this text before publication, drug information may change without notice and readers are advised to consult the manufacturer's packaging inserts before prescribing medications.

Reprints of chapters may be purchased from Lea & Febiger in quantities of 100 or more. Contact Sally Grande in the Sales Department.

PRINTED IN THE UNITED STATES OF AMERICA

Print number: 5 4 3 2 1

DEDICATION

To my grandmother, Irene, and my grandfather, Archie, in honor of that secret correspondence within our hearts; without their love my dreams would never have been realized.

Larry Patrick Tilley

To my parents Natalie and Sylvan, brother Scott, special son Simon, life partner Robin, and mentors Dr. David K. Detweiler, Dr. Robert B. Altman, and Dr. Larry P. Tilley, all of whom have shown me the incredible beauty of life in their hearts.

Michael S. Miller

To my grandmother Demi. Thank you for the valuable lessons about the purpose of life, the power of love, and the importance of family.

Francis W.K. Smith, Jr.

PREFACE

Canine and Feline Cardiac Arrhythmias: Self-Assessment is a companion volume to ***Essentials of Canine and Feline Electrocardiography: Interpretation and Treatment,*** third edition, by Dr. Larry P. Tilley. This self-assessment book is an important teaching aid for diagnosis and treatment of cardiac arrhythmias.

This textbook is personally gratifying for us, because it employs our special choice of teaching methods—the question-and-answer method of Socrates. We believe that this method of teaching stimulates the thinking process. The readers are presented with a challenge to their diagnostic ability and are stimulated to initiate the logical process of deductive reasoning.

The main focus of this book is diagnosis of arrhythmias. Although many textbooks offer detailed and complete coverage of the topic, they rarely allow for reader interaction in the learning process. This book encourages reader interaction and provides feedback regarding the reader's ability to recognize and treat arrhythmias. The question-and-answer case format allows the reader to work at an individualized pace. A single case can be completed in several minutes. Two hundred cases are included to provide in-depth coverage of arrhythmias encountered in clinical practice. Cases are arranged randomly by rhythm diagnosis, but may progress from simple to complex. This arrangement keeps the reader challenged and allows the reader to use information learned in earlier cases to solve the more difficult cases.

Much of the material in this book is a compilation of our personal experience gained over the past 10 years, during which we evaluated thousands of transtelephonic electrocardiograms. This experience has been greatly enhanced by the extensive literature that has accumulated during these years. If one faithfully reads the introductory chapter on electrocardiography in this book or studies some of the basic electrocardiographic textbooks recommended in our reference list, a working knowledge of ECG interpretation will be gained. The reader is challenged to perfect his interpretation skills. The 200 tracings in this book provide the opportunity to practice, practice, and practice these skills.

In clinical practice, an electrocardiogram must be evaluated in conjunction with a complete data base. The cardiovascular data base consists of history, physical examination, and laboratory tests. The laboratory profile includes electrocardiogram and thoracic radiographs, and analysis of blood, urine, and extravascular fluids. Other diagnostic techniques that may be indicated for evaluation of a particular cardiovascular abnormality include cardiac catheterization, angiocardiography, echocardiography, and blood pressure determination. For organizational purposes, the cases in the book are presented in a standard format. On the front page of each case, the cardiovascular data and specific questions about the lead II ECG rhythm strip are given. The reverse side of the page gives our interpretation of the labeled tracing so that the reader can assess his ECG diagnosis. The diagnostic pearls, arrhythmia mechanisms, clinical significance, and therapeutic guidelines are included.

The electrocardiograms are presented as full-size tracings. Our hope is that the reader will gain real experience in interpreting electrocardiograms by being presented with them in much the same way as they are presented to veterinarians in a clinical setting. For quick recognition and easy understanding, we use identifying marks and arrows to draw attention to important points. Another important feature is that all electrocardiograms have been painstakingly retraced to improve clarity.

The interpretation of some electrocardiograms can be difficult. It is not uncommon to find that even after prolonged and careful studies, many practitioners and even cardiologists differ considerably in their interpretation of the same electrocardiogram. This we expect and accept. We hope that such differences of opinion will be made known to us, so that they may be evaluated and, where appropriate, introduced into subsequent editions.

An electrocardiogram has much to offer as a safe, simple, inexpensive test for the diagnosis and treatment of cardiac disease. This textbook attempts to eliminate the aura of mystery that surrounds the diagnostic and therapeutic principles of electrocardiography. The teaching principles that are presented will allow even the novice to make an intelligent assessment of an electrocardiogram. The textbook will be useful to a wide audience, and is comprehensive enough to serve as a reference for the advanced student and the veterinarian with expertise in cardiology.

We are in debt to the practicing veterinarians and their technicians who have provided us with hundreds of thousands of electrocardiograms. They have taught and stimulated us to become better students and teachers of internal medicine and cardiology. In addition to thanking veterinarians who have referred cases to us, we would like to express our gratitude to each of the veterinary students, interns, and residents who we have had the privilege of teaching. All illustrations and retraced electrocardiograms in this edition are the work of Ms. Denise Donnell. We would especially like to thank Ms. Christine MacMurray for her editorial supervision of the entire manuscript. We gratefully acknowledge the assistance of the Word Processors and Technicians of Cardiopet, Inc. Thanks are also extended to Carroll Cann and his staff at Lea & Febiger.

Floral Park, New York

Larry Patrick Tilley
Michael S. Miller
Francis W.K. Smith, Jr.

Contents

Diagnosis and Management of Cardiac Arrhythmias: Basic Concepts

Diagnosis and Management of Cardiac Arrhythmias: Basic Concepts

*To make no mistakes is not in the power of man; but from their errors and mistakes the wise and good learn wisdom for the future.**

PLUTARCH

The purpose of this self-assessment textbook is to provide the reader with an opportunity to evaluate his ability to diagnose arrhythmias by electrocardiography. Each tracing is accompanied by a short history and question on interpretation. The tracing is then shown again on the reverse side of the page with appropriate labelling and interpretation. The section on self-assessment is preceded by this review of the basic concepts of diagnosing and managing cardiac arrhythmias. We recommend that this section be reviewed first.

In general, the person best qualified to read an electrocardiogram is the clinician who is taking care of the animal. Any other person who reads the electrocardiogram should become a consultant and discuss the clinical picture with the clinician before the first interpretation is made.

The electrocardiogram must be evaluated in conjunction with a complete data base. For an evaluation of the cardiovascular system, this data base ideally consists of history, physical examination, radiographic studies and laboratory profile. The history should include age, breed, weight, medication (especially digitalis), and associated diseases. The laboratory profile should include any hematologic test-

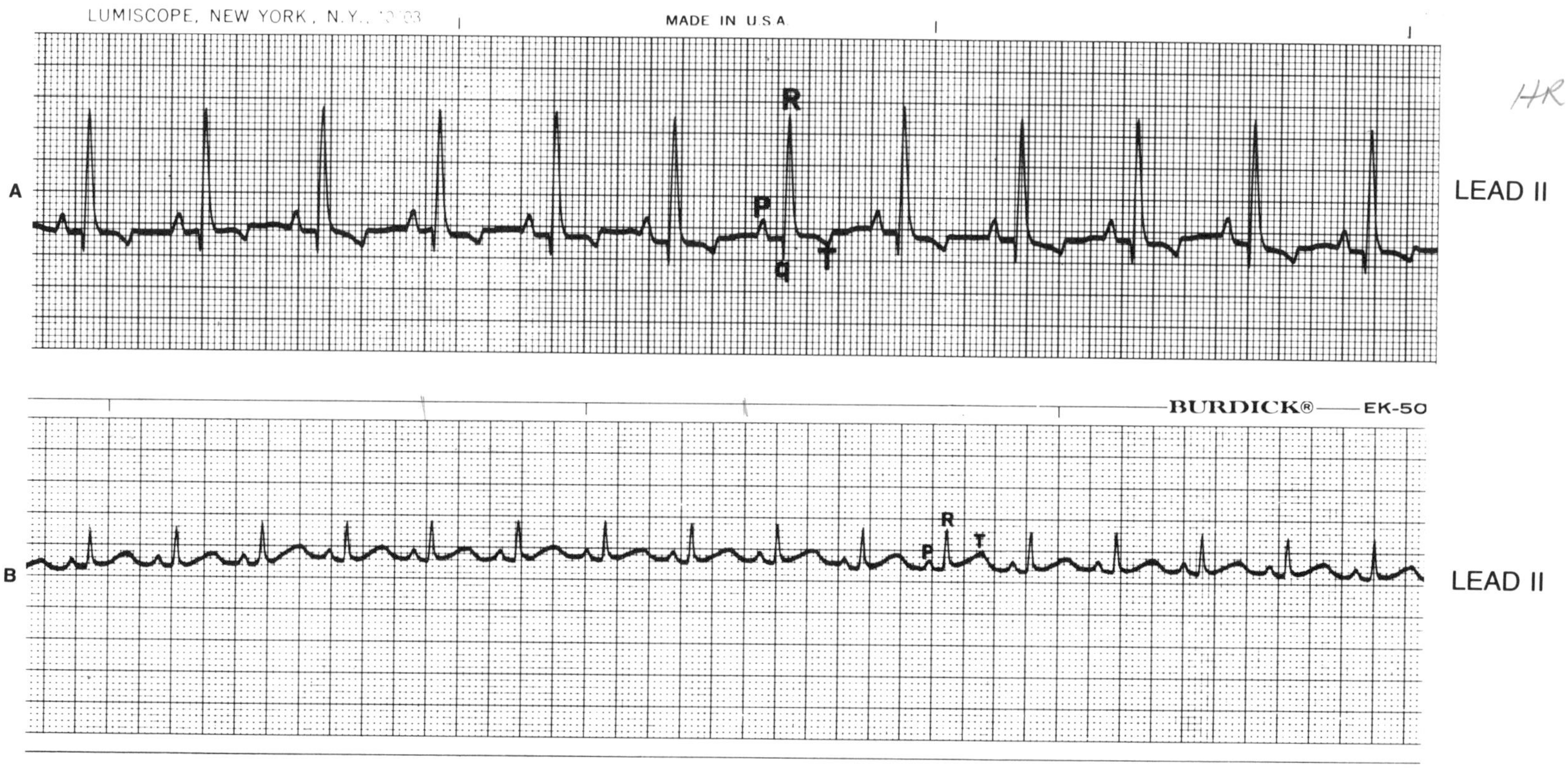

Fig. 1. A lead II rhythm strip taken at the end of a complete electrocardiographic recording is used in both dogs and cats for the first three steps in an analysis. The steps include (1) heart rate, (2) heart rhythm, and (3) complexes and intervals. The analysis of these two lead II electrocardiographic strips is normal. The clinician can readily see that the feline electrocardiographic **(B)** has a faster heart rate and smaller complexes when compared with the canine electrocardiogram **(A)**. Paper speed, 50mm/sec; standardization, 1 cm = 1 mv.

*Edwards, T. (Ed.): *The New Dictionary of Thoughts: A Cyclopedia of Quotations.* Standard Book Co., 1957.

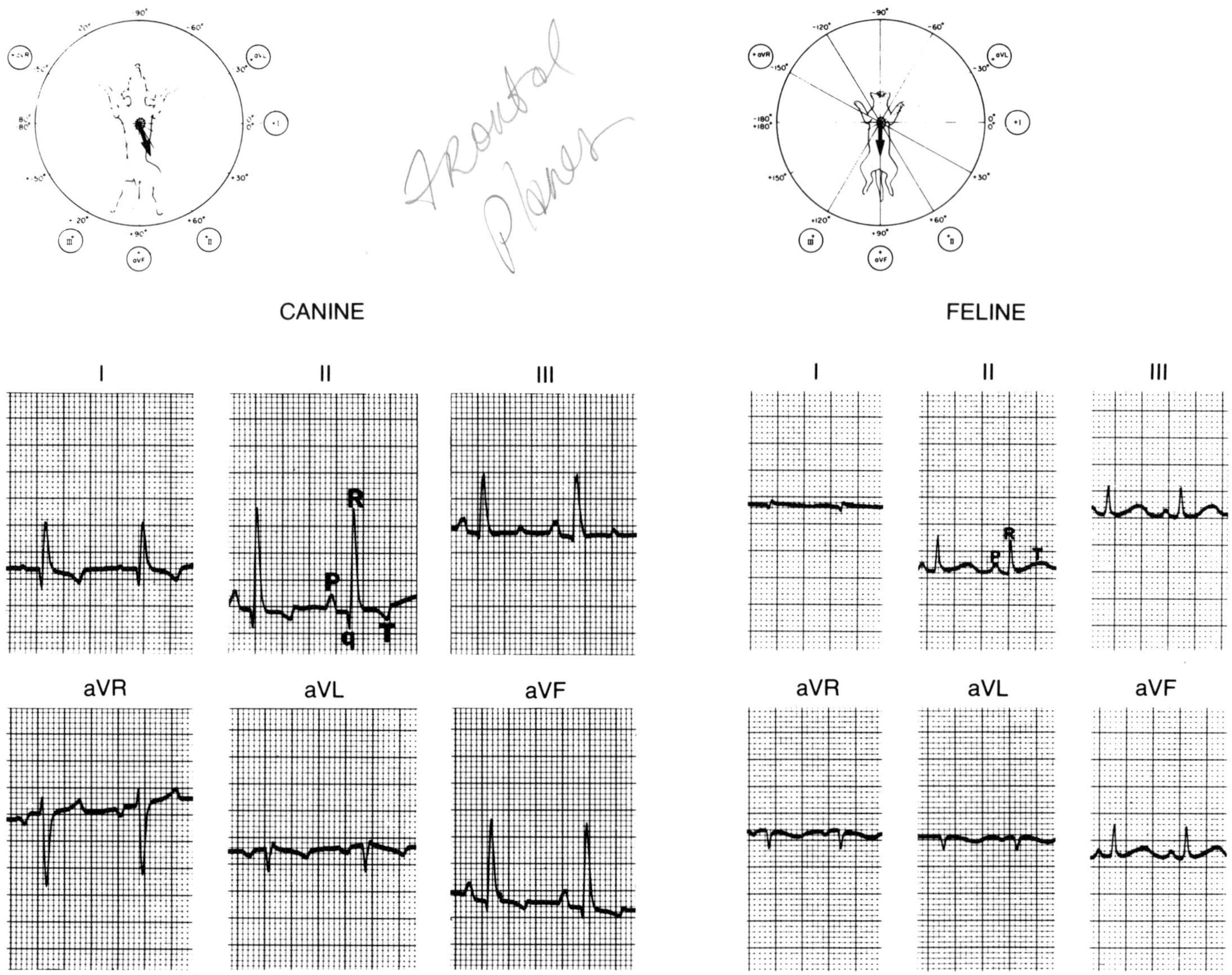

Fig. 2. For the systematic analysis of the direction and magnitude of the electrical axis of the heart, the six basis limb leads (*I, II, III, aVR, aVL,* and *aVF*) are arranged in a circular field according to the direction of each lead and the location of the positive electrodes. The mean electrical axis for this dog is +70°, and for this cat, approximately +90°.

ing, urinalysis, and evaluation of extravascular fluids. An echocardiographic study may also be necessary.

Before the electrocardiogram is examined, one should read the tracing before it is cut and mounted. Long strips of one lead must be studied for the accurate analysis of rhythm and heart rate. Lead II is usually used for the analysis of heart rate and heart rhythm and for measuring complexes and intervals.

ROUTINE APPROACH TO THE ELECTROCARDIOGRAM

The complete electrocardiogram should include at least 3 to 4 complexes of each bipolar standard lead (I, II, III), 3 augmented unipolar limb leads (aVR, aVL, aVF), and at least 15 to 20 inches of a lead II rhythm strip. The unipolar precordial chest leads (CV_5RL, also termed rV_2; CV_6LL, or V_2; CV_6LU, or V_4; and V_{10}) can also be recorded for added electrocardiographic accuracy in specific conditions. The minimum electrocardiographic recording includes a lead II rhythm strip (Fig. 1) and the 6 basic limb leads (Fig. 2).

After the complete electrocardiogram has been recorded, it must be analyzed to determine whether it is normal or abnormal. Such a determination is made measuring the various complex heights and interval lengths (Figs.3 and 4) and comparing them with normal values (Tables 1 and 2).

At least four features of every electrocardiogram should be examined systematically: heart rate, heart rhythm, P-QRS-T complexes and intervals, and mean electrical axis. The steps in analysis are as follows:

1. Calculate the heart rate.
2. Evaluate the heart rhythm.
3. Measure the complexes and intervals.
   a. P wave
   b. P-R interval
   c. QRS complex
   d. S-T segment
   e. T wave
   f. Q-T interval
   g. Basic limb leads (I, II, III, aVR, aVL, and aVF) (Fig. 2)
4. Determine the mean electrical axis.

ARRHYTHMIAS

An arrhythmia can be defined as (1) an abnormality in the rate, regularity, or site of origin of the cardiac impulse or (2) a disturbance in conduction of the impulse such that the normal sequence of activation of the atria and ventricles is altered. During normal sinus rhythm, the cardiac impulse originates in the sinoatrial (SA) node and spreads in an orderly fashion throughout the atria, through the atrioventricular (AV) node and His-Purkinje system, and throughout the ventricles.

Abnormalities of impulse formation or impulse conduction are the basic mechanisms that underlie arrhythmias and are the basis for the following classification:

Table 1. Canine

Rate
- 70 to 160 beats/min for adult dogs
- 60 to 140 beats/min for giant breeds
- Up to 180 beats/min for toy breeds
- Up to 220 beats/min for puppies

Rhythm
- Normal sinus rhythm
- Sinus arrhythmia
- Wandering SA pacemaker

Measurements (lead II, 50 mm/sec, 1 cm = 1 mv)
- P wave
  - Width: maximum, 0.04 sec (2 boxes wide)
    maximum, 0.05 sec (2½ boxes wide) in giant breeds
  - Height: maximum, 0.4 mv (4 boxes tall)
- P-R interval
  - Width: 0.06 to 0.13 sec (3 to 6½ boxes)
- QRS complex
  - Width: maximum, 0.05 sec (2½ boxes) in small breeds
    maximum, 0.06 sec (3 boxes) in large breeds
  - Height of R wave*: maximum, 3.0 mv (30 boxes) in large breeds
    maximum, 2.5 mv (25 boxes) in small breeds
- S-T segment
  - No depression: not more than 0.2 mv (2 boxes)
  - No elevation: not more than 0.15 mv (1½ boxes)
- T wave
  - Can be positive, negative, or diphasic
  - Not greater than one fourth amplitude of R wave
  - Amplitude range ±0.05 to 1.0 mv (½ to 10 boxes) in any lead
- Q-T interval
  - Width: 0.15 to 0.25 second (7½ to 12½ boxes) at normal heart rate; varies with heart rate (faster rates have shorter Q-T intervals and vice versa)

Electrical axis (frontal plane)
- +40° to +100°

Precordial chest leads (values of special importance)
- CV_5RL (rV_2): T wave positive, R wave not greater than 3.0 mv (30 boxes)
- CV_6LL (V_2): S wave not greater than 0.8 mv (8 boxes), R wave not greater than 3.0 mv (30 boxes)*
- CV_6LU (V_4): S waves not greater than 0.7 mv (7 boxes), R wave not greater than 3.0 mv (30 boxes)*
- V_{10}: negative QRS complex, T wave negative except in Chihuahua

* Not valid for thin deep-chested dogs under 2 years of age.

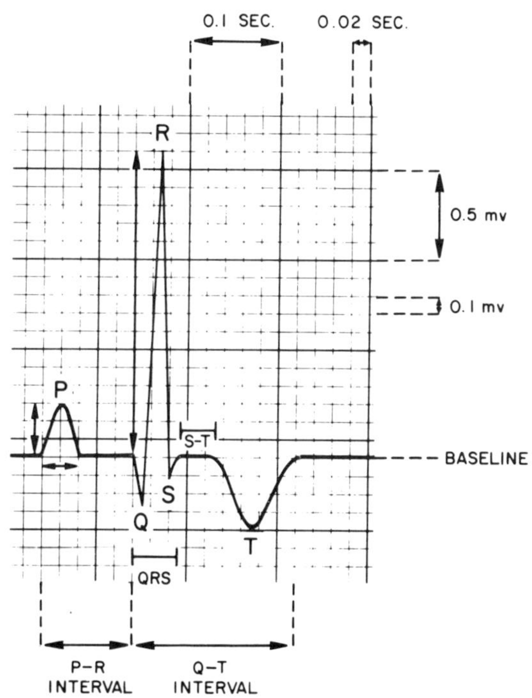

Fig. 3. Close-up of a normal canine lead II P-QRS-T complex with labels and intervals. *P*, 0.04 sec by 0.3 mv; *P-R*, 0.1 sec; *QRS*, 0.05 sec by 1.7 mv; *S-T* segment and *T* wave, normal; *Q-T*, 0.18 sec.

Sinus rhythm
- Normal sinus rhythm
- Sinus tachycardia
- Sinus bradycardia
- Sinus arrhythmia
- Wandering sinus pacemaker

Abnormalities of impulse formation
- Supraventricular
  - Sinus arrest
  - Artial premature complexes (APCs)
  - Atrial tachycardia
  - Atrial flutter
  - Atrial fibrillation
- Atrioventricular (AV) junction
  - AV junctional premature complexes
  - AV junctional tachycardia
  - AV junctional escape rhythm (secondary arrhythmia)
- Ventricular
  - Ventricular premature complexes (VPCs)
  - Ventricular tachycardia
  - Ventricular flutter
  - Ventricular fibrillation
  - Ventricular asystole
  - Ventricular escape rhythm (secondary arrhythmia)

Abnormalities of impulse conduction
- Sinoatrial block
- Persistent atrial standstill ("silent" atrium)
- Atrial standstill (hyperkalemia)
- AV block
  - First degree
  - Second degree
  - Third degree (complete heart block)

Abnormalities of both impulse formation and impulse conduction
- Pre-excitation (Wolff-Parkinson-White syndrome), reciprocal rhythm (re-entry)
- Parasystole
- Other complex rhythms

Knowledge of the anatomic and physiologic properties of the unique impulse-forming and impulse-conducting system of the atria, the AV junction, and the ventricles is essential for the accurate analysis of cardiac arrhythmias (Fig. 5).

Activation of heart muscle results from spontaneous discharge in a pacemaker and conduction of this impulse from cell to cell. The physiologic pacemaker is located in the SA node. The rate and rhythm of the heart are controlled by the SA node, so normal cardiac rhythm is termed *sinoatrial* or sinus rhythm (Fig. 5). The impulse originating there is propagated through the atria via preferential pathways leading

Table 2. Feline

Rate
- Range: 120 to 240 beats/min
- Mean: 197 beats/min

Rhythm
- Normal sinus rhythm
- Sinus tachycardia (physiologic reaction to excitement)

Measurements (lead II, 50 mm/sec, 1 cm = 1 mv)*
- P wave
  - Width: maximum, 0.04 sec (2 boxes wide)
  - Height: maximum, 0.2 mv (2 boxes tall)
- P-R interval
  - Width: 0.05 to 0.09 sec (2½ to 4½ boxes)
- QRS complex
  - Width: maximum, 0.04 sec (2 boxes)
  - Height of R wave: maximum, 0.9 mv (9 boxes)
- S-T segment
  - No depression or elevation
- T wave
  - Can be positive, negative, or diphasic; most often positive
  - Maximum amplitude: 0.3 mv (3 boxes)
- Q-T interval
  - Width: 0.12 to 0.18 sec (6 to 9 boxes) at normal heart rate (range 0.07 to 0.20 sec, 3½ to 10 boxes); varies with heart rate (faster rates, shorter Q-T intervals; and vice versa)

Electrical axis (frontal plane)
- 0 to ±160° (not valid in many cats)

Precordial chest leads
- CV_6LL (V_2): R waves <1.0 mv (10 boxes)
- CV_6LU (V_4): R wave not greater than 1.0 mv (10 boxes)
- V_{10}: T wave negative, R/Q wave >1.0

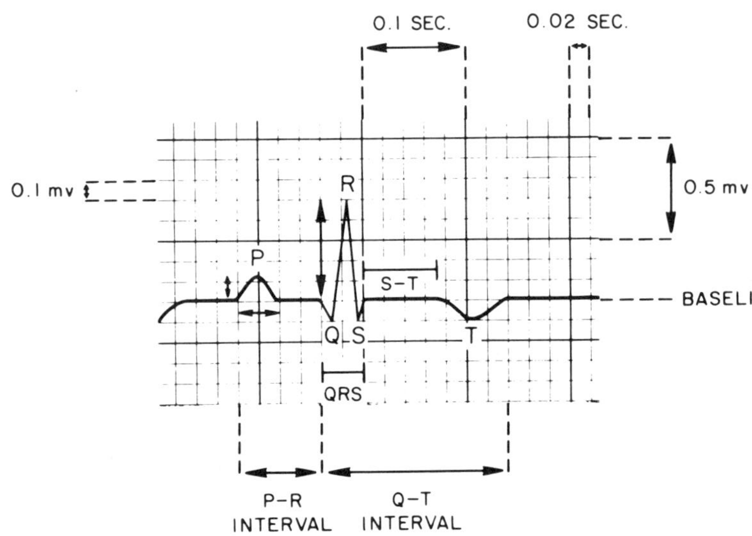

Fig. 4. Close-up of a normal feline lead II P-QRS-T complex with labels and intervals.

to the AV node. After a delay at the AV node, the impulse travels down the bundle of His, the bundle branches and their subsidiaries, and the Purkinje fiber system, which eventually comes in contact with the ventricular myocardium.

The heart has many potential pacemaking cells. The SA node has the fastest inherent discharge rate, whereas the cells in the rest of the conduction system exhibit a slower rate of impulse formation. The more distal a potential pacemaker is from the SA node, the slower is its inherent discharge rate. A normal pacemaker is under the influence of the autonomic nervous system. Its rate is constantly adjusted by autonomic impulses according to need.

RECOGNITION OF ARRHYTHMIAS—A SYSTEMATIC APPROACH

With the foregoing general knowledge of the normal anatomic and physiologic properties of the impulse-forming and impulse-conducting system of the heart (Fig. 5), and with the use of a systematic approach to the electrocardiographic strip, the accurate diagnosis of arrhythmias can be greatly simplified. A systematic approach to the accurate electrocardiographic analysis of a rhythm strip (usually lead II) for the diagnosis of arrhythmias includes the following steps.

Step 1. General Inspection of the Electrocardiogram. A determination should be made as to whether the arrhythmia is occasional, frequent, or continuous; regular or irregular; and repetitive or occurring with various combinations—in other words, whether the rhythm is normal sinus rhythm or characteristic of a cardiac arrhythmia. The heart rate should also be classified as rapid (tachycardia), slow (bradycardia), or normal.

Step 2. Identification of P Waves. This step should include determination of whether the atrial activity (P waves) is uniform or regular. The lead (usually lead II) with well-defined P waves should be used. The precordial chest leads often have P waves that are easy to see. A crucial part of the electrocardiographic examination is the identification and analysis of the P waves. Determining direction and shape of the P waves can also help in the analysis of the arrhythmia. A normal P wave (positive and rounded, as in lead II) usually indicates that the impulse is originating in the SA node. A P wave that differs from normal in shape and is upright may represent an ectopic pacemaker in the atrium. P waves that are inverted in leads I, II, III, and aVF most often indicate formation of the impulse in or near the AV junction. The absence of P waves usually signifies atrial fibrillation, atrial standstill, atrial activity of low voltage in the respective lead, or buried P waves in QRS complexes of AV junctional rhythms. In various supraventricular tachycardias, the P wave can be superimposed on a portion of the QRS complex, S-T segment, or T wave of the preceding cardiac cycle.

Step 3. Recognition of QRS Complexes. The QRS complexes should be characterized as to their morphology, uniformity, and regularity. A QRS complex of normal morphology and identical to those recorded before an arrhythmia usually indicates normal activation of

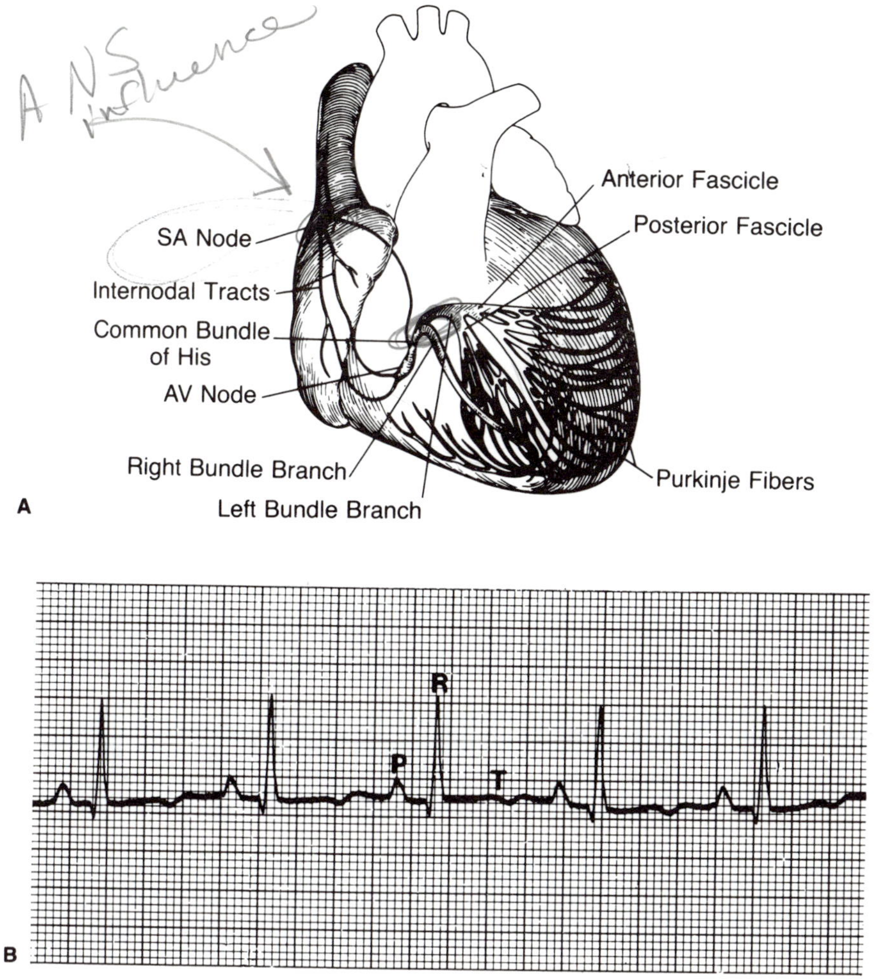

Fig. 5. A, Impulse-forming and impulse-conducting system of the heart. (From DeSanctis, R.W.: Disturbances of cardiac rhythm and conduction. In *Scientific American Medicine.* Edited by E. Rubinstein. New York, Scientific American, 1982, with permission.) **B,** The normal lead II electrocardiogram shows a normal cardiac rhythm, termed sinoatrial or sinus rhythm.

the ventricles. Such complexes may be the result of an impulse formed in the SA node or an abnormal impulse originating anywhere above the bundle of His. QRS complexes that appear normal can be categorized as "supraventricular." Wide QRS complexes with various configurations may indicate an ectopic pacemaker below the bundle of His (ventricular) or a lesion in the intraventricular conduction system.

Two other conditions associated with abnormal QRS complexes are *aberration* and *fusion* complexes. Aberration is a condition in which the impulse traveling from above the bundle of His finds a part of the ventricular conducting system still in a refractory phase. A common example of a fusion complex is the simultaneous activation of the ventricles that results when one impulse arrives from the SA node at the same time another arrives from a ventricular ectopic pacemaker.

Step 4. Relationship Between P Waves and QRS Complexes. The time from the onset of the P wave to the onset of the QRS complex is called the P-R interval, which is a measure of AV conduction. The P-R intervals are essentially constant in normal sinus rhythm.

P waves may precede normal QRS complexes by different time spans. An abnormally long P-R interval usually indicates an AV conduction delay or first-degree heart block. An abnormally short P-R interval may be seen in such conditions as accessory conduction around the AV node, or in AV junctional rhythms in which the P wave is positioned close to the QRS complex. When a P wave is not followed by a QRS complex, an AV block (also termed second-degree heart block) has occurred. The P-R interval can also lengthen gradually until the P wave occurs without a succeeding QRS complex (called Wenckebach AV block). When the P-R interval varies, the relationship of the atria and ventricles in the cardiac cycle should be determined. Complete heart block, a form of AV dissociation, represents an interrupted connection between the atria and the ventricles. One impulse-forming site is the SA node; the other is an independent ventricular escape rhythm.

By establishing the relationship of the P wave and QRS complex, the clinician can determine the dominant rhythm. The four major sites of the heart with pacemaker cells from which impulses may arise are the SA node, the atrial conduction tissue, the AV junction (AV node–His bundle region), and the ventricular conduction tissue (bundle branches and Purkinje fibers).

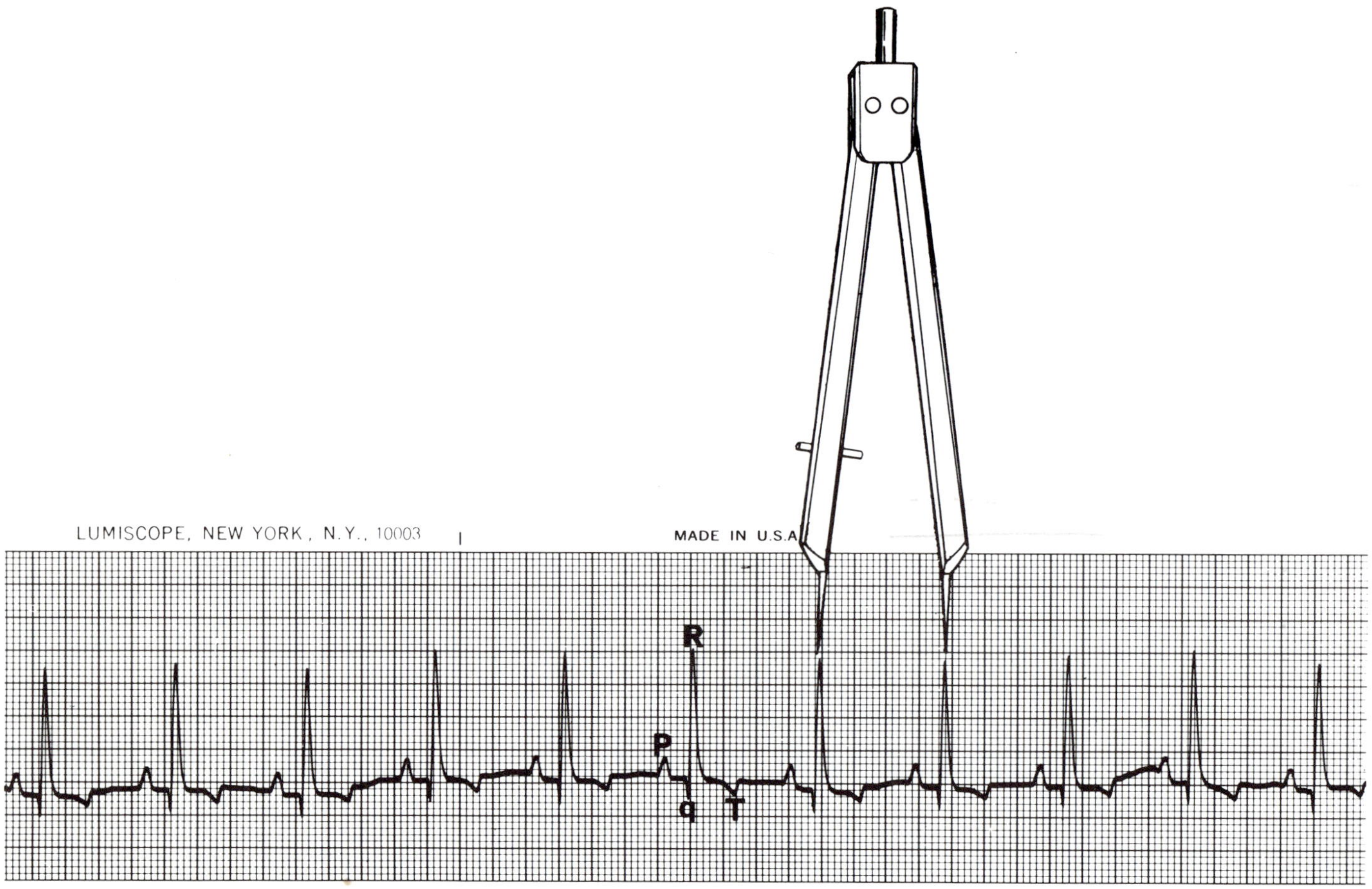

Fig. 6. Use of an electrocardiographic caliper for plotting P-P and/or R-R intervals to determine whether rhythm is regular or for locating P-QRS complexes. The QRS complexes occur at a regular rhythm in this canine electrocardiogram.

At each of these sites, impulses may originate at rates faster than, slower than, or the same as those of the normal sinus rate. Arrhythmias with rates slower than that of the sinus rate usually occur because of SA nodal depression, allowing "escape" of other pacemakers from its influences. These slow cardiac rhythms are called passive or escape rhythms. By contrast, a normally functioning SA node may not be able to act as the pacemaker because other pacemakers are abnormally forming impulses at a faster rate. These arrhythmias are then "active." Both types of abnormal impulse formation may be intermittent or persistent, repetitive, or occurring in varying combinations.

The clinician can also use electrocardiographic calipers for plotting intervals (Fig. 6). The needle points of each of the two legs are positioned over the apex of two successive P waves (or QRS complexes). If calipers are not available, a simple method is to place a card immediately beneath the apex of the P waves (or QRS complexes) that are recognized (Fig. 7), and then to make a mark on the card in conjunction with each apex of two or three P waves (or QRS complexes). The card (or caliper) can be shifted to the right or left so that the first mark falls on the next P wave (or QRS complex). When the rhythm is regular, all the marks on the card or two needle points fall under the appropriate complexes. This method often can be used to find P waves in arrhythmias in which some P waves are hidden in the QRS complexes.

Step 5. Summary of Findings and Final Classification of the Arrhythmia. By following the preceding four steps, the clinician can gather sufficient information to answer the following questions and thus determine the final interpretation of the arrhythmia.

a. What is the dominant rhythm? The dominant rhythm for most arrhythmias is sinus impulses from the SA node. An ectopic rhythm may also be dominant, such as in atrial tachycardia. Occasionally the dominant rhythm changes from the SA node to an ectopic focus (atrial, AV junction, or ventricular) on the same strip. The dominant rhythm also may change from one ectopic to another ectopic rhythm on the same strip (e.g., from atrial fibrillation to ventricular tachycardia).

b. Is the arrhythmia an abnormality of impulse formation or of impulse conduction or both? If either or both, what is the site of abnormality?

When these basic questions are answered, the final classification of the arrhythmia can be made. The terminology for arrhythmias is standard. In terms used for abnormalities of impulse formation, the first word is usually the site of the dominant rhythm (sinus, atrial, AV junction, or ventricular), and the second word indicates the rhythm or rate (e.g., "atrial tachycardia"). In terms used for abnormalities of impulse conduction, the first word is the site of the conduction defect, and the second word is the defect (e.g., "sinoatrial block").

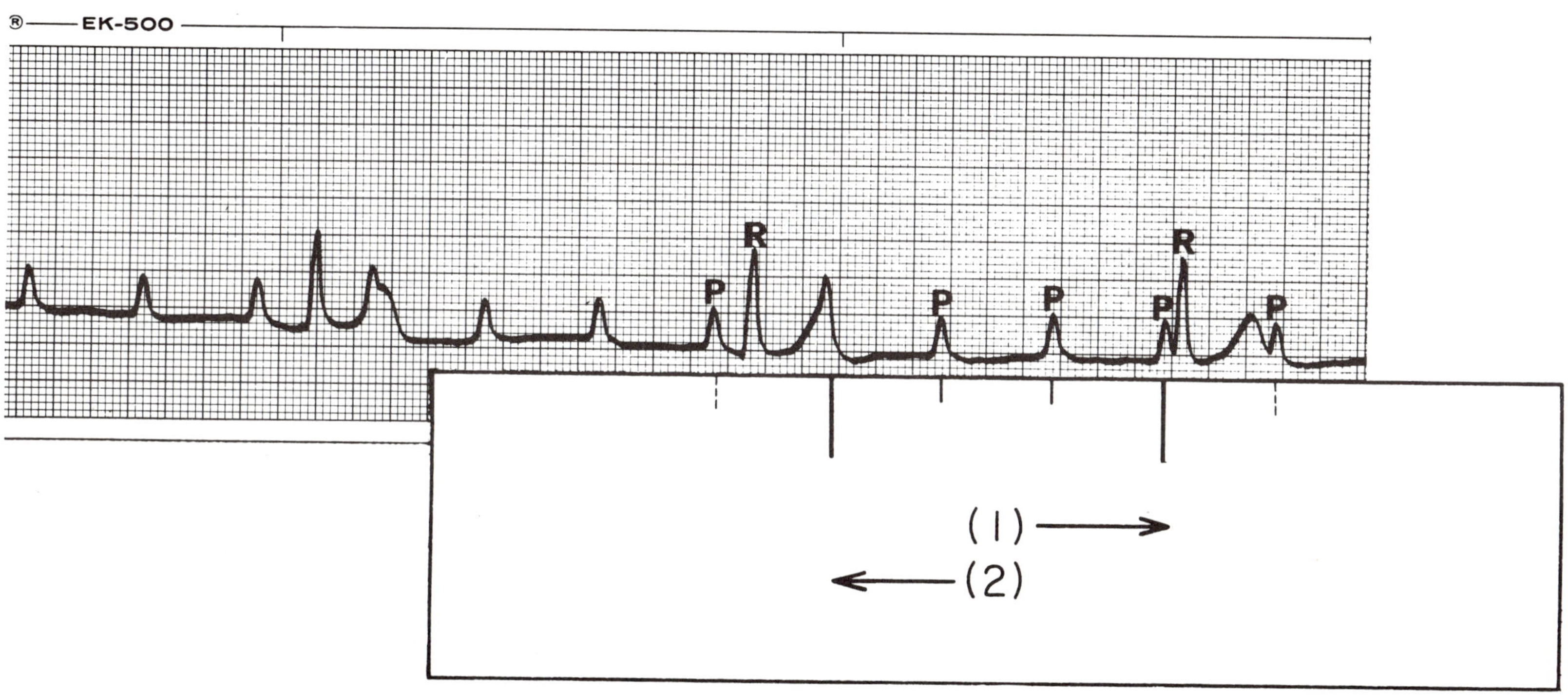

Fig. 7. Card method for examining arrhythmias. A card has been marked at two places (small dark lines) beneath the apex of two waves. By moving the card to the right *(1)*, the examiner can see that a P wave (heavy dark line) falls within an R wave. By moving the card to the left *(2)*, one determines that a P wave (heavy dark line) falls within a T wave (explaining its increased amplitude). This electrocardiogram shows an example of complete heart block.

In summary, a systematic method for accurate electrocardiographic analysis of a rhythm strip (usually lead II) for identifying arrhythmias includes the following steps:

Step 1. General inspection: heart rate and rhythm.
Is the rhythm normal sinus or characteristic of a type of cardiac arrhythmia? The heart rate should also be classified as rapid, slow, or normal.

Step 2. Identification of P waves.
Is the atrial activity regular and the shape uniform?

Step 3. Recognition of QRS complexes.
The QRS complexes should be characterized according to their morphology, uniformity, and regularity.

Step 4. Relationship between P waves and QRS complexes.

Step 5. Summary of findings and final classification of the arrhythmia.

What is the predominant rhythm? Is the arrhythmia an abnormality of impulse formation or of impulse conduction or both? If either or both, what is the site of the abnormality?

COMPLEX ARRHYTHMIAS—USING A LADDER DIAGRAM

The ladder diagram technique (Figs. 8 and 9), which is used commonly in human beings, enhances the clinician's understanding of arrhythmias. Ladder diagrams are a valuable teaching and interpretive tool and should be used in the field of veterinary cardiology. They are used primarily to explain the more complex arrhythmias when illustrating the underlying mechanisms would otherwise be difficult. Clinicians, however, should feel free to apply the ladder diagram technique to any of the arrhythmias.

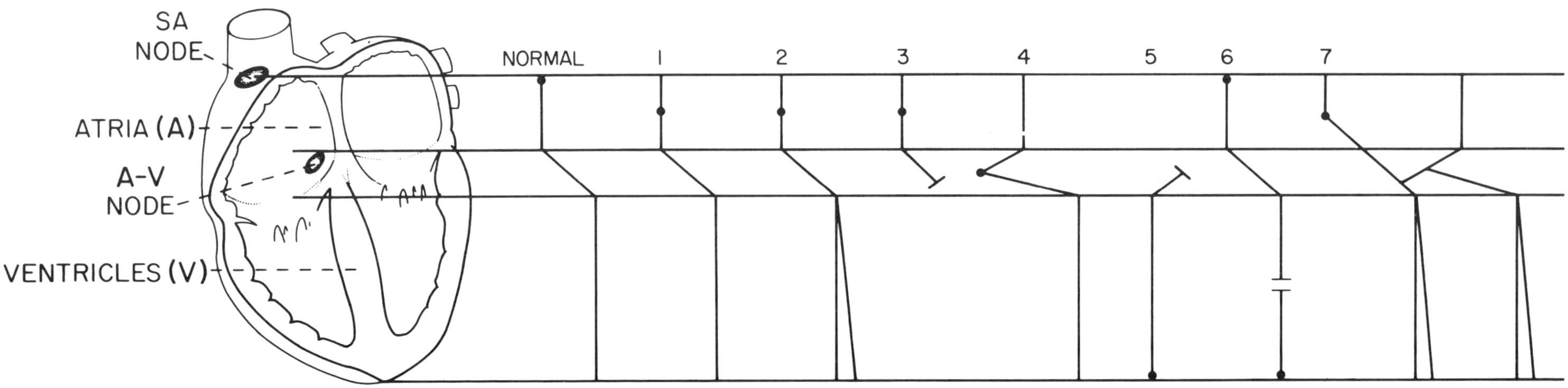

Fig. 8. Representative examples of the AV ladder diagram: **1**, Atrial premature complex (APC) with normal conduction; **2**, APC with aberrant ventricular conduction (also used to illustrate left and right bundle branches); **3**, APC not conducted; **4**, AV junctional premature complex with anterograde ventricular and retrograde atrial conduction; **5**, ventricular premature complex (VPC) with partial penetration of the AV junction; **6**, ventricular fusion complex between a sinus impulse and an ectopic ventricular impulse; **7**, APC and one reciprocal complex (re-entry) with aberrant ventricular conduction.

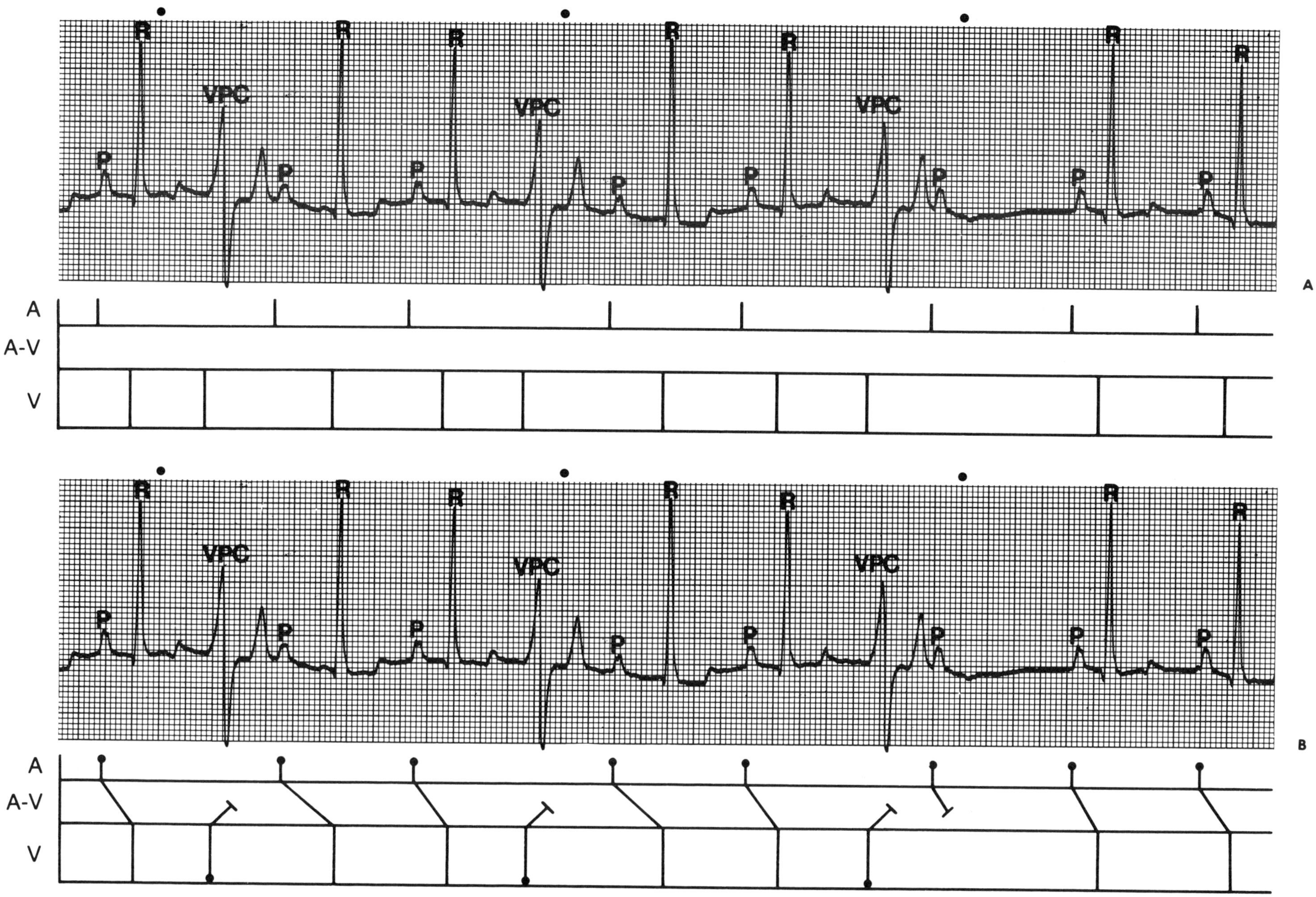

Fig. 9. How to use the AV ladder diagram. **A**, First draw the lines for the P waves (A level) and QRS complexes (V level); the lines should coincide with the beginning of the P wave and the QRS complex, respectively. **B**, Then draw a line between the A and V levels to indicate AV conduction. The site of impulse formation can be represented by a dot.

The ladder diagram easily explains the prolonged P-R interval after the first two VPCs, as well as the blocked P wave after the third VPC. The first two interpolated VPCs have penetrated the AV junction and caused the subsequent P-R interval to be prolonged. The third VPC has rendered the AV junction completely refractory, blocking the next sinus P wave. A compensatory pause exists after the third VPC.

TREATMENT

With proper electrocardiographic diagnosis and establishment of cause, most cardiac arrhythmias can be managed. Because of the growing range of possible diagnostic techniques and treatment modes, the risk of choosing the wrong therapeutic approach or even of overtreatment has increased. One must determine if the animal has been administered cardiac drugs, especially digitalis. Digitalis can cause almost every arrhythmia reported. Antiarrhythmic drugs are often more effective when the underlying cause of the arrhythmia is treated. For example, the correction of hypoxia or acid-base or electrolyte imbalance alone may eliminate an arrhythmia or make the specific antiarrhythmic drug effective. The treatment of congestive heart failure by the usual methods often terminates the existing arrhythmia.

For a complete and detailed review of the treatment of cardiac arrhythmias in dogs and cats, the interested reader is encouraged to refer to the recently published textbook and companion volume to this book, entitled *Essentials of Canine and Feline Electrocardiography, Interpretation and Treatment* by L.P. Tilley. The pathophysiologic basis of cardiac arrhythmias is discussed in Chapter 8. A detailed discussion of the use of antiarrhythmic drugs in dogs and cats can be found in Chapter 11, by Dr. John D. Bonagura and Dr. William W. Muir. Chapter 14, Cardiopulmonary Drug Formulary, by Dr. Francis W.K. Smith, Jr., contains extensive cardiopulmonary drug tables (indications, dosages, side effects, contraindications, drug interactions), digoxin dosage tables, and constant rate infusion calculation equations. Special methods for analyzing arrhythmias are discussed in Chapter 10 by Dr. Michael S. Miller and Dr. Clay A. Calvert. Chapter 12, by Dr. Philip R. Fox, reviews the special methods for treating arrhythmias, cardiopulmonary arrest and resuscitation, and pacemaker therapy.

SELF-ASSESSMENT: HELPFUL HINTS

Your approach to the electrocardiogram should be similar to the investigative methods of Sherlock Holmes. Holmes's sentences are representative of the analytic procedure needed to study the surface electrocardiogram:

"It was invisible. I only saw it because I was looking for it."

"As a rule, the more bizarre a thing is, the less mysterious it proves to be."

"I have trained myself to see what others overlook."

"Never trust upon general impressions, but concentrate yourself upon details."*

*Conan Doyle, A.: *The Illustrated Sherlock Holmes Treasury: A Facsimile of the Original Publications in Strand Magazine, 1901-1905.* New York, Avenue Books, 1976.

These quotations will be useful when you start to test yourself on the series of case studies in this textbook. Electrocardiographic diagnosis can be deduced from simple observation and logical analysis of the electrical events.

If you have faithfully read this introductory review of electrocardiography or have studied some of the basic electrocardiographic textbooks recommended in the reference list, you should have gained a working knowledge of ECG interpretation. You must now perfect your interpretative skills. The 200 tracings in this book give you the opportunity to practice, practice, practice these skills.

Because these tracings are a self-test, you can measure your progress and determine your strengths and weaknesses. If your answer disagrees with the given answer, re-evaluate your measurements and learn from your mistakes. Remember, some of the interpretations may be open to debate. Interpretation of surface electrocardiograms is not an exact science. Prominent cardiologists have been known to disagree over the interpretation of some tracings.

After you have determined the correct electrocardiographic diagnoses, answer the questions on diagnosis and treatment. Only by answering all these questions can this self-assessment teaching approach be useful. The ECG interpretation, when integrated with pertinent clinical findings and results of other diagnostic procedures, enables one to arrive confidently at a diagnosis.

This book should only be the beginning. You must constantly practice the skills you have learned here to perfect your interpretative abilities. **Remember, throughout the book, except where noted, electrocardiograms are lead II and were recorded at a paper speed of 50 mm/sec and a standard amplitude of 1 cm = 1 mv.**

RECOMMENDED TEXTBOOK READINGS

1. Allen, D.G., and Kruth, S.A.: *Small Animal Cardiopulmonary Medicine.* Toronto, B.C. Decker, 1988.
2. Bonagura, J.D. (Ed.): *Contemporary Issues in Small Animal Practice; Cardiology.* Volume 7. New York, Churchill Livingstone, 1987.
3. Chung, E.K.: *Manual of Cardiac Arrhythmias.* New York, York Medical Books, 1986.
4. Collet, M., and LeBobinnec, G.: *Electrocardiographie et rhythmologie canines.* Paris, Editions du Point Veterinaire, 1991.
5. Detweiler, D.K.: The dog electrocardiogram: A critical review. In *Comprehensive Electrocardiography: Theory and Practice in Health and Disease.* Edited by P.W. MacFarland and T.D.V. Lawrie. New York, Pergamon Press, 1988.
6. Edwards, N.J.: *Bolton's Handbook of Canine and Feline Electrocardiography.* 2nd Edition. Philadelphia, W.B. Saunders, 1987.
7. Ettinger, S.J., and Suter, P.F.: *Canine Cardiology.* Philadelphia, W.B. Saunders, 1970.
8. Fish, C.: *Electrocardiography of Arrhythmias.* Philadelphia, Lea & Febiger, 1990.
9. Fox, P.S. (Ed.): *Canine and Feline Cardiology.* New York, Churchill Livingstone, 1990.
10. Friedman, H.H.: *Diagnostic Electrocardiography and Vectorcardiography.* 3rd Edition. New York, McGraw-Hill, 1985.
11. Gompf, B., Tilley, L.P., and Harpster, N. (Eds.): *Nomenclature and Criteria in Diseases of the Heart and Vessels (Small Animal Medicine).* Denver, American Animal Hospital Association and The Academy of Veterinary Cardiology, 1986.

12. Hamlin, R.L. (Guest Ed.): Efficacy of cardiac therapy. Vet. Clin. North Am. (Small Anim. Pract.), *21(5)*: 1991.
13. Horwitz, L.N.: *Current Management of Arrhythmias.* Philadelphia, B.C. Decker, 1991.
14. Liu, S-k., Hsu, F.S., and Lee, R.C.T.: *An Atlas of Cardiovascular Pathology.* Taiwan, Wonder Enterprise, 1989.
15. Mandel, W.J.: *Cardiac Arrhythmias: Their Mechanisms, Diagnosis, and Management.* Philadelphia, J.B. Lippincott, 1987.
16. Marriott, H.J.L., and Conover, M.B.: *Advanced Concepts in Arrhythmias.* 2nd Edition. St. Louis, C.V. Mosby, 1989.
17. Miller, M.S., Tilley, L.P., and Detweiler, D.K.: Cardiac electrophysiology. In *Duke's Physiology.* 11th Edition. Edited by M.J. Swenson. Ithaca, N.Y., Cornell University, 1993 (in press).
18. Murtaugh, R.J., and Kaplan, P.M.: *Veterinary Emergency and Critical Care Medicine.* St. Louis, Mosby Yearbook, 1991.
19. Pick, A., and Langendorf, R.: *Interpretation of Complex Arrhythmias.* Philadelphia, Lea & Febiger, 1979.
20. Tilley, L.P. (Guest Ed.): Cardiopulmonary diagnostic techniques. Vet. Clin. North Am. (Small Anim. Pract.) *13(2)*: 1983.
21. Tilley, L.P.: *Essentials of Canine and Feline Electrocardiography. Interpretation and Treatment.* 3rd Edition. Philadelphia, Lea & Febiger, 1992.
22. Tilley, L.P. (Guest Ed.): Feline cardiology. Vet. Clin. North Am. (Small Anim. Pract.), *7(2)*: 1977.
23. Tilley, L.P., and Owens, J.M.: *Manual of Small Animal Cardiology.* New York, Churchill Livingstone, 1985.
24. Tilley, L.P., Smith, F.W.K., and Miller, M.S.: *Cardiology Pocket Reference.* 2nd Edition. Denver, American Animal Hospital Association, 1993.

Case 1

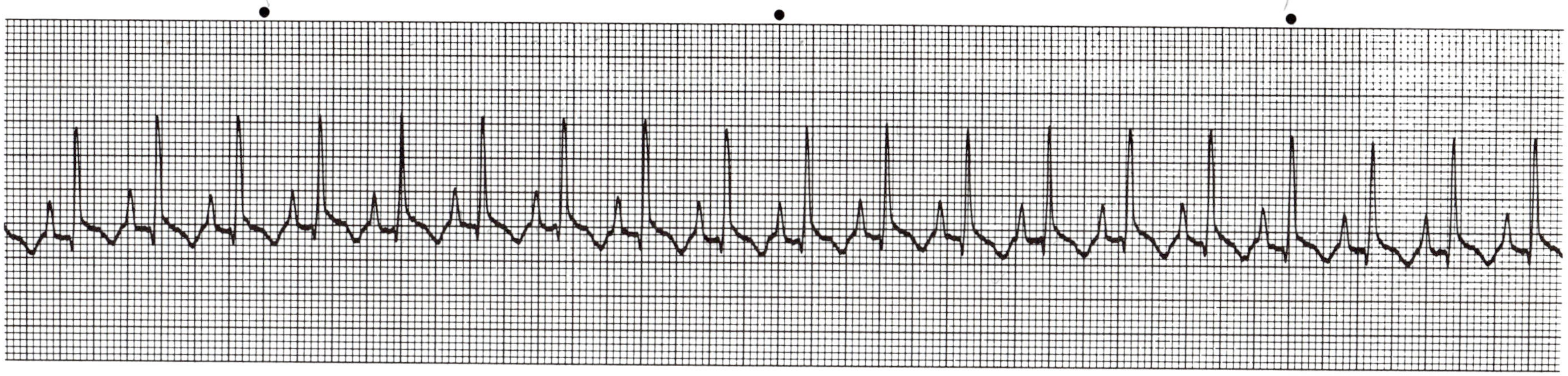

Question: This rhythm strip was recorded from a dog with a fever.

1. What is the rhythm diagnosis?
2. What is the best therapeutic approach?

Case 2

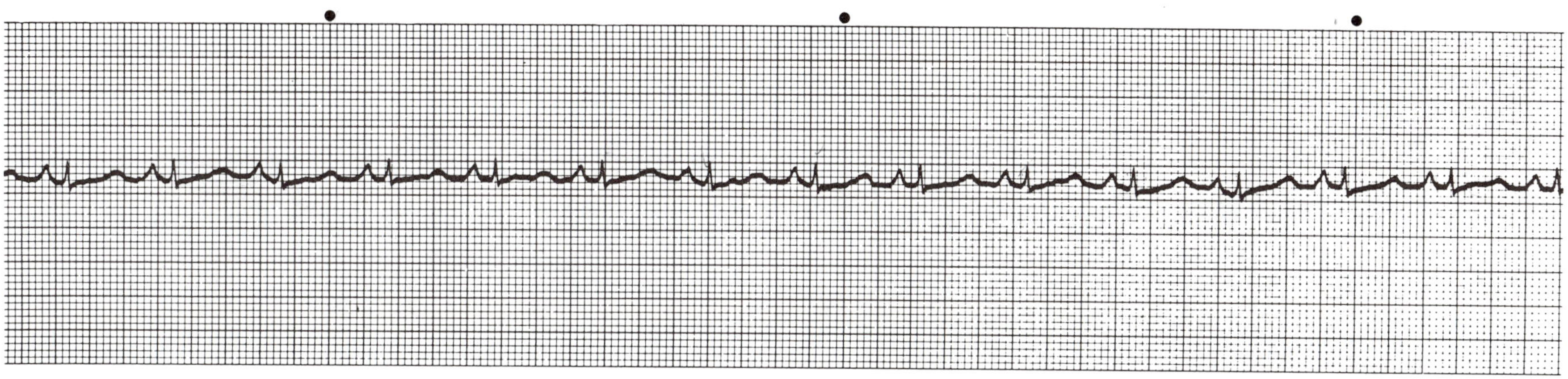

Question: This tracing was recorded from a cat that was undergoing evaluation for surgery.

1. What is the rhythm diagnosis?

Case 1

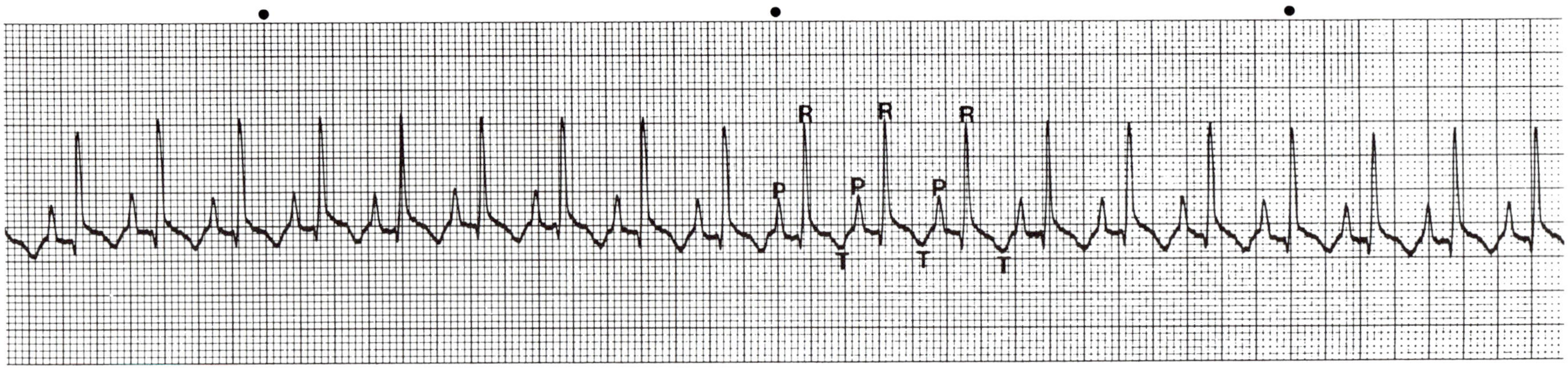

Answer: Sinus tachycardia. Heart rate is 260 beats/min. Approximate rate determined by counting the approximate number of R-R intervals between 2 sets of dots and multiplying by 20, i.e., $13 \times 20 = 260$. This arrhythmia should be approached by simply identifying and eliminating the underlying factor. For example, antibiotics were administered to the dog for a bacterial infection that was causing the fever. The infection and accompanying sinus tachycardia eventually were eliminated. If the sinus tachycardia is a result of congestive heart failure, digoxin to control the heart rate is indicated. The short P-R interval and increase in amplitude of the P wave can be normal variants in fever, anemia, hyperthyroidism, and other heightened adrenergic states.

Case 2

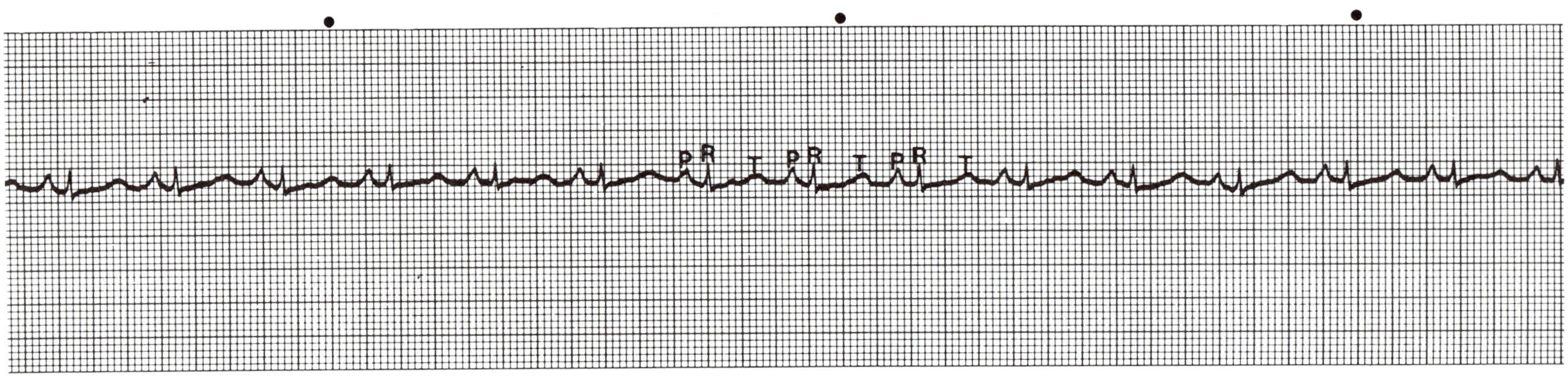

Answer: Normal sinus rhythm. Heart rate is 190 beats/min ($9\frac{1}{2}$ R-R intervals between 2 sets of dots $\times 20 = 190$). By way of review, the following steps should be used for analyzing any rhythm strip: (1) general inspection of the electrocardiogram—heart rate (normal on strip) and rhythm (regular on this strip; sinus arrhythmia rare in cats), (2) identification of the P waves, (3) recognition of the QRS complexes (R normally small), (4) the relationship between P waves and QRS complexes (constant in this strip), and (5) summary of findings with final classification of the arrhythmia (normal sinus rhythm).

Case 3

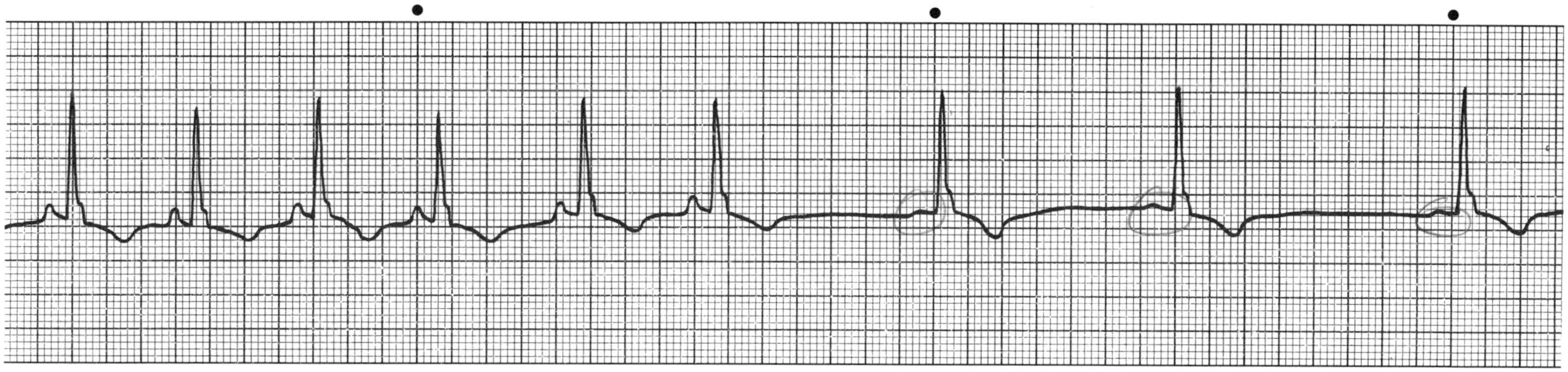

Question: This lead II ECG was obtained from a 12-year-old Miniature Poodle with no clinical signs. A grade IV/VI holosystolic murmur was heard over the left fifth intercostal space. → Mitral ?

1. What is the rhythm diagnosis? SINUS ARRHYTHMIA
2. What is the best therapeutic approach? WORK UP the Heart murmur – this rhythm is probably a NON - issue

HR = 100

IRRegular R→R interval
Short P→R interval
Smaller P waves w/ prolonged interval beats

Case 4

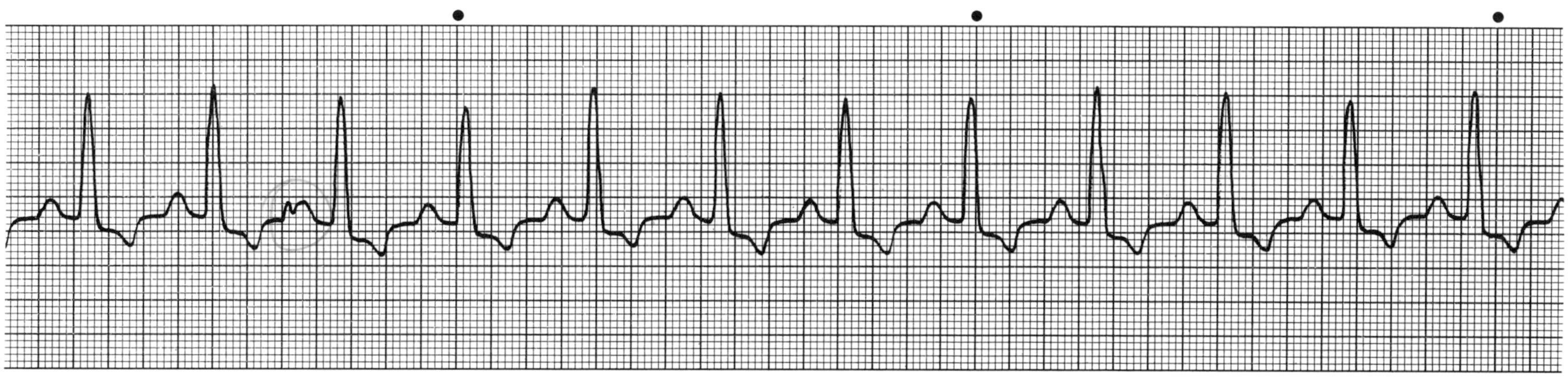

Question: This lead II ECG was obtained from a 3-year-old Labrador Retriever with no clinical signs. A loud murmur was heard on auscultation during routine physical examination.

1. What is the rhythm diagnosis? Normal Sinus Rhythm
2. What is the most likely underlying disorder? Atrial enlargement or mild pathology
3. What is the best therapeutic approach? Work up the murmur

HR = 180
Regular R→R

One notched P wave ~ abnormal atrial conduction?

Case 3

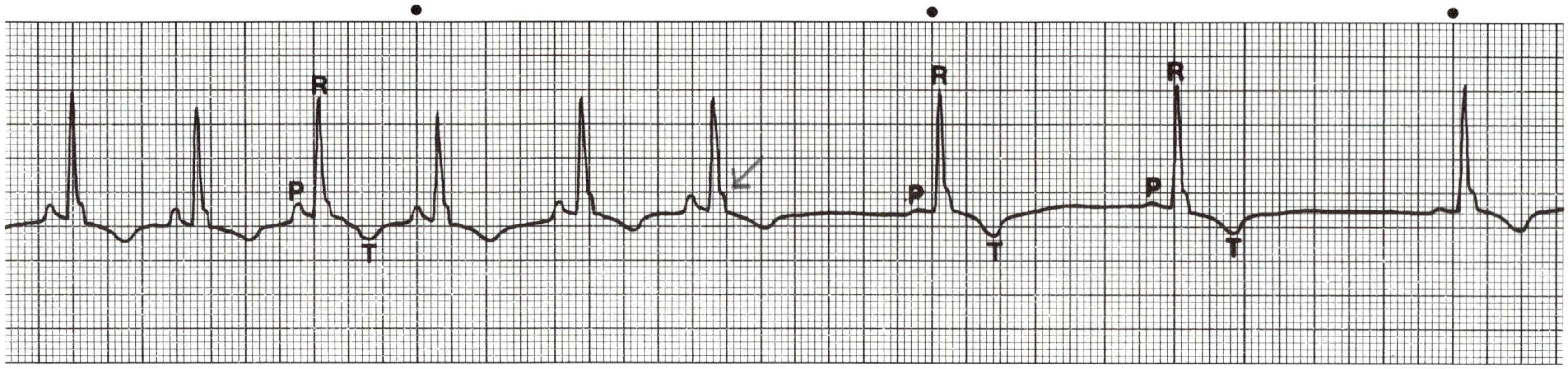

Answer: Sinus arrhythmia with a wandering sinus pacemaker. Heart rate is 100 to 110 beats/min. Sinus arrhythmia and a wandering sinus pacemaker (change in P wave amplitudes) are both normal variants caused by changing levels of vagal tone. Sinus arrhythmia represents alternating periods of slower and more rapid heart rates, usually related to respiration. The heart rate increases with inspiration and decreases with expiration. Respiratory sinus arrhythmia is a normal finding in dogs. A wandering sinus pacemaker is a shift of the pacemaker from within the SA node or from the SA to the AV node. This is a frequent normal finding in dogs, and does not require treatment. The notching on the downslope of the QRS complex is thought to result from myocardial fibrosis caused by a microscopic intramural myocardial infarction, which does not require treatment. Myocardial infarction caused by a blockage of the main coronary arteries and involving large areas of the myocardium is common in humans, but is uncommon in dogs.

Case 4

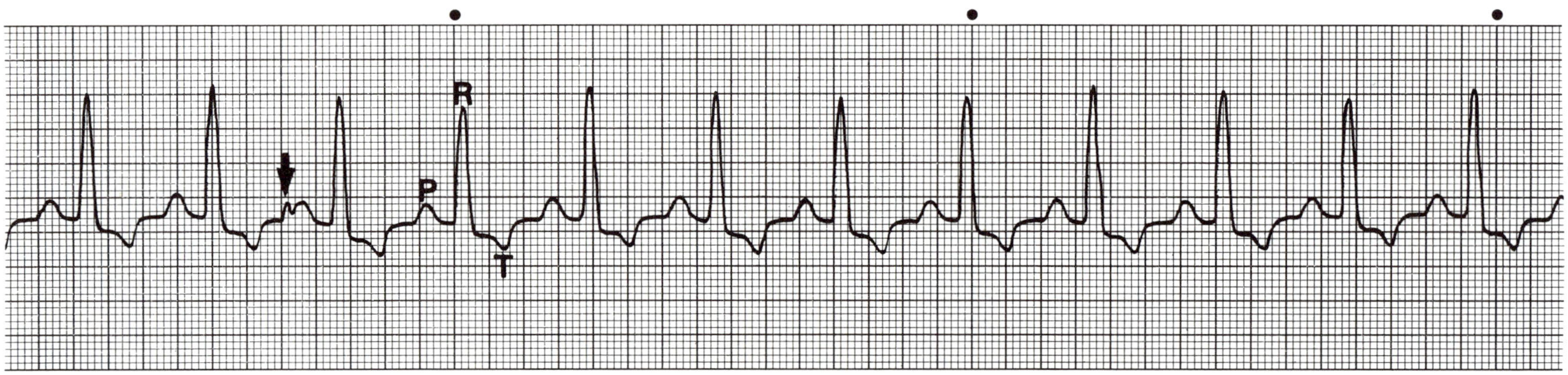

Answer: Sinus rhythm. Heart rate is 165 beats/min. The complex marked with an arrow is an artifact. The artifact does not interrupt the normal sinus P-QRS-T complexes. Artifacts are common and are caused by patient movement, electrical interference, and poor ECG electrode contact with the skin. An artifact can be confused with an active ECG abnormality, and if not recognized, this confusion can result in unnecessary treatment. No treatment is required in this dog. Notice the increased width of the P waves (p mitrale), which is probably correlated with left atrial dilation. A follow-up ECG should be done in 1 to 2 months, because the wide P waves may be a harbinger of atrial arrhythmias, including atrial fibrillation.

Case 5

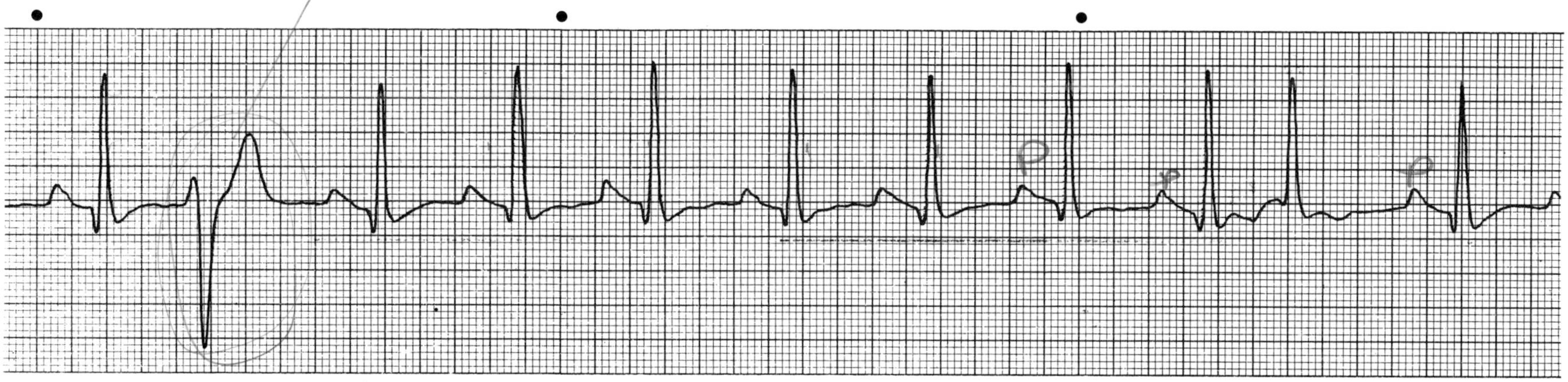

Question: This rhythm strip was obtained from an 8-year-old Poodle with a grade V/VI holosystolic mitral valvular murmur and a history of nocturnal coughing.

1. What is the rhythm diagnosis?
2. What is the most likely underlying disorder?
3. What is the best therapeutic approach?
4. What rhythm disturbance should be anticipated?

Case 6

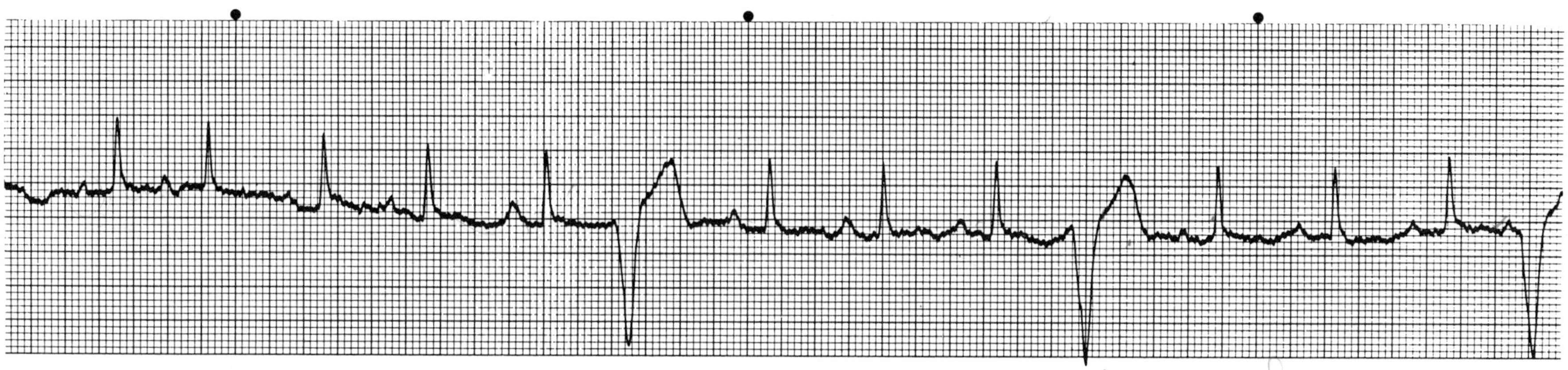

Question: This rhythm strip was recorded from a cat with hypertrophic cardiomyopathy and heart failure.

1. What is the rhythm diagnosis?
2. What is the best therapeutic approach?

Case 5

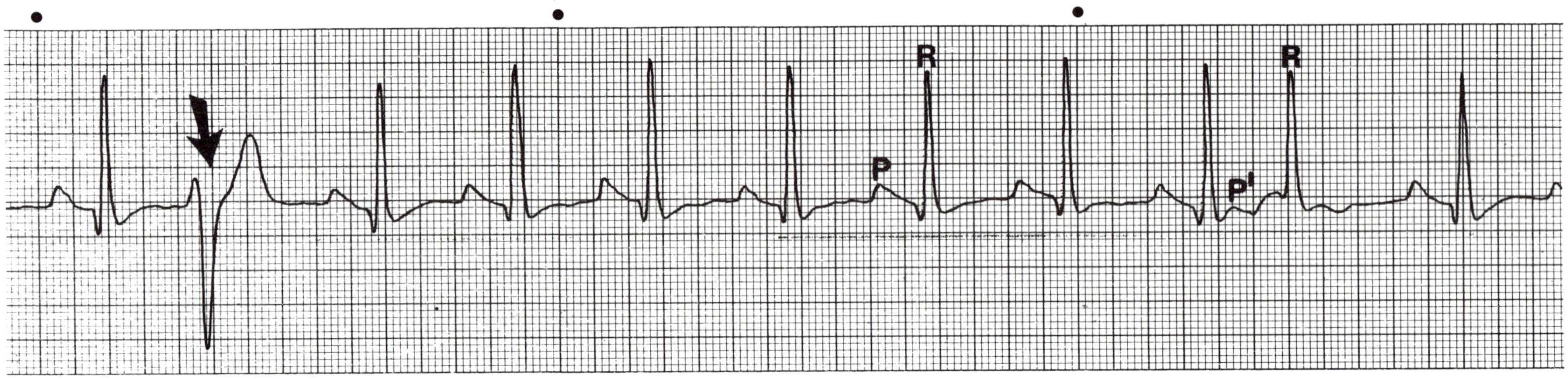

Answer: Sinus rhythm with one ventricular premature complex and one atrial premature complex. Heart rate is 160 beats/min. The atrial premature complex is probably caused by left atrial distention, a supposition supported by the extremely wide P waves (0.06 sec). Atrial enlargement is probably the result of degenerative valve disease in this small-breed dog. The atrial premature complex can be distinguished from a ventricular premature complex (arrow) by the presence of a P′ wave (labeled) in the S-T segment of the preceding complex. The morphology of the atrial premature complex is also similar to that of the sinus QRS complexes. The arrhythmias do not occur with sufficient frequency to warrant antiarrhythmic therapy at this time. If edema is present, the dog should be treated with diuretics and probably vasodilators. This combination therapy should decrease atrial dimensions, decrease wall stress on the ventricle, and indirectly abolish the arrhythmias. This dog should be closely monitored by frequent ECGs. The prolongation of the P waves raises concern that the dog will go into atrial fibrillation in the near future.

Case 6

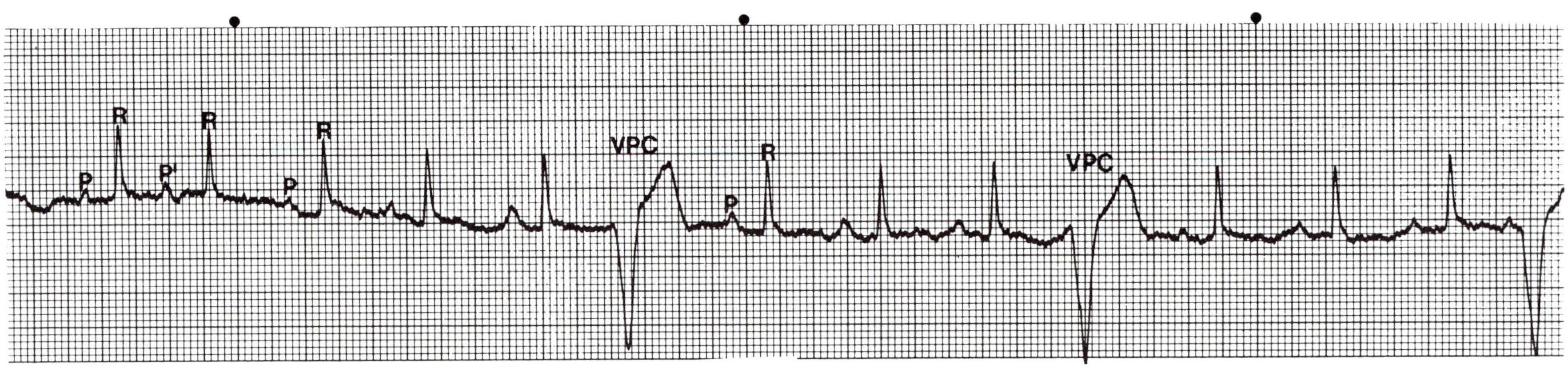

Answer: Normal sinus rhythm with three ventricular premature complexes (VPCs) of probable left ventricular origin (pattern similar to right bundle-branch block) and one atrial premature complex. Heart rate is approximately 175 beats/min. A rhythm strip should always be evaluated from left to right while constantly looking for premature complexes or pauses in the rhythm. The second complex is an atrial premature complex. The P′ wave and the QRS complex are both premature. The QRS complexes of the ventricular premature complexes are wide and bizarre. They also are not associated with P waves. These arrhythmias disappeared after the heart failure was treated with cage rest and diuretics. The presence of some minor artifact is indicated by the jagged baseline. Good electrode contact with the skin was probably not obtained.

Case 7

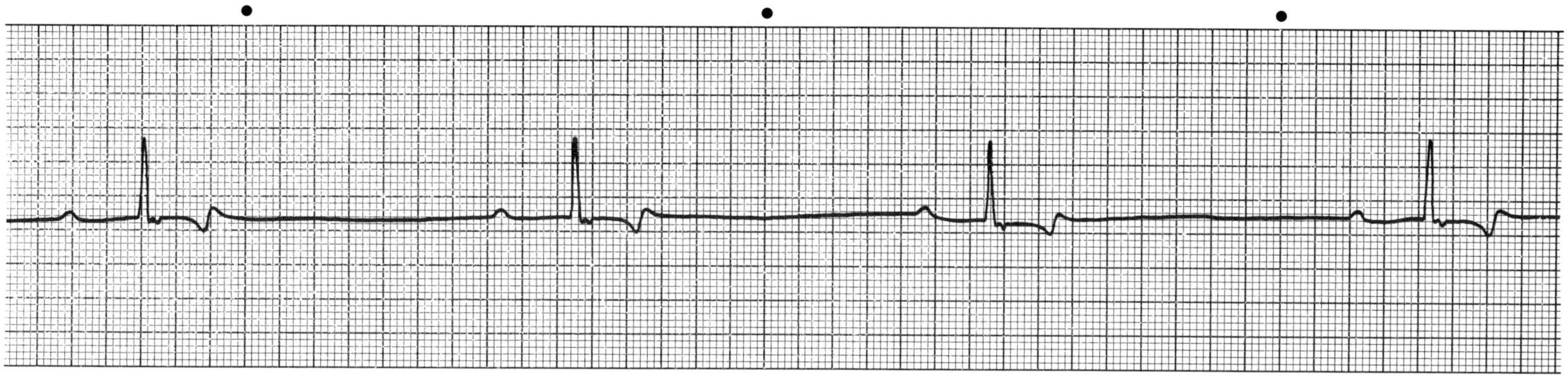

Question: This rhythm strip was recorded from a 12-year-old Boston Terrier. The dog had no clinical signs. The ECG was obtained as part of a geriatric workup.

1. What is the rhythm diagnosis?
2. What are common causes of this arrhythmia?
3. What is the best therapeutic approach?
4. What advice should be given to the owners?

Case 8

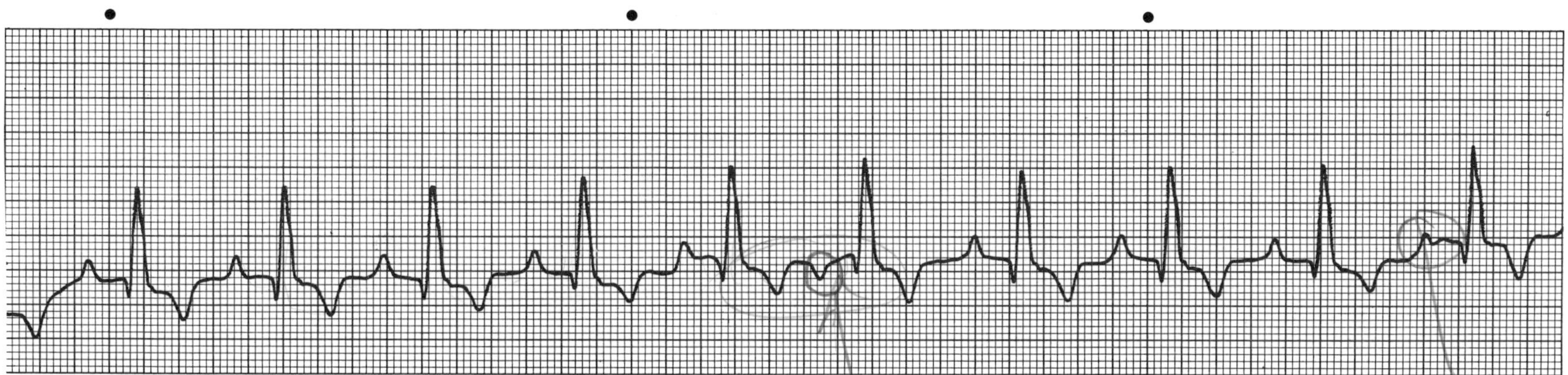

Question: This lead II ECG was obtained from a 7-year-old Miniature Schnauzer with no clinical signs. An irregular heart rhythm was heard on auscultation.

1. What is the rhythm diagnosis?
2. What is the best therapeutic approach?

Case 7

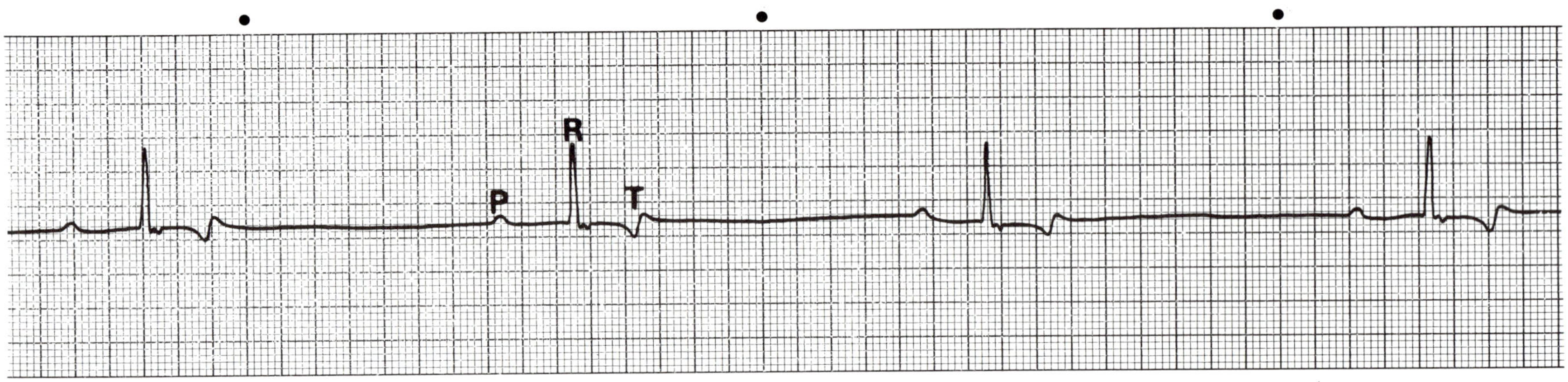

Answer: Sinus bradycardia with first-degree AV block. Heart rate is approximately 50 beats/min. Common causes of sinus bradycardia include sinus node disease, conditions that increase vagal tone, hypothyroidism, hypothermia, and drug therapy. First-degree AV block (P-R interval >0.13 sec) is associated with degeneration and fibrosis of the AV node, increased vagal tone, and drug therapy. Treatable causes of bradycardia, such as hypothyroidism, should be ruled out. Animals show great variation in the degree of bradycardia necessary to elicit clinical signs. While this dog had no clinical signs and a heart rate of 50, another animal might be weak or syncopal. Treatment should be dictated by clinical signs and not by the heart rate. This dog does not require treatment. The owners should be alerted to watch for signs of exercise intolerance, weakness, and collapse. If signs develop, a trial course of anticholinergic therapy with propantheline or isopropamide would be recommended.

Case 8

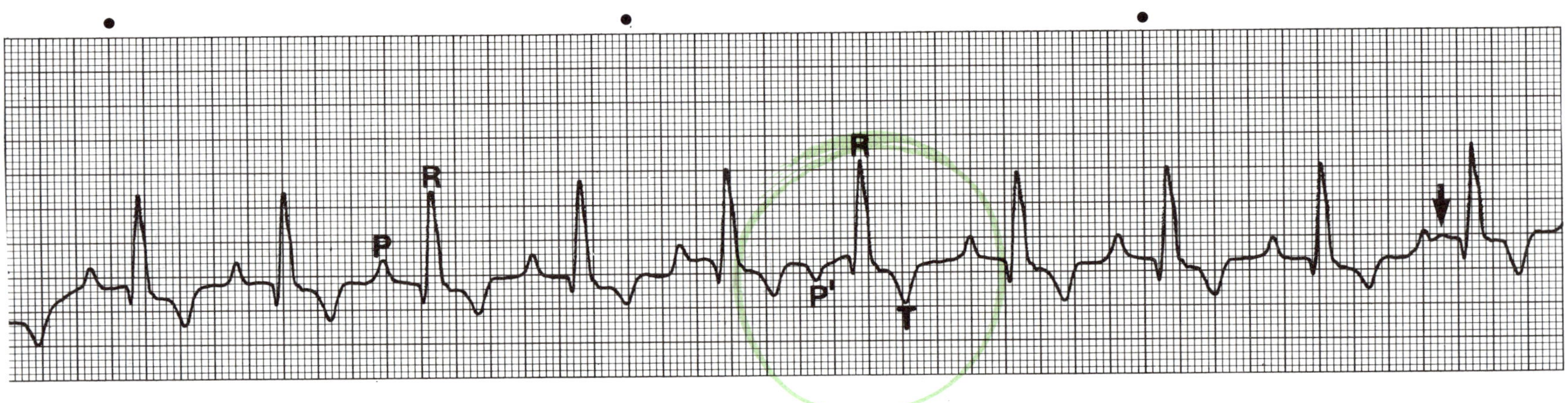

Answer: Sinus rhythm with one atrial premature complex. Heart rate is 130 beats/min. The dog has no clinical signs; thus, treatment is not required initially. The QRS complex after the premature P′ wave is similar to the QRS complexes of the sinus beats, one of the important criteria for atrial premature complexes. Because the atrial premature complex (negative P′ wave) cannot be distinguished from an atrial ectopic complex arising from a low atrial focus, the term "supraventricular premature complex" can be used. The seemingly ectopic complex marked with an arrow is artifact, because it does not interrupt the cardiac rhythm and is too close to the QRS complex to allow double depolarization of the ventricles.

Case 9

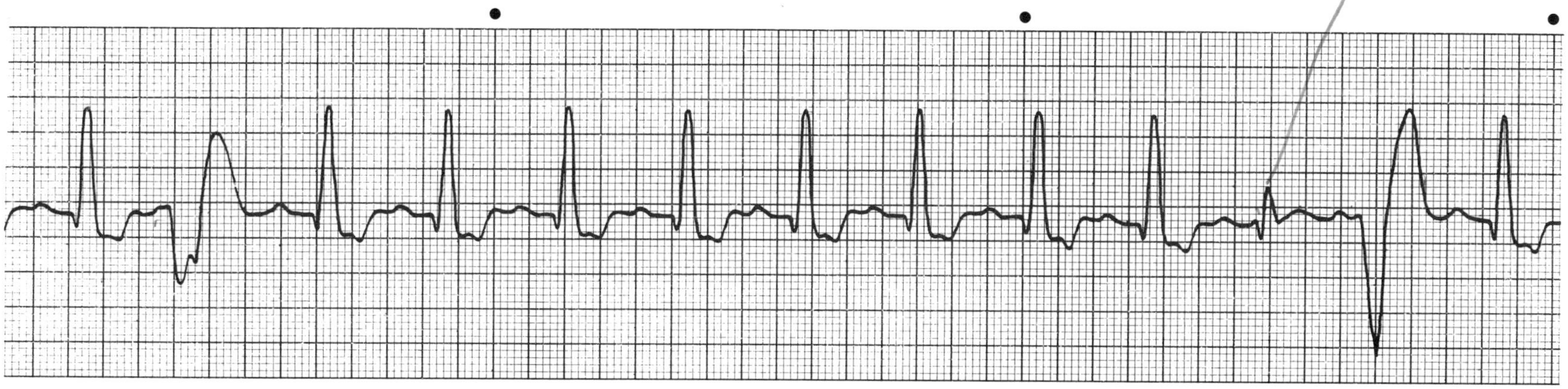

Question: This rhythm strip was recorded from a 6-year-old King Charles Spaniel with a history of congestive heart failure that was being treated with furosemide and enalapril. The dog was examined because of lethargy.

1. What is the rhythm diagnosis?
2. What is the best therapeutic approach?

Case 10

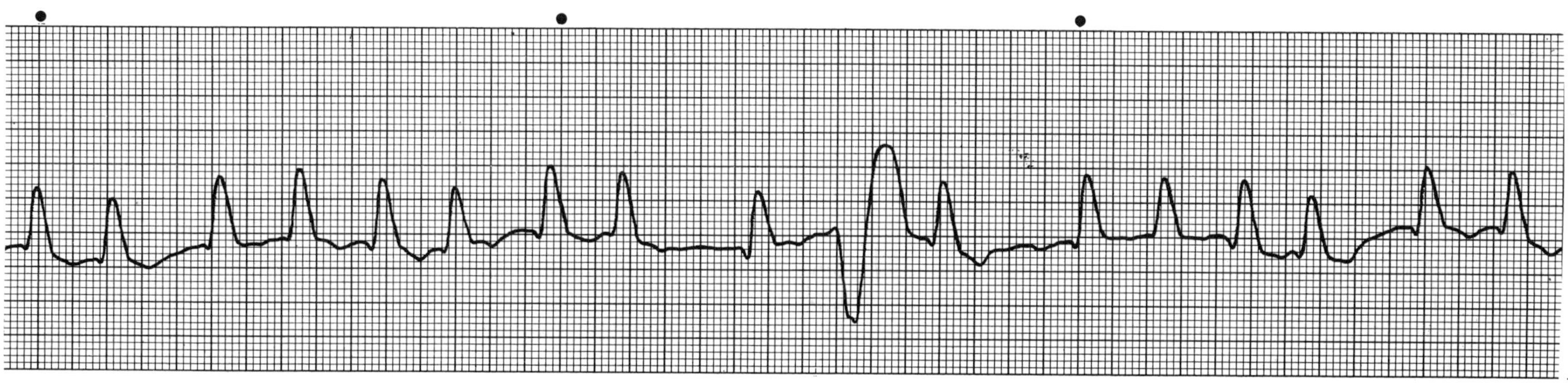

Question: This lead II ECG was obtained from a 3-year-old Great Dane that had echocardiographic signs typical of idiopathic dilated cardiomyopathy.

1. What is the rhythm diagnosis?
2. What is the most likely underlying disorder?
3. What is the best therapeutic approach?

Case 9

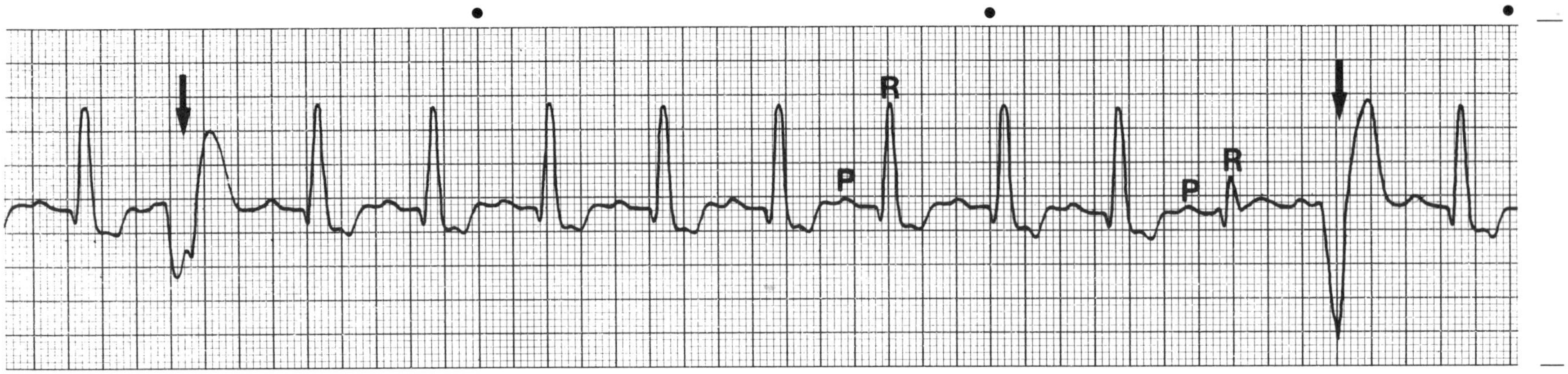

Answer: Sinus rhythm with two ventricular premature complexes (arrows) and a fusion beat. Heart rate is 180 beats/min. The QRS complexes of the ventricular premature complexes are wide and bizarre and are not associated with P waves. The third complex from the end is the fusion beat. The morphology of a fusion beat is intermediate between that of the sinus complexes and that of the ventricular premature complexes. A fusion beat has a P-R interval similar to that of the sinus complexes and initial forces that are the same as those of the sinus complexes. The amplitude of the complexes is midway between that of the sinus complexes and of the ventricular premature complexes, however, and the T waves have the same polarity as that of the ventricular premature complexes. If lethargy is believed to be associated with the arrhythmia, procainamide, quinidine, or tocainide should be prescribed. An ECG is re-evaluated in 2 to 3 days.

Case 10

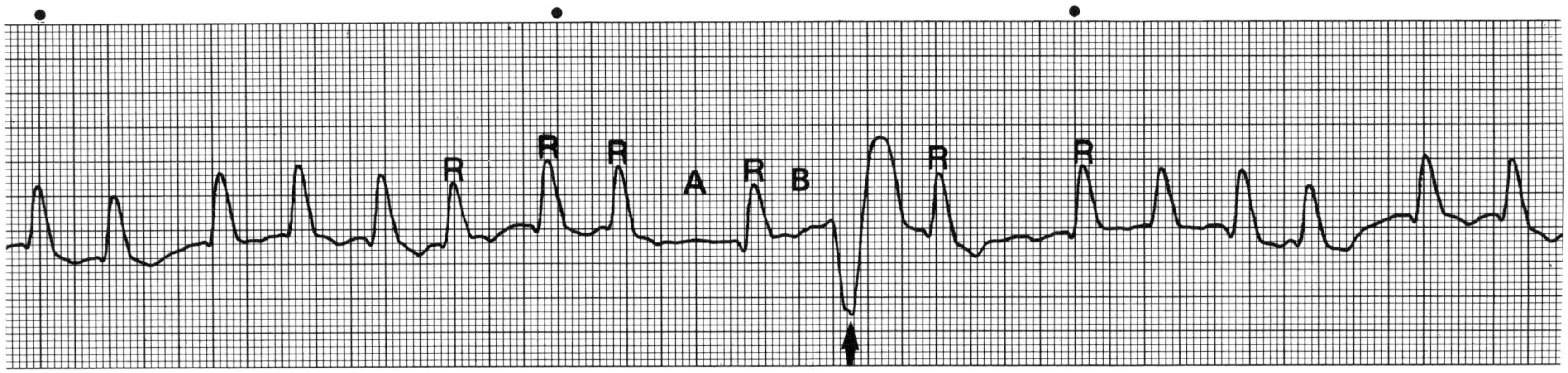

Answer: Atrial fibrillation. Heart rate is 220 beats/min. Dilated cardiomyopathy is the most common cause of atrial fibrillation. Digoxin is the preferred drug for this arrhythmia, especially in dogs with echocardiographic evidence of dilated cardiomyopathy (e.g., poor left ventricular contractility) or signs of congestive heart failure. Notice that the negative, wide QRS complex (arrow) resembles a ventricular premature complex; however, deduction and applied electrocardiographic criteria suggest that it may be a supraventricular beat with aberrant ventricular conduction. The term "aberrant ventricular conduction" is used when alteration of a supraventricular impulse occurs in the ventricles. Such alteration results in a change in the QRS complex amplitude, polarity (+ or −), and duration (width) when compared with the QRS complex of the normally conducted beats. The occurrence of aberrancy depends critically on a long R-R cycle (A) and short R-R cycle (B) preceding the wide complex (arrow). The electrophysiologic basis of aberrant conduction is refractoriness of the specialized conduction tissues that is dependent on cycle length (heart rate). Commonly, when a short cycle (B) follows a longer cycle (A), the supraventricular impulse is conducted aberrantly in a right bundle-branch block pattern (Ashman's phenomenon). Right bundle-branch Purkinje fibers typically have a refractory period longer than that of left bundle-branch fibers at normal heart rates. Ashman's phenomenon is common in animals with atrial premature complexes, atrial fibrillation, and at the onset of paroxysmal supraventricular tachycardia. The coupling interval of the premature complex and length of the preceding cycle determine the onset of aberrant conduction, also called functional bundle-branch block. Aberrantly conducted beats are often confused and improperly treated as ventricular premature complexes.

Case 11

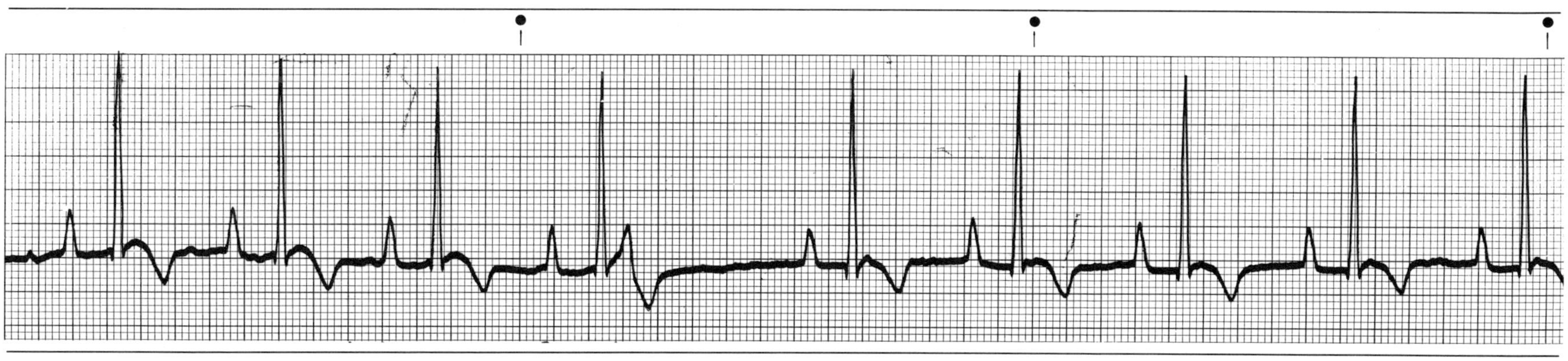

Question: This rhythm strip was recorded from a dog with a chronic cough. The dog had been given digoxin for a suspected cardiac insufficiency.

1. What is the rhythm diagnosis?
2. What is the most likely underlying disorder?

Case 12

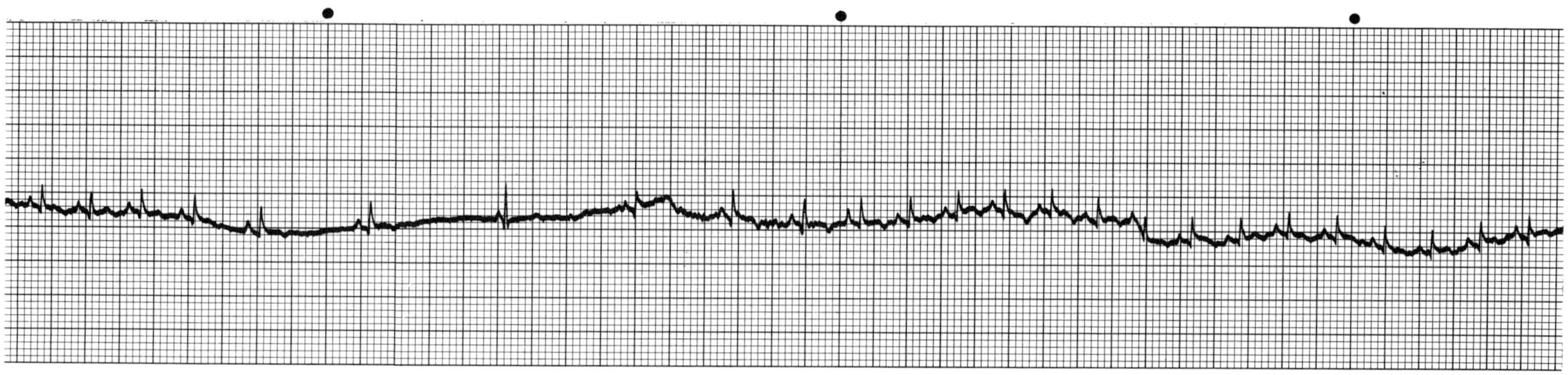

Question: This ECG was recorded from a cat with a severe upper respiratory infection. An abnormality in rhythm was auscultated. Paper speed: 25 mm/sec.

1. What is the rhythm diagnosis?
2. What is the most likely underlying disorder?

Case 11

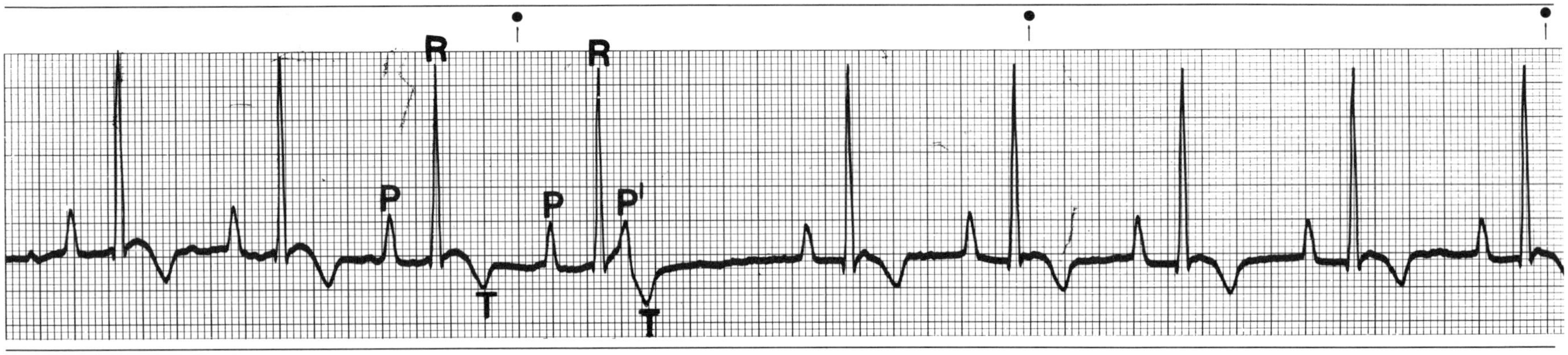

Answer: Sinus rhythm and a non-conducted atrial premature complex. Heart rate is 120 beats/min. The premature P′ wave is so early that the AV junction has not totally recovered, i.e., the impulse is not conducted to the ventricles. The premature P′ wave is superimposed on the S-T segment of the previous QRS complex. The tall peaked P′ waves, indicative of right atrial enlargement, were compatible with secondary pulmonary hypertension from a collapsed trachea on thoracic radiographs. Atrial premature complexes are associated with atrial enlargement or any atrial disease (e.g., neoplasia), or are secondary to drugs (e.g., digoxin). By way of review, the following steps should be used to analyze any rhythm strip: (1) general inspection of the electrocardiogram—heart rate (normal on this strip) and rhythm (regular with a pause on this strip), (2) identification of the P waves (P′-shaped complex deforming the S-T segment of the QRS complex before the pause), (3) recognition of the QRS complexes (appear normal), (4) the relationship between P waves and QRS complexes (no QRS complex following P′ wave, thus explaining the noncompensatory pause in rhythm; other P waves associated with the QRS complexes), and (5) summary of findings with final classification of the arrhythmias (sinus rhythm with a non-conducted atrial premature complex).

Case 12

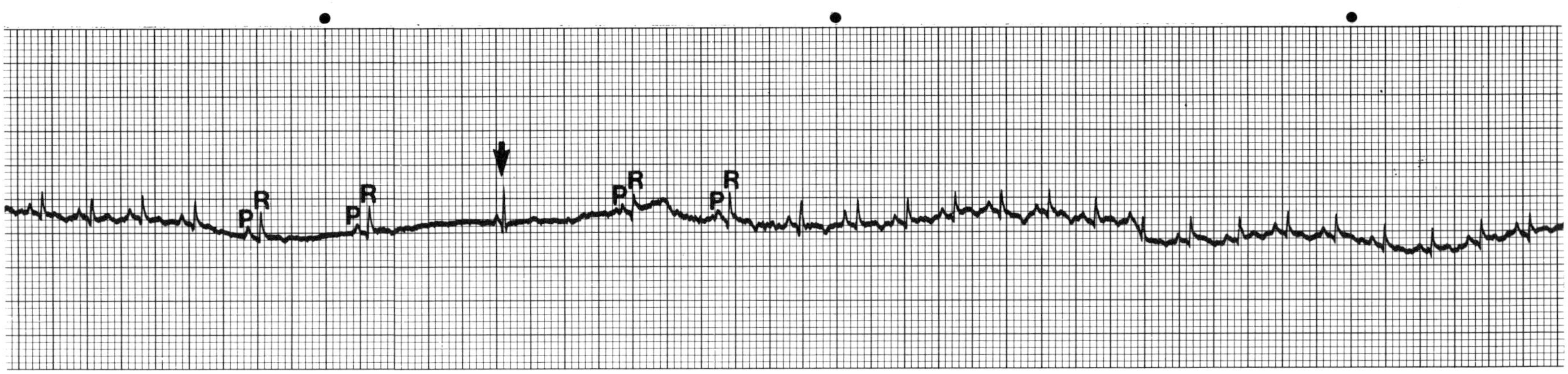

Answer: Intermittent sinus arrest or sinoatrial block. Heart rate is variable. After the first six sinus complexes, a pause occurs followed by an escape complex (arrow). A sinus P wave just happens to precede the complex at a short P-R interval. Sinus arrest is the failure of impulses to be formed within the SA node because the automaticity in the node has been depressed. Sinoatrial block is due to exit block of impulse out of the SA node. The rhythm is irregular with pauses demonstrating a lack of P-QRS-T complexes. The pauses are twice or greater than twice the normal R-to-R interval. Sinus arrest is rare in the cat. Associated conditions include either irritation of the vagus nerve or pathologic conditions involving the atria. Irritation of the vagus nerve can result from surgical manipulation, thoracic neoplasms, severe respiratory disorders, and vomiting. Atrial diseases include dilation, fibrosis of the SA node, cardiomyopathy, drug toxicity, and electrolyte imbalances. As with many arrhythmias, the underlying cause should be treated.

Case 13

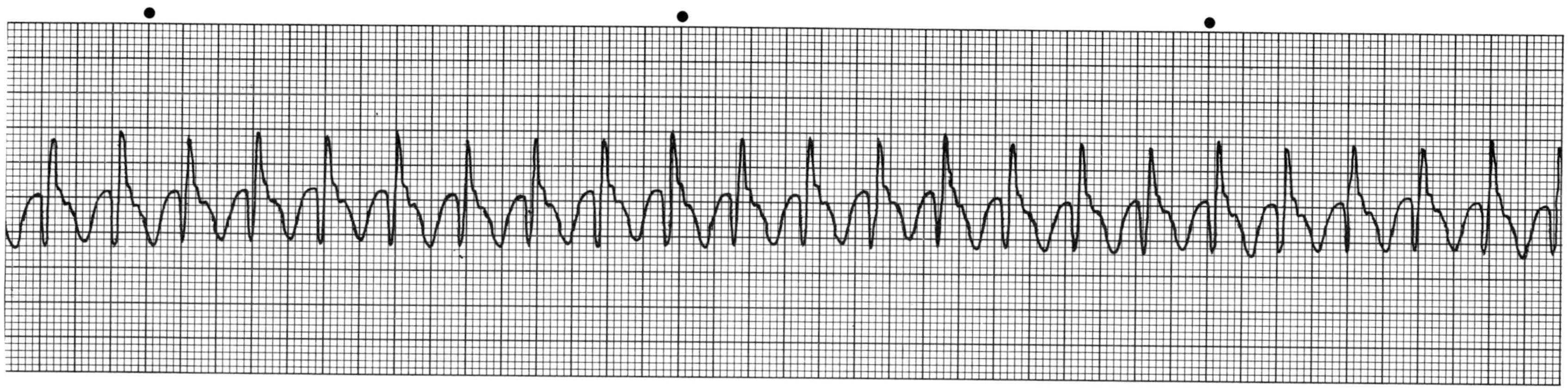

Question: This rhythm strip was recorded from a 5-year-old Golden Retriever with a history of syncope.

1. What is the rhythm diagnosis?
2. What are common causes of this arrhythmia?
3. What is the best therapeutic approach?

Case 14

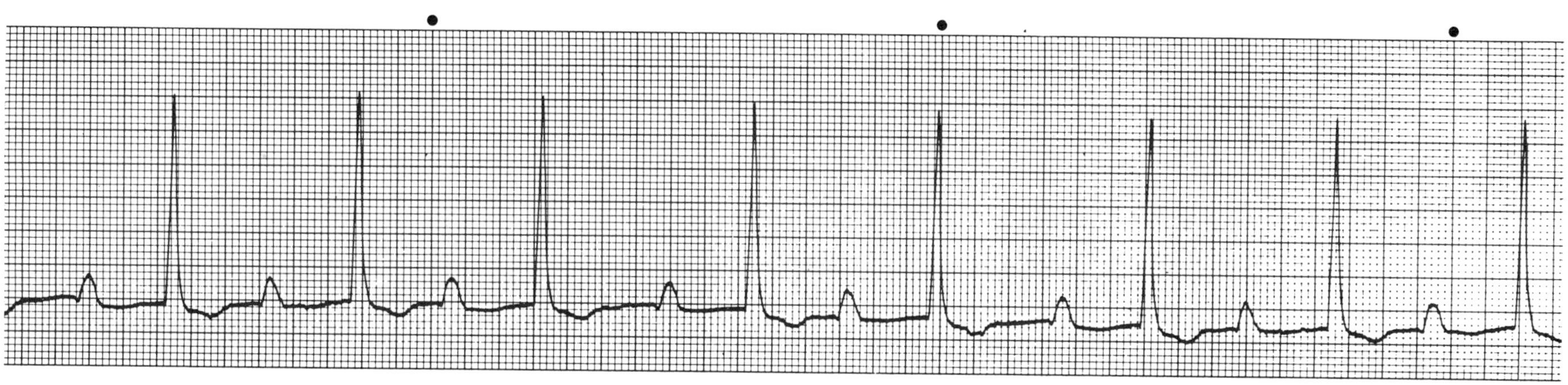

Question: This rhythm strip was obtained from a dog with chronic mitral valvular insufficiency that was being treated with digoxin. Severe vomiting and diarrhea had been present for 2 days.

1. What is the rhythm diagnosis?
2. What is the most likely underlying disorder?
3. What is the best therapeutic approach?

Case 13

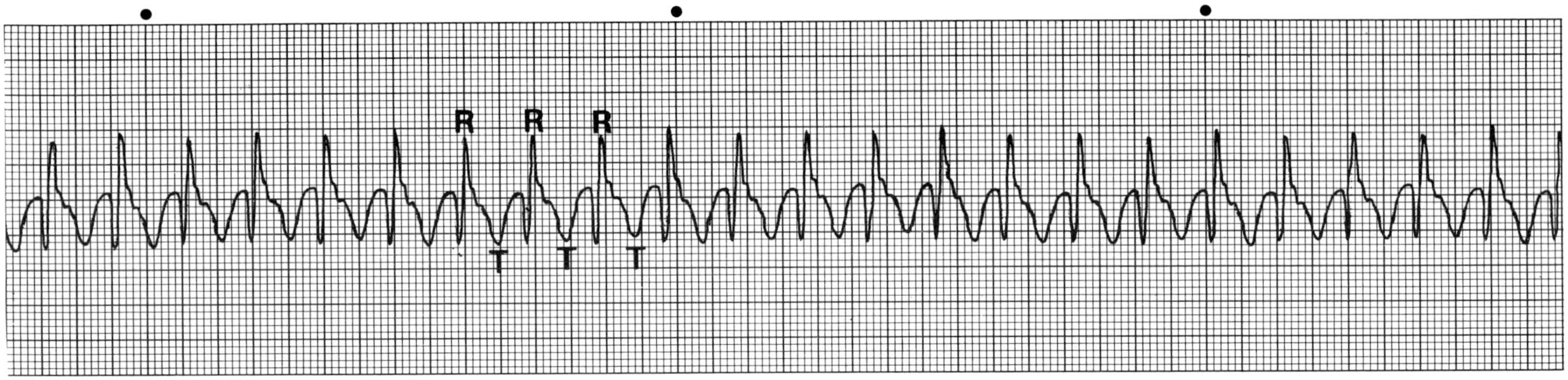

Answer: Supraventricular tachycardia. Heart rate is 300 beats/min. The narrow complex tachycardia supports a diagnosis of supraventricular tachycardia. Differential diagnosis includes sinus tachycardia, atrial tachycardia, and atrial flutter. Ventricular tachycardia should also be considered. Atrial tachycardia is associated with atrial distention or disease and can also occur secondary to a systemic disturbance. Dilated cardiomyopathy is a common cause of this arrhythmia in a large-breed dog. A vagal maneuver should be performed to try to break the tachycardia. If unsuccessful, propranolol, diltiazem, verapamil, or adenosine should be administered to terminate or control the arrhythmia. If dilated cardiomyopathy is documented or suspected, long-term therapy with digoxin also should be instituted.

Case 14

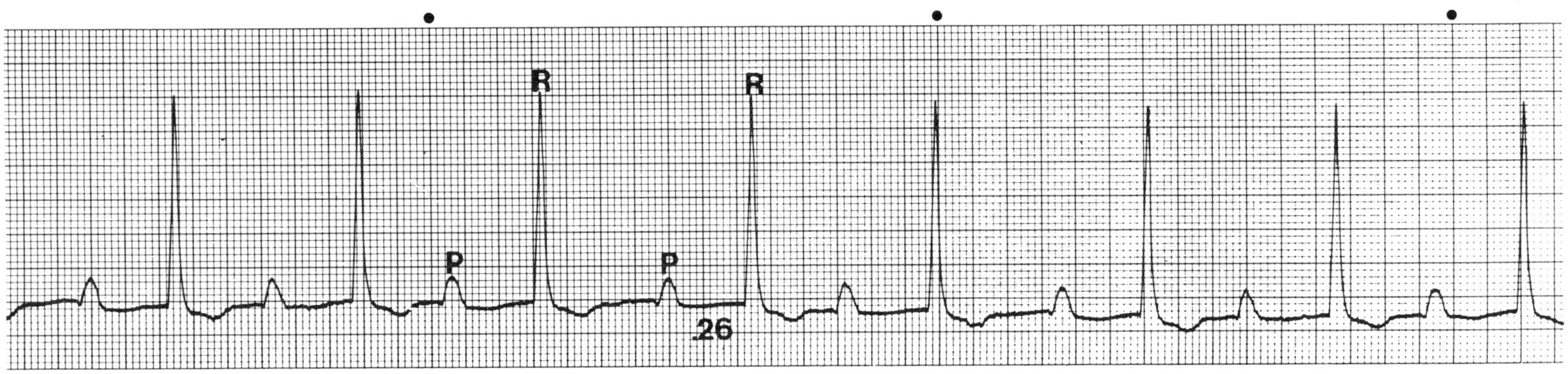

Answer: Sinus rhythm with severe first-degree AV block. Heart rate is 110 beats/min. The P-R interval is 0.26 sec, or 13 boxes (normal not greater than 0.13 sec or 6½ boxes). The wide P waves (0.06 sec) indicate probable left atrial enlargement. Digoxin toxicity is a common cause of first-degree AV block. Prevention of digoxin toxicity is the safest approach. Discontinuation of the drug is the treatment of choice until all toxic signs are resolved, which may take several days. The dosage of digoxin then should be reduced. An electrocardiogram should be obtained at least 3 or 4 times a day during the period of toxicity because arrhythmias are often intermittent. Remember, digitalis can cause any cardiac arrhythmia.

Case 15

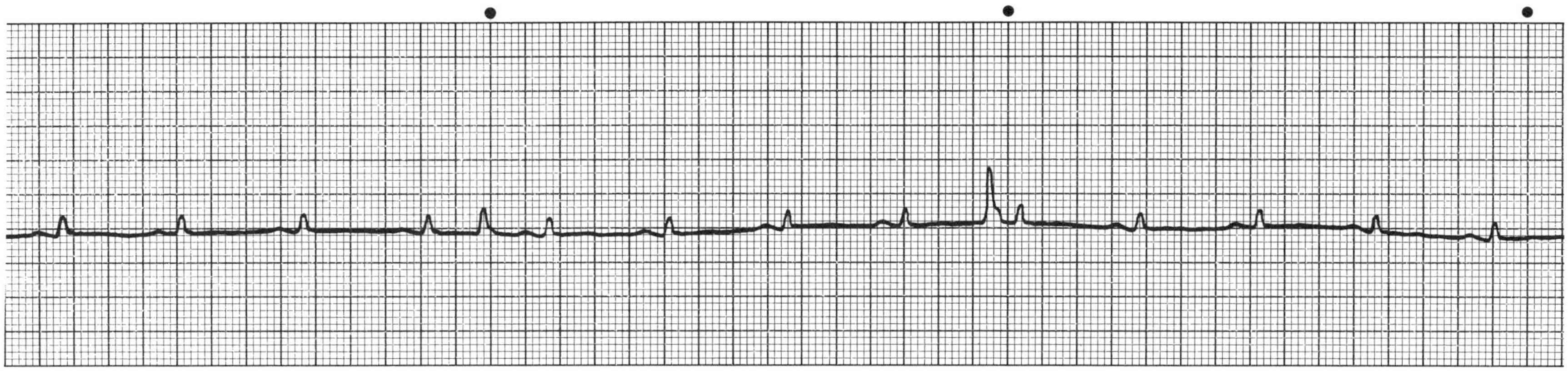

Question: This rhythm strip was recorded from a cat during a preoperative evaluation for a dental procedure.

1. What is the rhythm diagnosis?
2. Should any special preoperative measures be taken?

Case 16

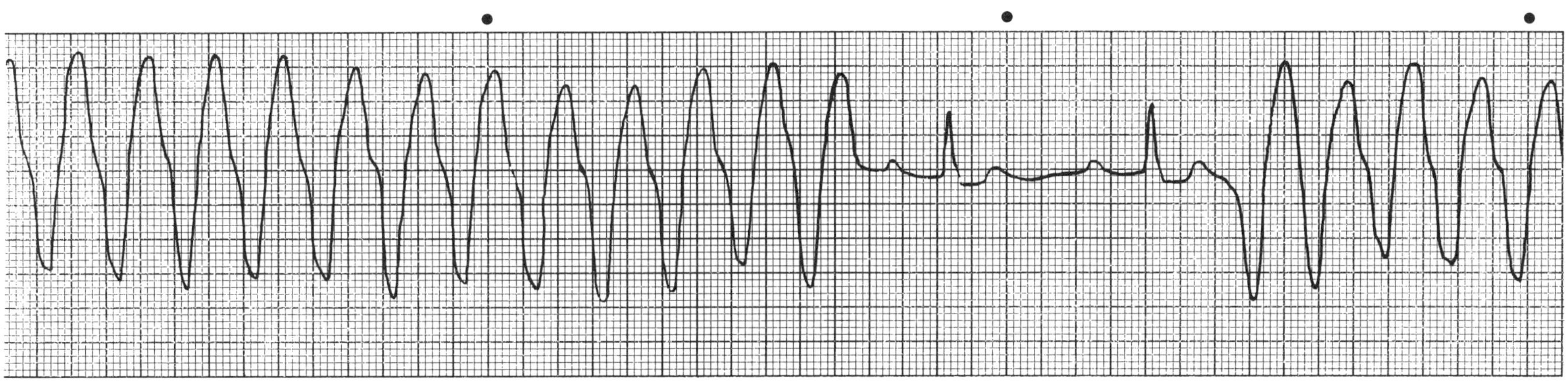

Question: This lead II ECG strip was obtained 2 days after a 5-year-old Golden Retriever had been hit by a car. The dog was hospitalized and treated for shock and hemorrhage.

1. What is the rhythm diagnosis?
2. What is the best therapeutic approach?

Case 15

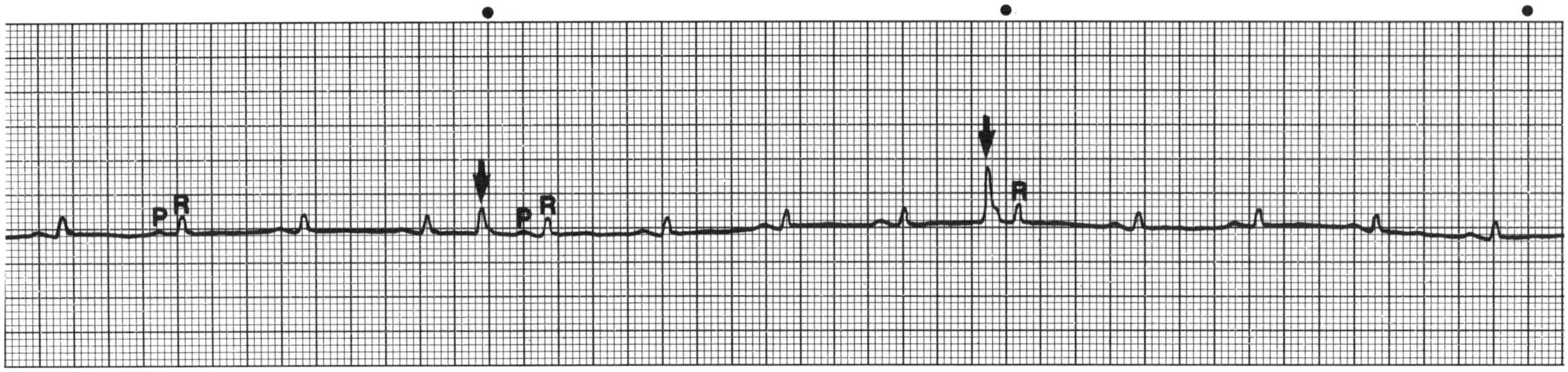

Answer: Artifact simulating atrial and/or ventricular ectopic complexes. Heart rate is approximately 175 beats/min. The artifact (arrows) occurred when the cat jerked its leg. The artifact simulates an ectopic complex, but does not interrupt the normal sinus P-QRS-T complexes. Other factors that are useful in differentiating artifact from arrhythmias include the rhythm of the artifact (usually irregular), the rate of the artifact (usually variable), and the lack of a T wave following the artifact complex. There are no major cardiac arrhythmias or conduction disturbances to pose a problem during anesthesia.

Case 16

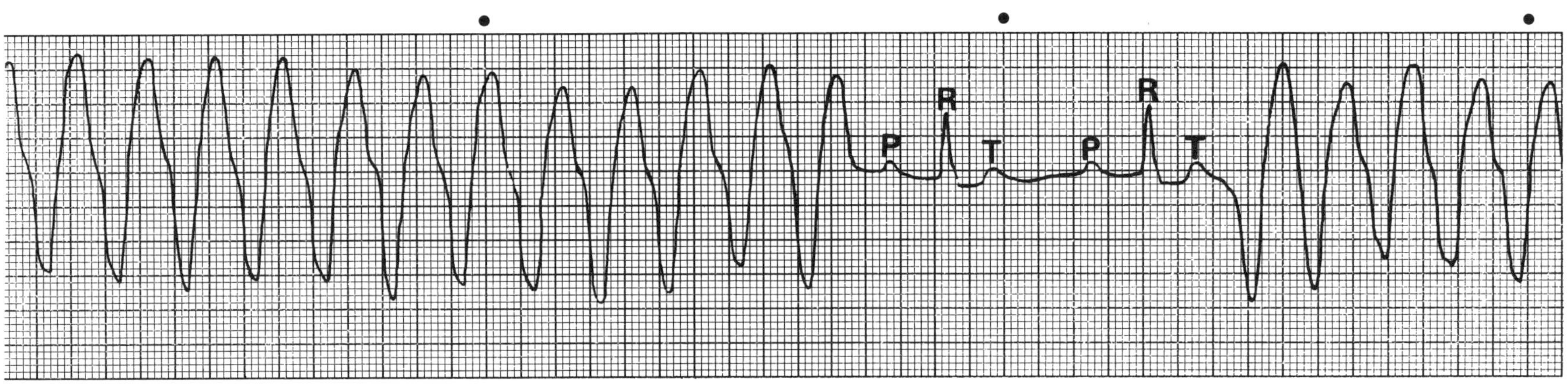

Answer: Sinus rhythm with paroxysmal ventricular tachycardia. Heart rate is 300 beats/min during the tachycardia. A lidocaine bolus should be administered to determine if the tachyarrhythmia can be terminated with this drug. Lidocaine can be administered as many as 4 times in 2 mg/kg boluses at 10-min intervals. If the response is favorable, a lidocaine infusion can be continued until the dog is stable enough to be started on procainamide or quinidine orally. Normal acid base and electrolyte status is important to ensure the success of lidocaine. If the response to the lidocaine bolus is inadequate, procainamide can be administered intravenously. Successive, premature, wide, and bizarre QRS complexes, with no association to the underlying atrial rhythm (P waves), are the hallmark of ventricular tachycardia. Therapeutic goals are to prevent progression of this electrically unstable tachycardia to ventricular fibrillation and to stabilize the hemodynamic status of the dog. The slight irregularity in the interval between successive ventricular premature complexes can be explained by variations in conduction within the ventricle or exit block. With exit block, the ventricular premature complexes may originate in the intraventricular Purkinje system, and conduction speed between the Purkinje system and ventricular myocardium can vary.

Case 17

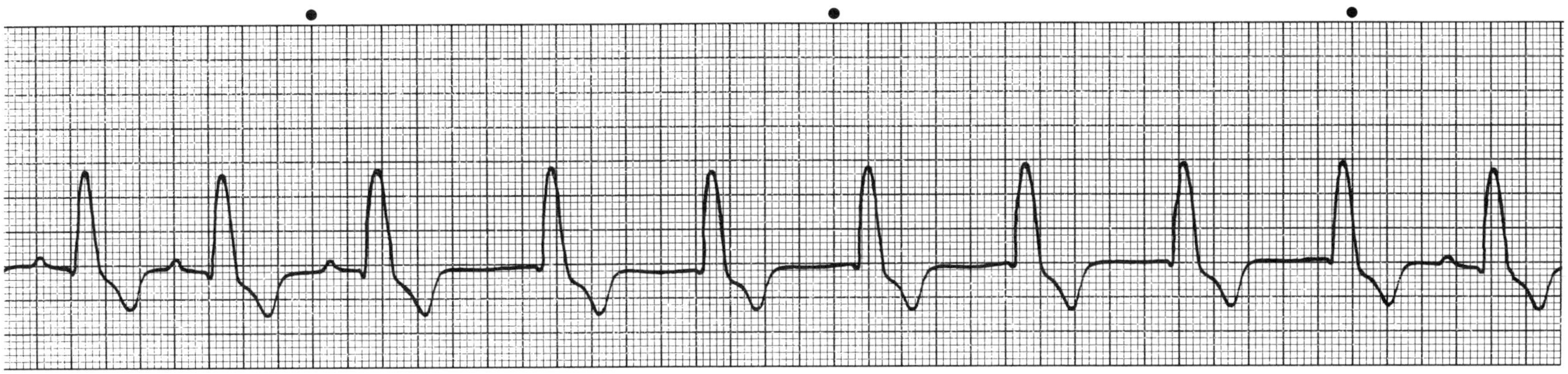

Question: This lead II ECG was recorded from an 8-year-old Poodle with dental disease. The ECG was obtained as part of a preanesthetic evaluation. The dog exhibited no clinical signs of cardiac disease.

1. What is the rhythm diagnosis?
2. What is the most likely underlying disorder?
3. What is the best therapeutic approach?

Case 18

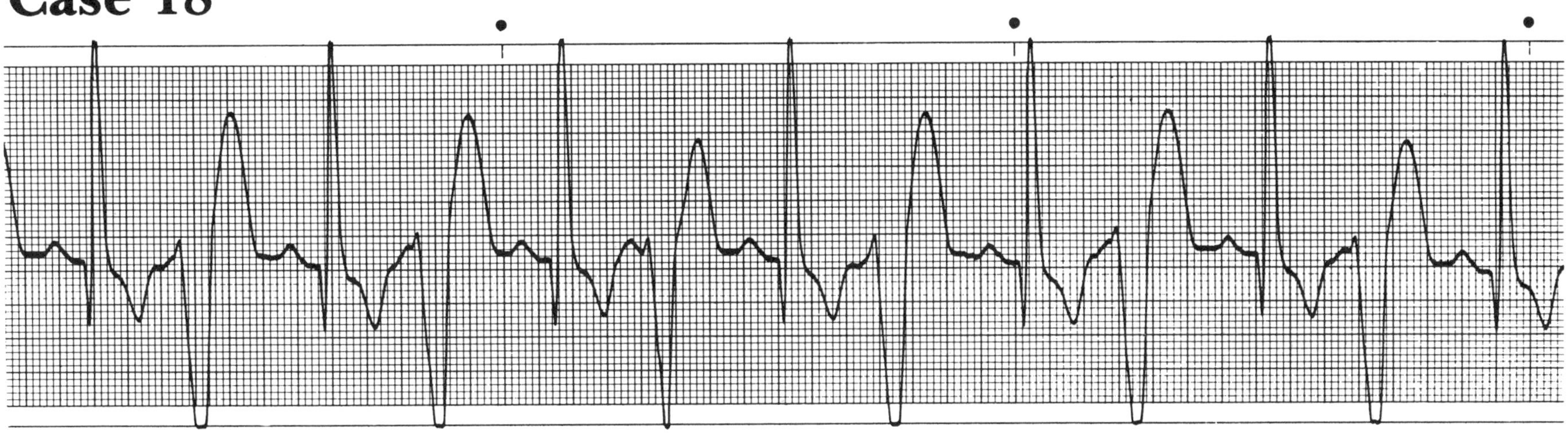

Question: This tracing was recorded from an 8-month-old Collie with congestive heart failure and a machinery murmur on auscultation.

1. What is the rhythm diagnosis?
2. What is the most likely underlying disorder?
3. What is the best therapeutic approach?

Case 17

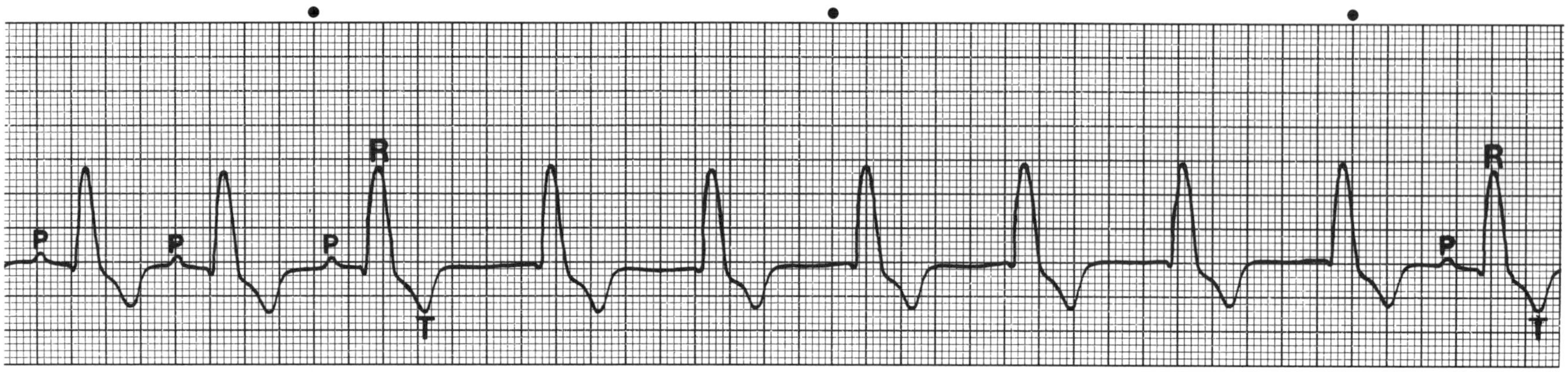

Answer: Sinus arrhythmia with a wandering sinus pacemaker. Heart rate is 140 beats/min. Sinus arrhythmia is present. The P waves vary in amplitude and at times are not visible in the baseline. Wandering sinus pacemaker, a variant of sinus arrhythmia, is a shift of the pacemaker from within the SA node or from the SA node to the AV node. This results in variation in the amplitude of the P waves. This ECG variant is normal in dogs and can be accentuated by conditions that increase vagal tone. The QRS complexes are extremely wide (0.08 sec). This characteristic is seen in dogs with left ventricular enlargement. Left bundle-branch block is a more likely diagnosis, because this dog has no history of heart disease. The absence of left ventricular enlargement on thoracic radiographs lends support to a diagnosis of left bundle-branch block. Left bundle-branch block can sometimes be confused with ventricular arrhythmia. The constant P-R interval supports a diagnosis of sinus rhythm. These ECG changes do not pose a contraindication to general anesthesia and do not require treatment.

Case 18

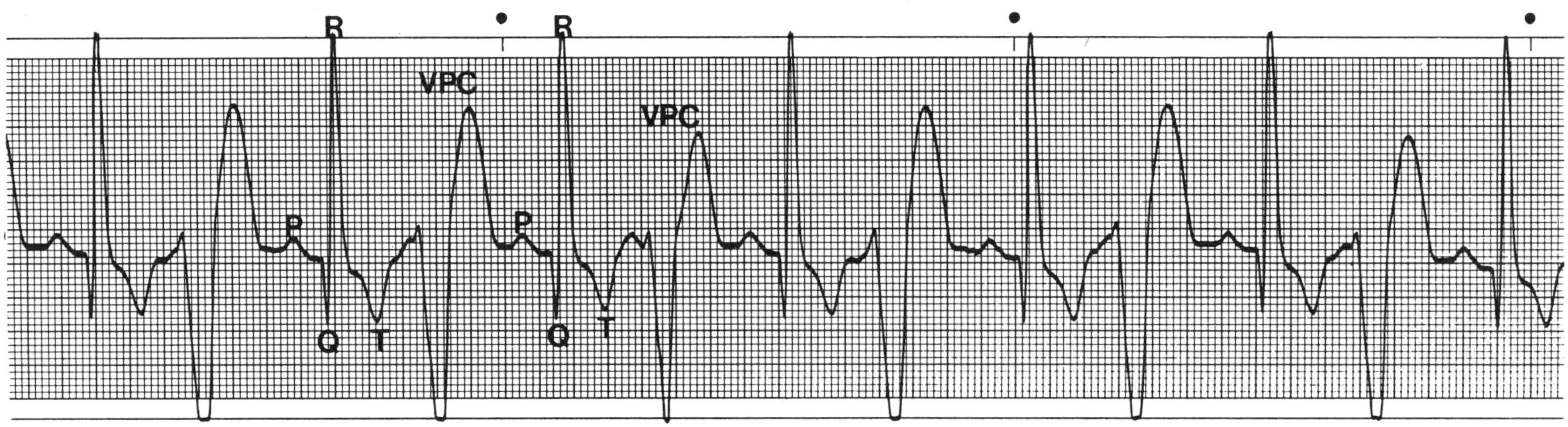

Answer: Ventricular bigeminy, left ventricular premature complexes (VPCs) alternating with normal sinus complexes. Heart rate is approximately 180 beats/min. The wide P waves and the tall and wide QRS complexes indicate left atrial and left ventricular enlargement. Thoracic radiographs were compatible with a patent ductus arteriosus and left-sided heart failure. Digoxin and diuretics were used to treat the heart failure. Lidocaine followed by procainamide was used to control the ventricular arrhythmia. The underlying condition, the heart failure and accompanying cause, must be treated. Surgical correction of the defect was later performed.

Case 19

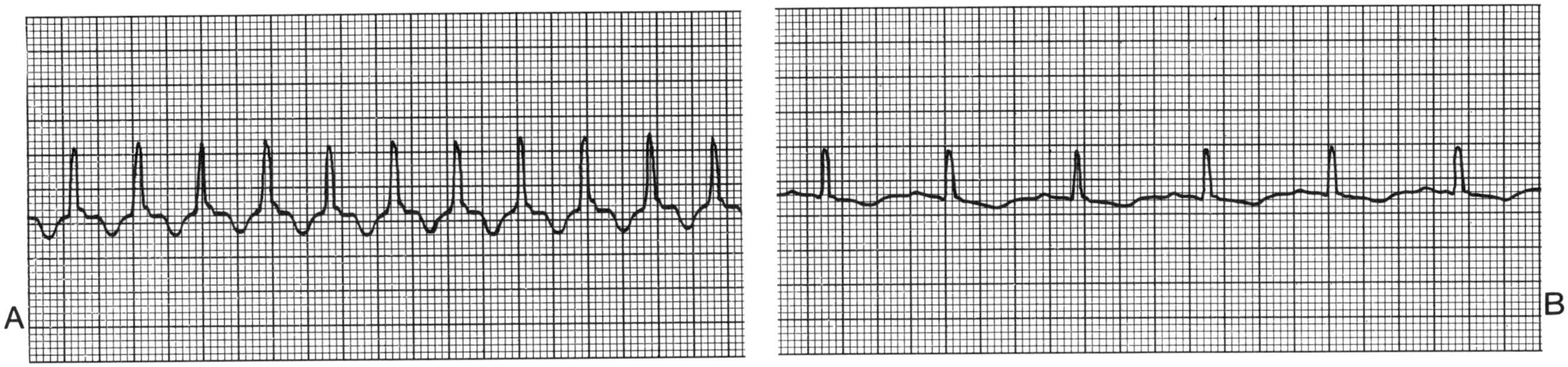

Question: This rhythm strip was obtained from a 10-year-old domestic shorthair cat with a history of lethargy and anorexia.
1. What is the rhythm diagnosis?
2. What is the best therapeutic approach?

Case 20

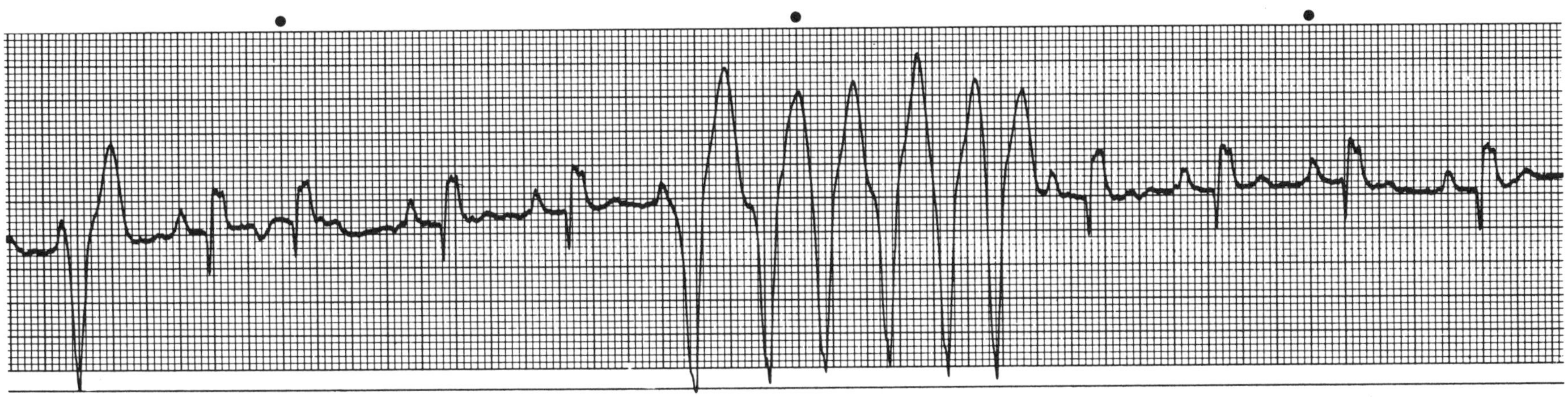

Question: This rhythm strip was recorded from a dog with mitral valvular insufficiency and pulmonary edema.
1. What is the rhythm diagnosis?
2. What is the best therapeutic approach?

Case 19

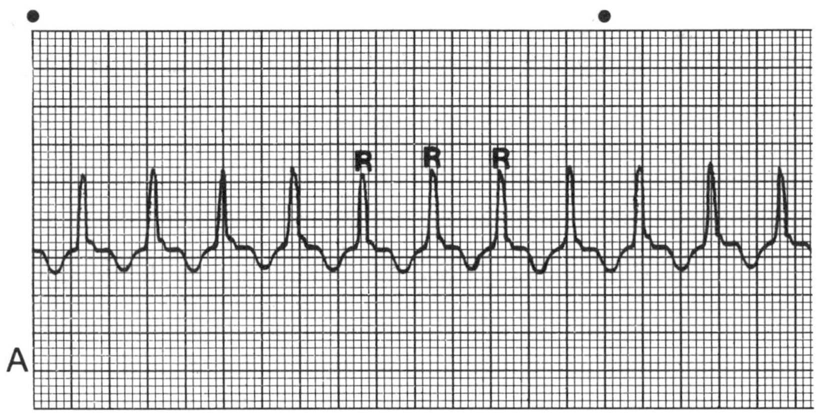

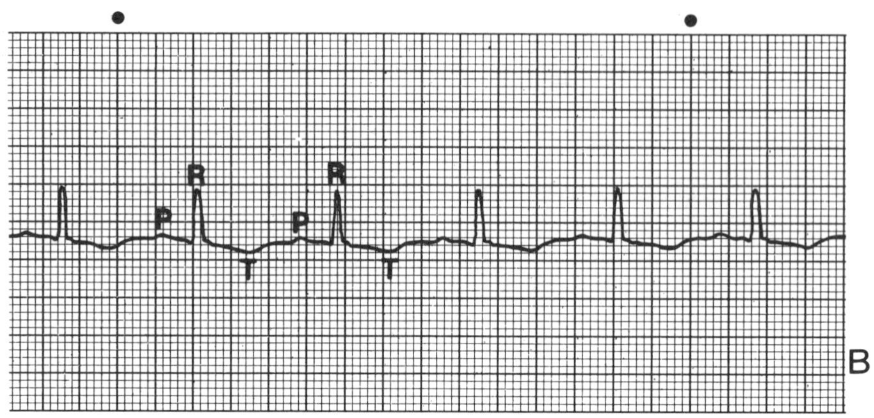

Answer: A. Atrial tachycardia. Heart rate is 330 beats/min. B. Sinus rhythm. Heart rate is 160 beats/min. The initial rhythm is extremely rapid. The complexes are narrow and positive in lead II, thereby suggesting a supraventricular rhythm (sinus, atrial, or junctional tachycardia). A high ventricular tachycardia cannot be ruled out completely. Treatment should be initiated quickly to slow the heart rate. Options include diltiazem and propranolol. Digoxin is also effective for supraventricular arrhythmias, but its onset of action is relatively slow. Diltiazem was administered to this cat, and a follow-up ECG was obtained 2 hours later. The expanded data base included thoracic radiographs and an echocardiogram. Hypertrophic cardiomyopathy was diagnosed, and the cat was maintained on diltiazem.

Case 20

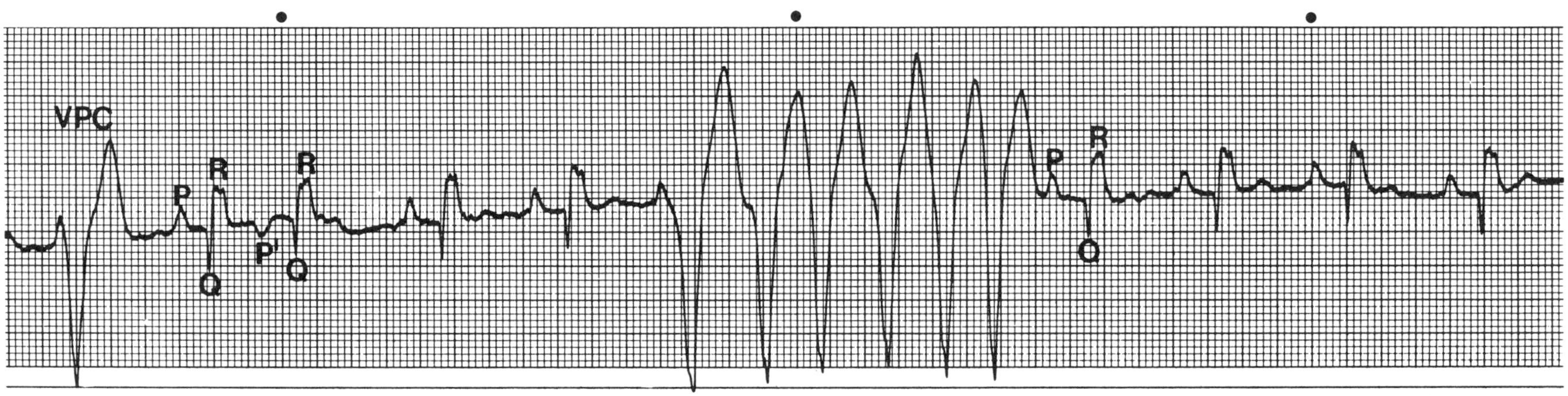

Answer: Paroxysmal ventricular tachycardia (midsection of strip) with one ventricular premature complex (VPC) and one supraventricular ectopic complex (P′-QR). Heart rate is variable. The ectopic P′ wave is inverted, thereby indicating that the atrial focus is in the lower portion of the atria near the AV junction. Supraventricular complexes commonly occur in severe mitral valvular insufficiency. The ventricular tachycardia most likely results from severe heart failure and secondary myocardial hypoxia. Cage rest, diuretics, and oxygen eliminated the ventricular arrhythmia. If paroxysms of ventricular tachycardia persist, procainamide or quinidine may also be needed. Ventricular tachycardia can cause a marked fall in cardiac output. The low-voltage sinus complexes are probably caused by the pulmonary edema.

Case 21

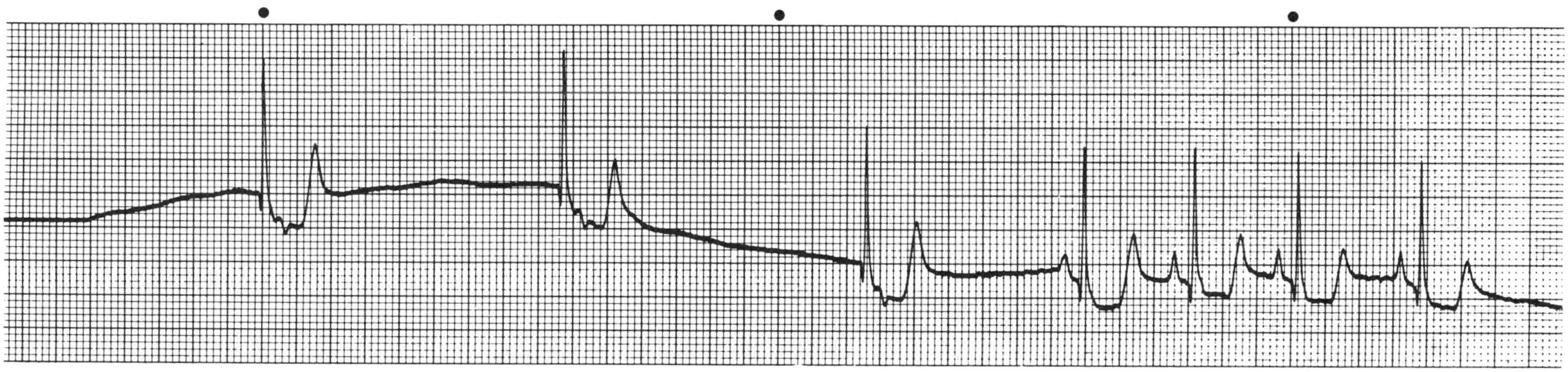

Question: This rhythm strip was recorded from a Miniature Schnauzer with episodes of syncope.

1. What is the rhythm diagnosis?
2. What is the most likely underlying disorder?
3. What is the best therapeutic approach?

Case 22

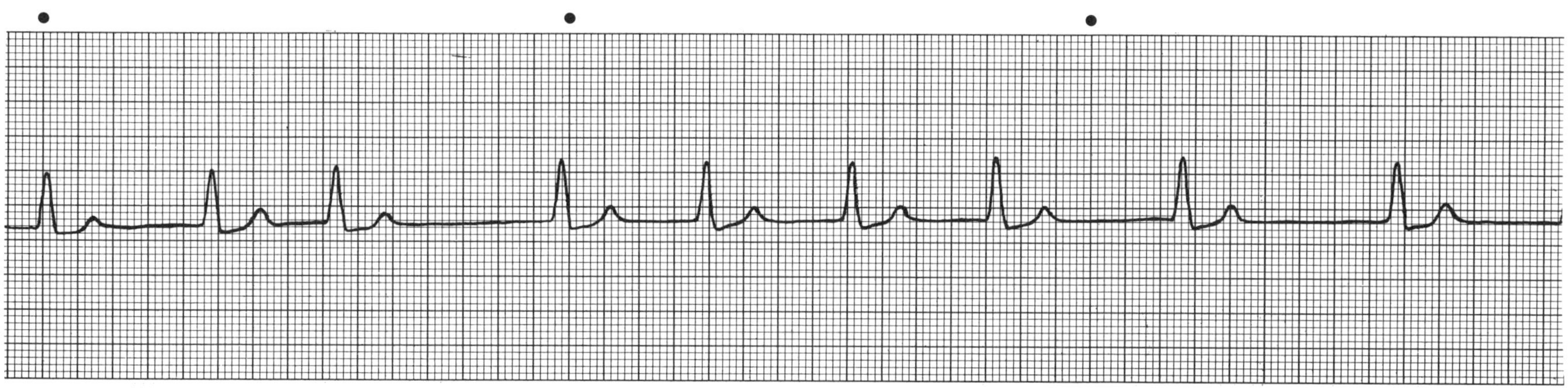

Question: This lead II ECG was obtained from a 4-year-old Labrador Retriever 24 hours after gastric dilatation had been relieved by insertion of a stomach tube.

1. What is the rhythm diagnosis?
2. What is the most likely underlying disorder?
3. What is the best therapeutic approach?

Case 21

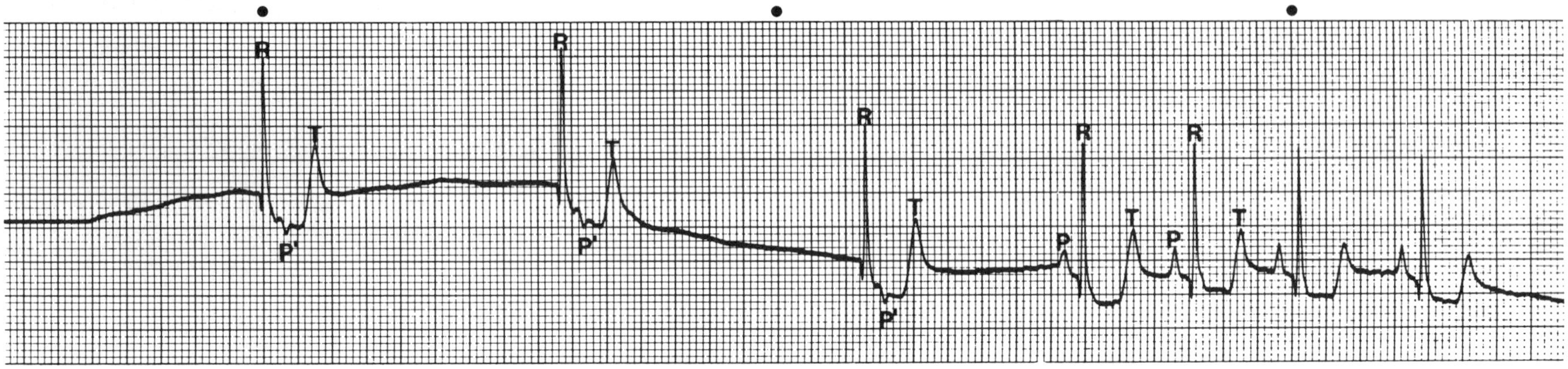

Answer: Junctional escape rhythm (the first three complexes) and a period of sinus arrest or block. Heart rate is variable. The escape rhythm represents a safety or rescuing mechanism that operates when a pause occurs in the heart rhythm. Inverted P′ waves follow each of the QRS complexes. The negative P′ waves in junctional complexes may precede, be superimposed on, or follow the QRS complex. The rhythm returns to a normal sinus rhythm at the end of the strip. The electrocardiographic pattern is compatible with sick sinus syndrome. Large T waves and S-T segment depression may indicate myocardial hypoxia. This SA node abnormality is frequently found in Miniature Schnauzers. Drugs, such as atropine, are usually of limited value in advanced cases. Insertion of an artificial pacemaker is probably the only guaranteed successful therapy for symptomatic sick sinus syndrome.

Case 22

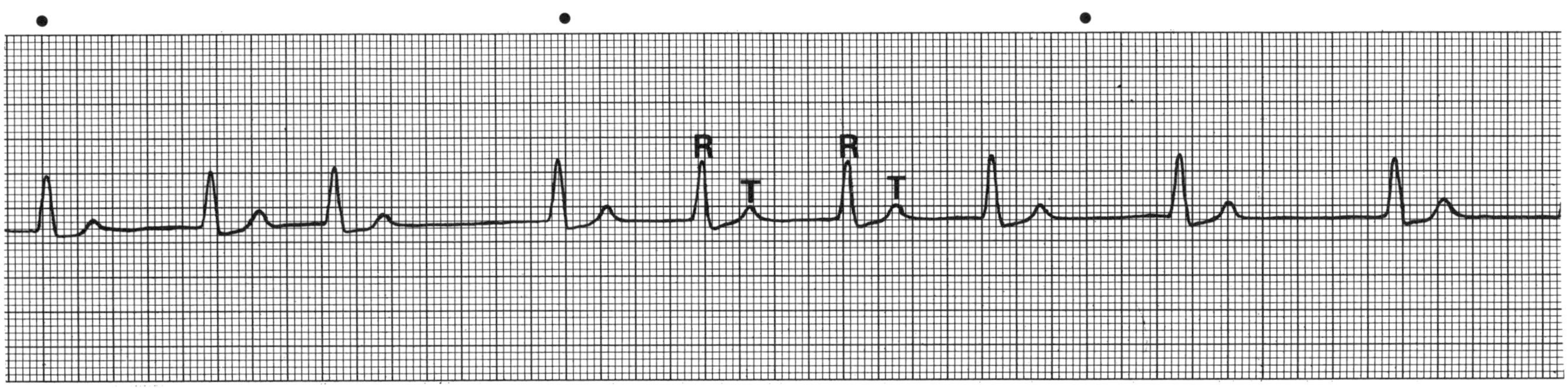

Answer: Atrial fibrillation. Heart rate is 120 beats/min. Atrial fibrillation occasionally develops after gastric dilatation, although ventricular arrhythmias are more common. Evidence of dilated cardiomyopathy may be evident on thoracic radiographs or echocardiogram. Intramuscular administration of quinidine gluconate can be used to convert atrial fibrillation back to sinus rhythm, provided no evidence exists of dilated cardiomyopathy or congestive heart failure. On the basis of the relatively slow heart rate, digoxin is not advised. Atrial fibrillation is characterized by the lack of visible P waves and by an irregularly irregular cardiac rhythm. Because of the slow atrial fibrillation rate (< 160 beats/min), electrolyte abnormalities and hypothyroidism should also be considered.

Case 23

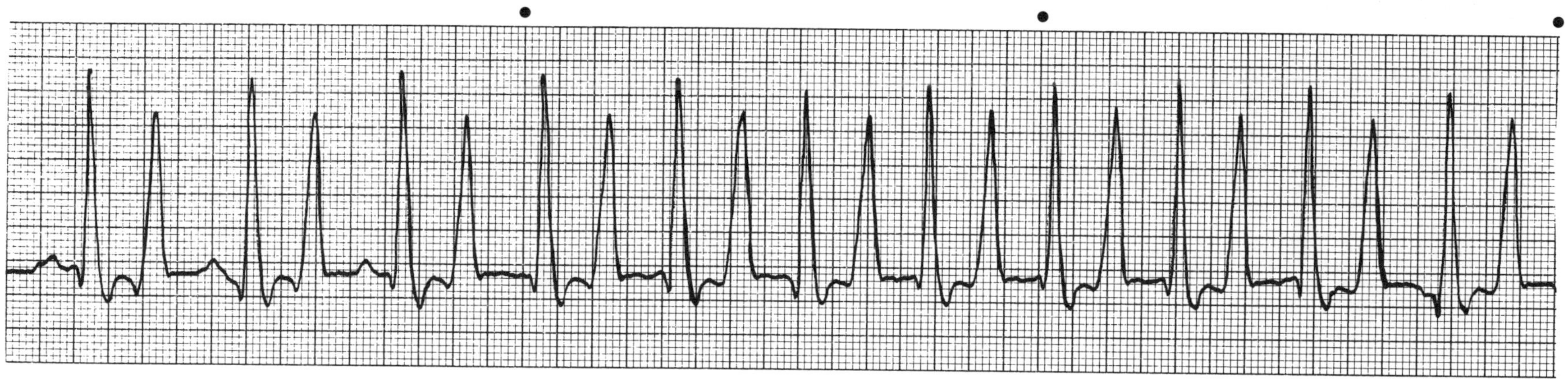

Question: This lead II ECG was obtained from a 10-year-old Keeshond that was being examined because of severe dyspnea and cyanosis.

1. What is the rhythm diagnosis?
2. What is the best therapeutic approach?

Case 24

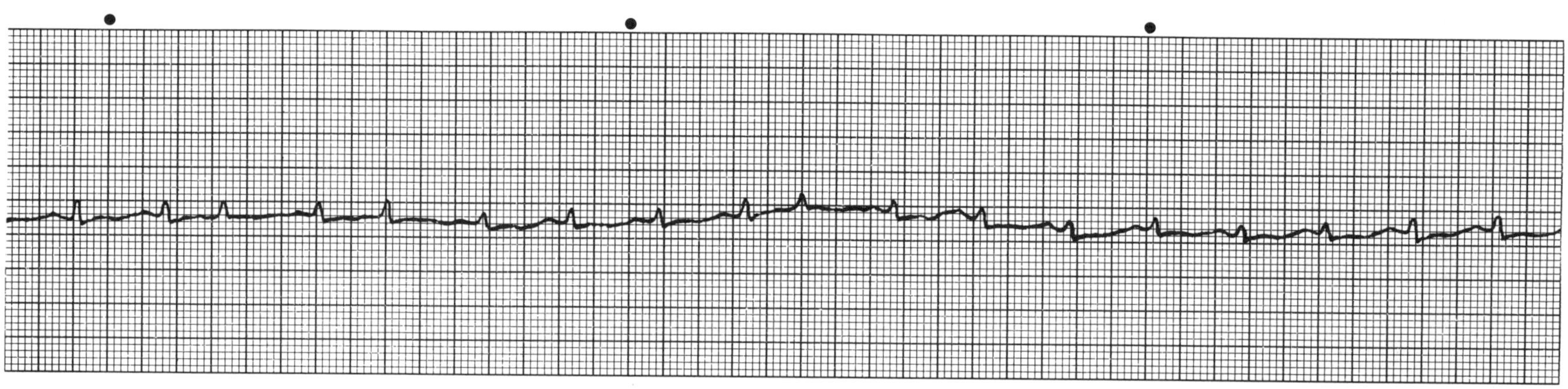

Question: This rhythm strip was obtained from a 10-year-old Siamese cat as part of a geriatric profile.

1. What is the rhythm diagnosis?
2. What is the best therapeutic approach?

Case 23

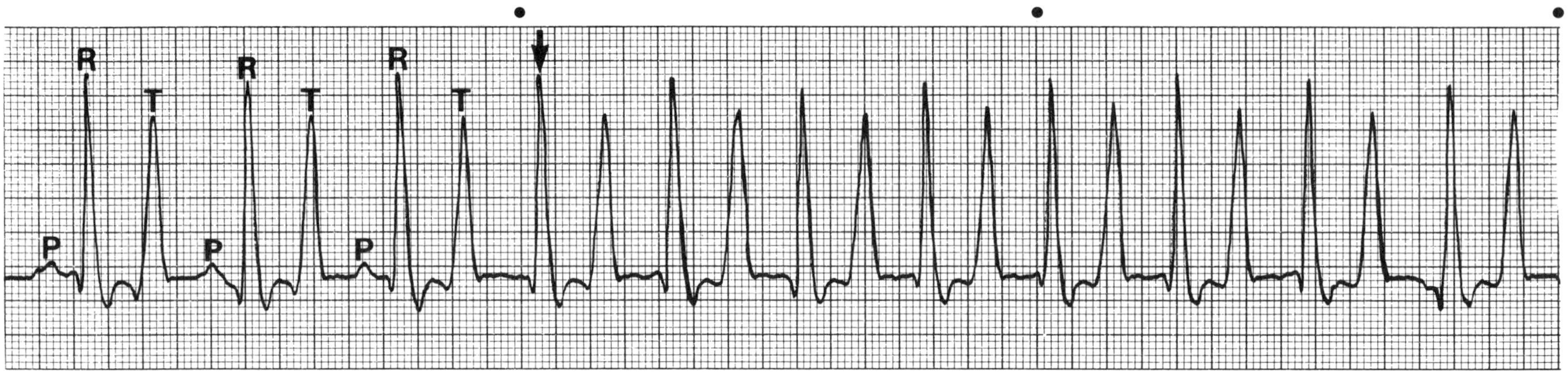

Answer: Sinus rhythm with paroxysmal supraventricular tachycardia. Heart rate is 160 beats/min during the tachycardia. Thoracic radiographs and blood tests are essential to differentiate primary heart disease (e.g., cardiomyopathy) from secondary heart disease caused by systemic problems. If signs are caused by congestive heart failure, digoxin should be used to control the atrial arrhythmia. If signs are not related to congestive heart failure, diltiazem would be another choice of antiarrhythmic drug. Diltiazem would control the arrhythmia more rapidly than digoxin and may be safer if myocardial hypoxia is present. Notice the huge T waves following the QRS complexes. The T wave abnormality may be caused by myocardial hypoxia, hyperkalemia, or metabolic disease. The T waves can be confused with ventricular premature complexes, but the lack of subsequent T waves eliminates ventricular premature complexes from the differential diagnosis. The premature QRS complexes (third through eighth starting at the arrow) resemble those of the sinus beats, thus supporting a diagnosis of atrial arrhythmia. The location of the ectopic atrial focus is not established. Whether the P waves precede the premature QRS complexes or are fused with preceding T waves is not clear.

Case 24

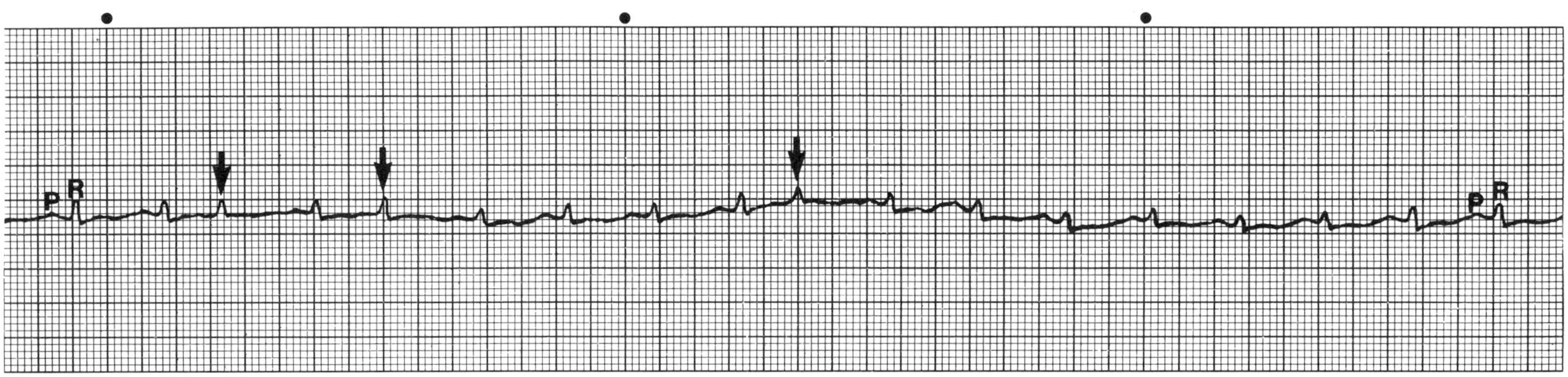

Answer: Sinus rhythm with atrial premature complexes (arrows). Heart rate is approximately 240 beats/min. The rhythm is irregular, being interrupted by premature complexes that appear similar to the sinus complexes. This finding suggests atrial premature complexes. The diagnosis is further supported by the presence of a noncompensatory pause. A noncompensatory pause results when the R-R interval of two normal sinus complexes enclosing a premature atrial complex is less than the R-R intervals between three consecutive sinus complexes. Atrial premature complexes in an animal with no clinical signs rarely require treatment. Their presence does raise concern about underlying cardiac disease. Thoracic radiographs are recommended in this cat. If the heart is enlarged, echocardiography would be indicated.

Case 25

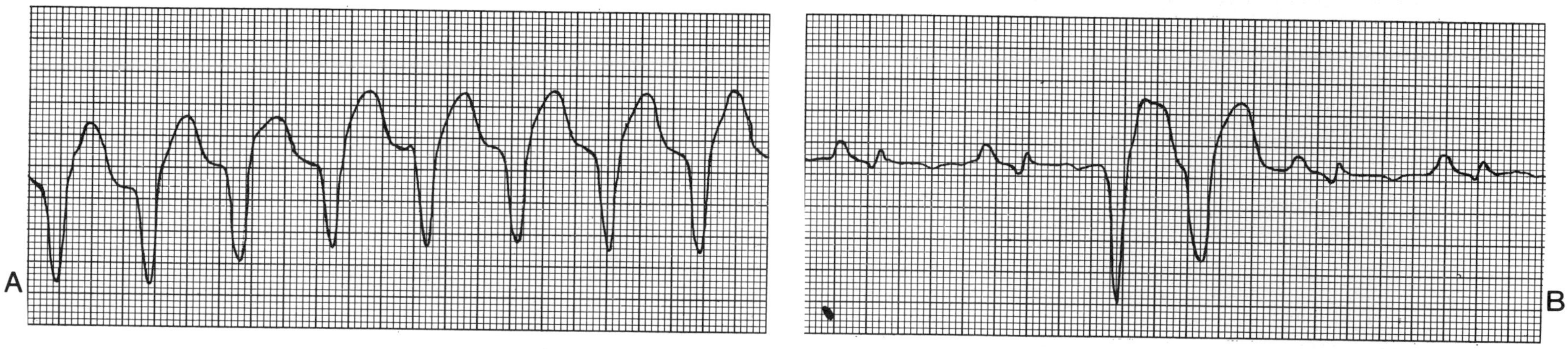

Question: This lead II rhythm strip was recorded from a 5-year-old Bulldog that had collapsed.

1. What is the rhythm diagnosis?
2. What is the most likely underlying disorder?
3. What is the best therapeutic approach?

Case 26

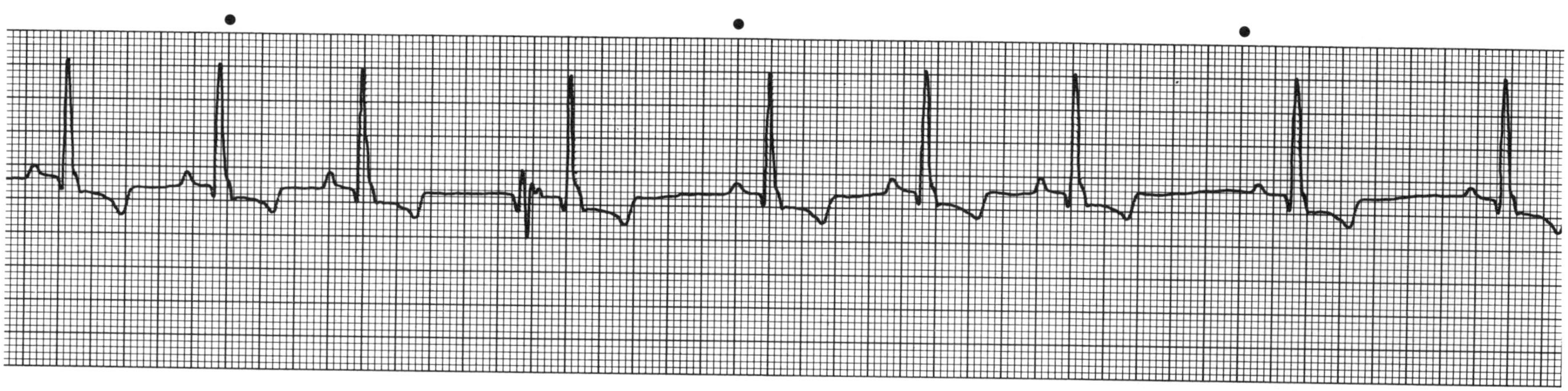

Question: This lead II ECG was obtained from a 10-year-old Wire-haired Fox Terrier that had no clinical signs during geriatric examination.

1. What is the rhythm diagnosis?
2. What is the best therapeutic approach?

Case 25

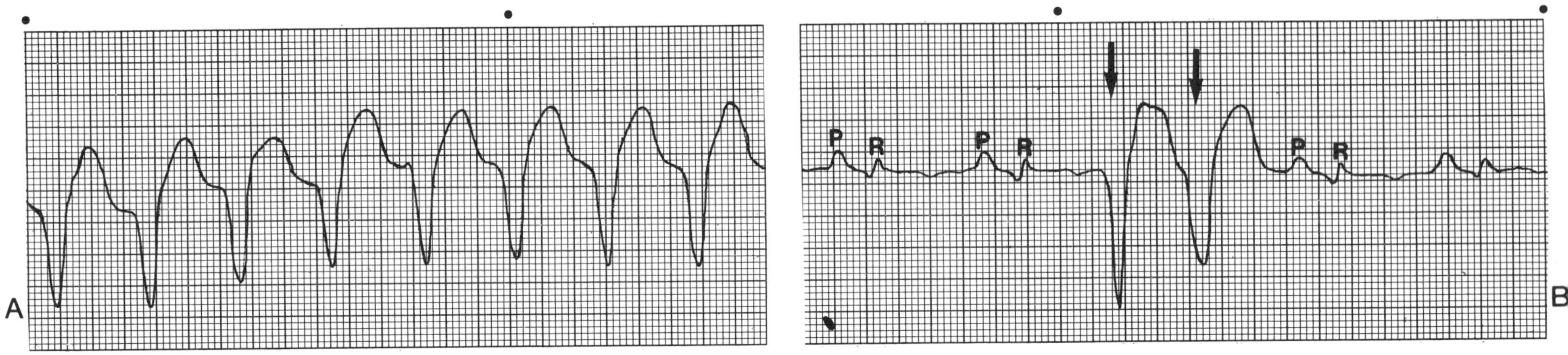

Answer: A. Ventricular tachycardia. Heart rate is 200 beats/min. B. Sinus rhythm with one couplet of ventricular premature complexes (arrows). The rapid heart rate, regular rhythm, and wide negative complexes in lead II support a diagnosis of ventricular tachycardia. Lidocaine was administered. The rhythm became predominantly sinus with occasional ventricular premature complexes. Notice how the sinus QRS complexes in strip B differ from the ventricular premature complexes in strip B and the tachycardia in strip A. The sinus complexes have extremely wide P waves, supporting a finding of left atrial enlargement. The differential diagnosis includes cardiomyopathy, myocarditis, neoplastic infiltration, drug toxicity, and trauma. Thoracic radiographs and possibly ultrasound evaluation of the heart are indicated. The dog was placed on a lidocaine infusion and started on procainamide. Other treatment options include quinidine, tocainide, and mexiletine.

Case 26

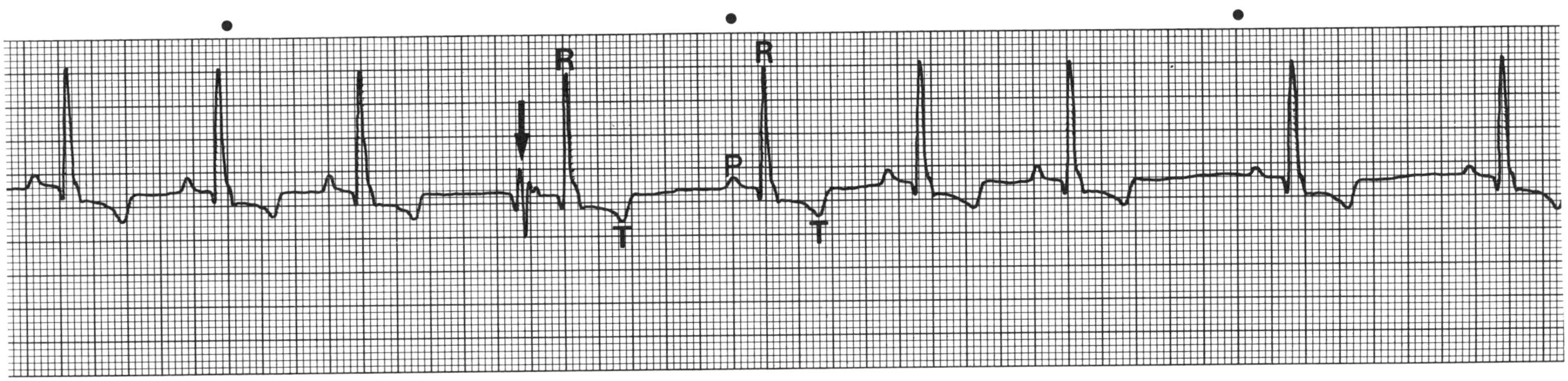

Answer: Sinus arrhythmia. Motion artifact (arrow). Heart rate is 120 beats/min. No treatment is required. The complex marked with an arrow is artifact. This complex does not interrupt the normal heart rhythm, nor is it followed by a T wave. Patient movement and electrical interference are common causes of artifacts on ECGs.

Case 27

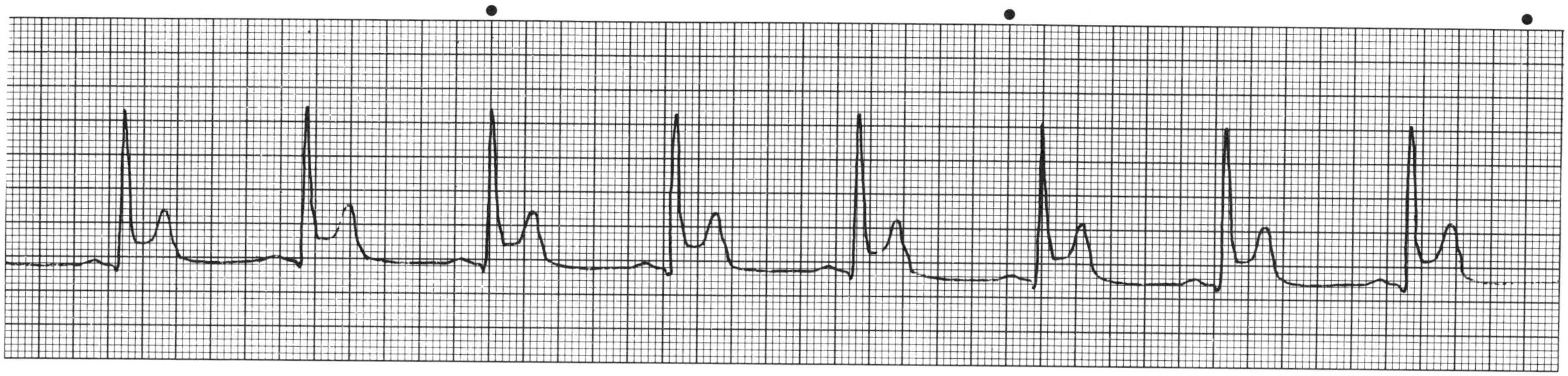

Question: This lead II ECG was obtained from a 16-year-old mixed breed dog that was examined because of weakness and persistent crying.

1. What is the rhythm diagnosis?
2. What is the most likely underlying disorder?
3. What is the best therapeutic approach?

Case 28

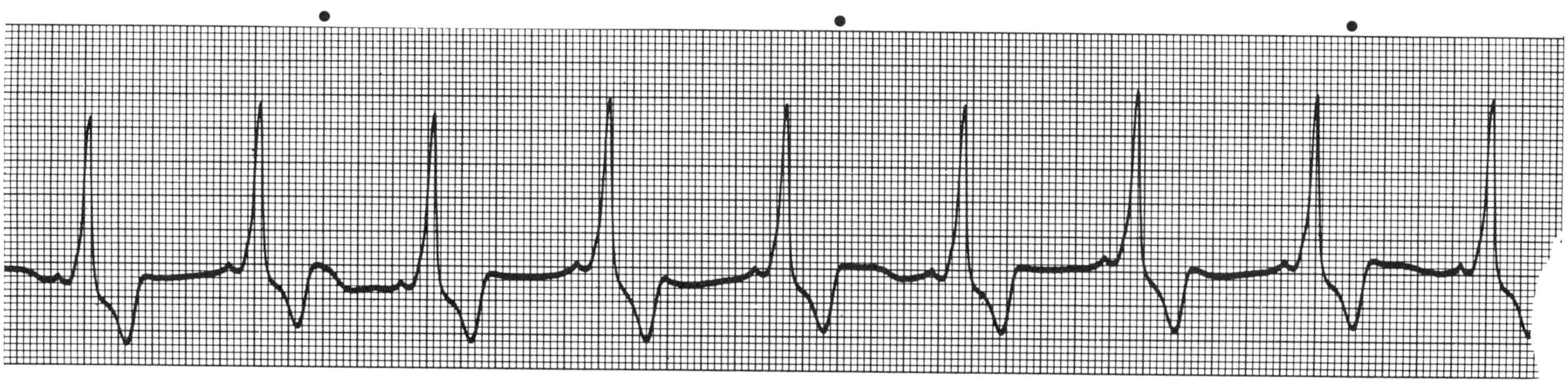

Question: This tracing was obtained from a dog that was undergoing evaluation for surgery. There were no signs of cardiac disease.

1. What is the rhythm diagnosis?
2. What is the most likely underlying disorder?
3. What is the best therapeutic approach?

Case 27

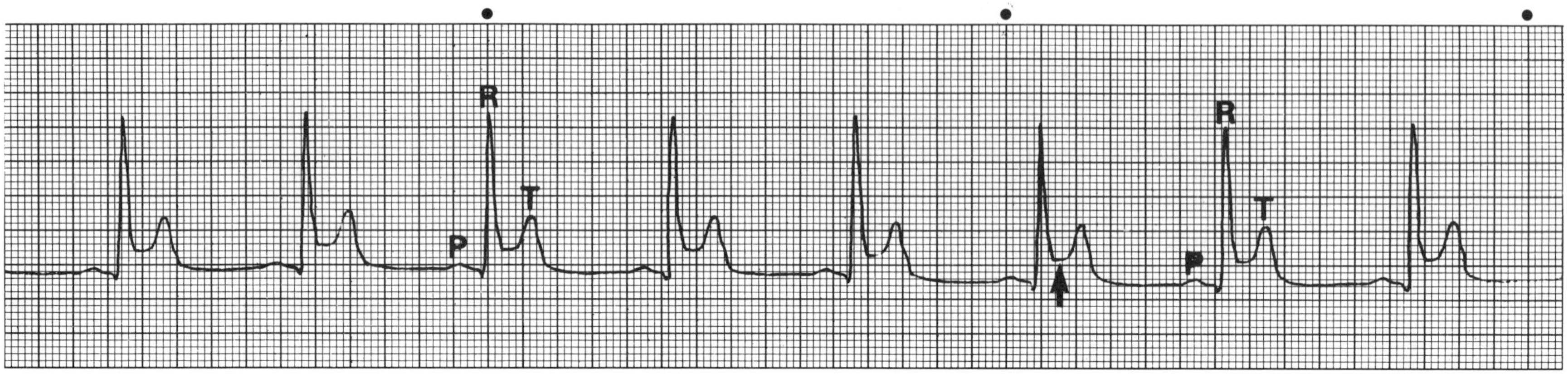

Answer: Sinus rhythm with a marked S-T segment elevation (arrow). Heart rate is 110 beats/min. Myocardial infarction is the most likely underlying disorder. Therapeutic guidelines for myocardial infarction include administration of analgesics, treatment for shock, stabilization of heart failure, and administration of anticlotting drugs and coronary artery vasodilators (nitrates). Serial ECGs to detect development of arrhythmias are also important. S-T segment elevation is the most common finding in humans after myocardial infarction. Although myocardial infarction is rare in dogs, coronary artery thrombosis associated with atherosclerosis may occur in old or hypothyroid dogs. S-T segment elevation caused by localized epicardial or myocardial injury may also be seen in dogs with pericarditis, pericardial effusion, and severe myocardial hypoxia.

Case 28

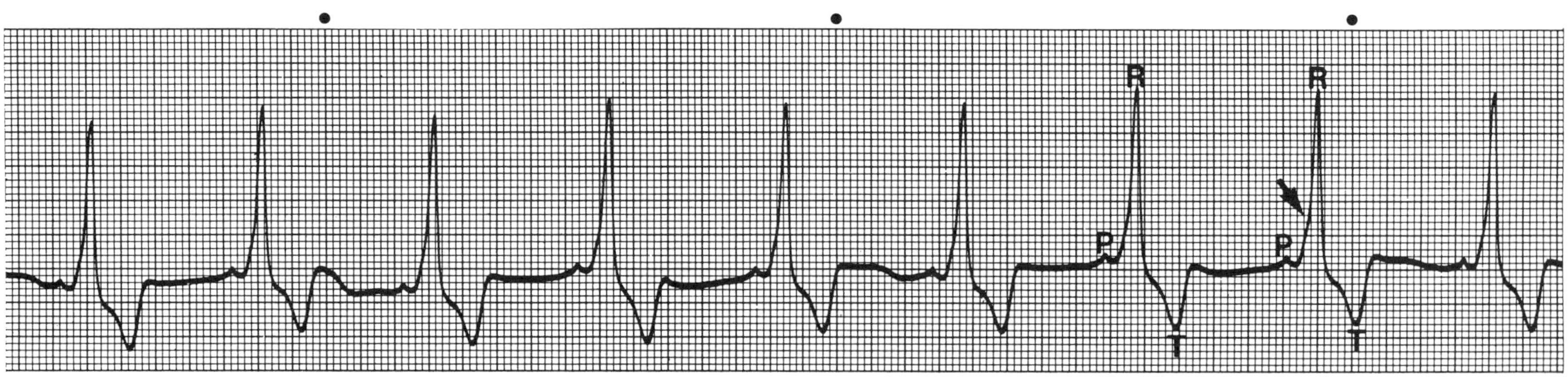

Answer: Ventricular pre-excitation. Heart rate is 120 beats/min. Ventricular pre-excitation occurs when impulses originating in the SA node or atrium activate a portion of the ventricles prematurely through an accessory pathway bypassing the AV node. Electrocardiographic features include a shortened P-R interval and a widened QRS complex with slurring or notching (arrow) (delta wave) of the upstroke of the R wave. The underlying disorder either may be an isolated congenital defect or may be associated with other congenital cardiac defects (e.g., atrial septal defect, tricuspid dysplasia). The dog should be closely monitored during surgery, and atropine should not be given. Paroxysmal tachycardia associated with ventricular pre-excitation (Wolff-Parkinson-White syndrome) can be a common occurrence.

Case 29

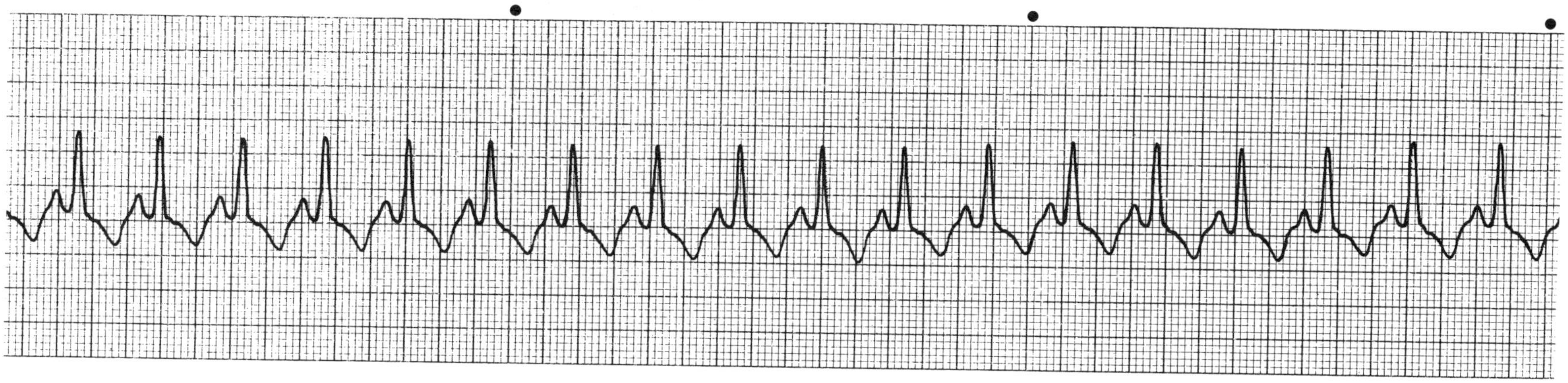

Question: This lead II rhythm strip was recorded from a 7-year-old male Persian cat with dyspnea.

1. What is the rhythm diagnosis?
2. What is the most likely underlying disorder?
3. What is the best therapeutic approach?

Case 30

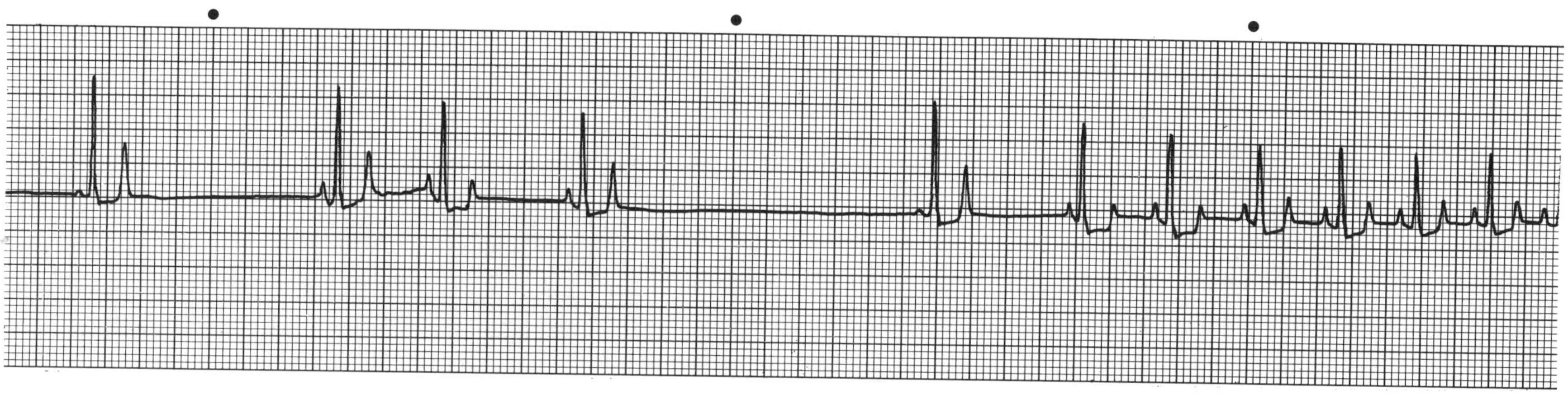

Question: This lead II ECG was obtained from a 3-year-old Pug with no clinical signs. An irregular rhythm was heard on auscultation. Paper speed: 25 mm/sec.

1. What is the rhythm diagnosis?
2. What is the best therapeutic approach?

Case 29

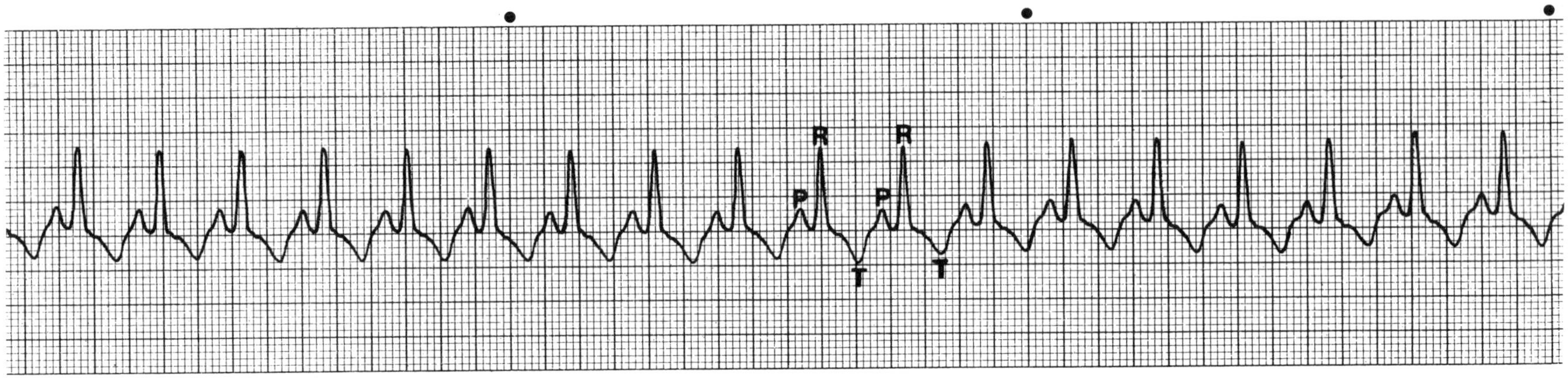

Answer: Sinus tachycardia. Heart rate is 250 beats/min. Sinus tachycardia in cats is associated with fever, stress, pain, hypotension, anemia, hyperthyroidism and heart failure. The tall and wide QRS complexes may indicate left ventricular enlargement. The history and ECG evidence of heart enlargement in this cat suggest cardiac failure. Thoracic radiographs and determination of serum thyroxine concentrations are recommended. Echocardiography may be necessary for a definitive diagnosis. If radiographs confirm heart failure, treatment to slow the heart rate should be instituted. Appropriate drugs for treating hypertrophic cardiomyopathy include diltiazem and propranolol. For hyperthyroidism, propranolol and methimazole (Tapazole) should be prescribed. Diuretics should be used for pulmonary edema or pleural effusion.

Case 30

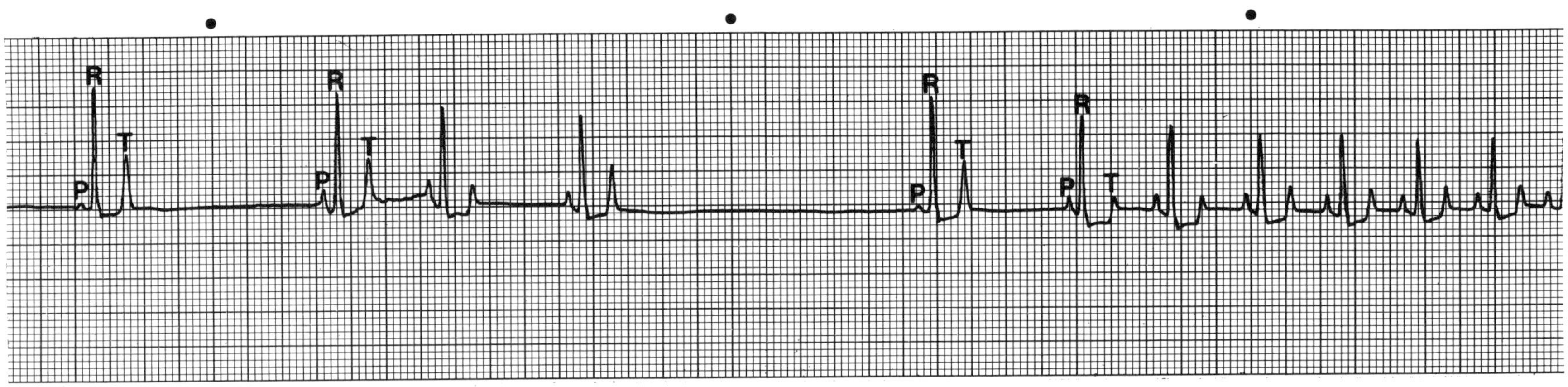

Answer: Pronounced sinus arrhythmia with sinus arrest or block. Heart rate is 50 to 70 beats/min. Sinus arrhythmia is characterized by a P wave-to-P wave interval with a variation greater than 10%. Varying levels of parasympathetic (vagal) tone to the sinus node that correlate with respiration are normal in resting dogs. Sinus arrhythmia is more pronounced in brachycephalic breeds and requires no treatment. Sinus arrest or block is defined as a pause of greater than twice the normal R-R interval. It may reflect increased levels of vagal tone or underlying sinus node disease. Sinus arrest or block requires no treatment in animals with no clinical signs. Notice the varying amplitudes of the P waves, termed "a wandering pacemaker," which are often associated with sinus arrhythmia. Also, notice the variation in amplitude of the QRS complexes and T waves. The distance between electrodes can change with thoracic wall motion during inspiration and expiration. The rate also increases during inspiration and decreases during expiration.

Case 31

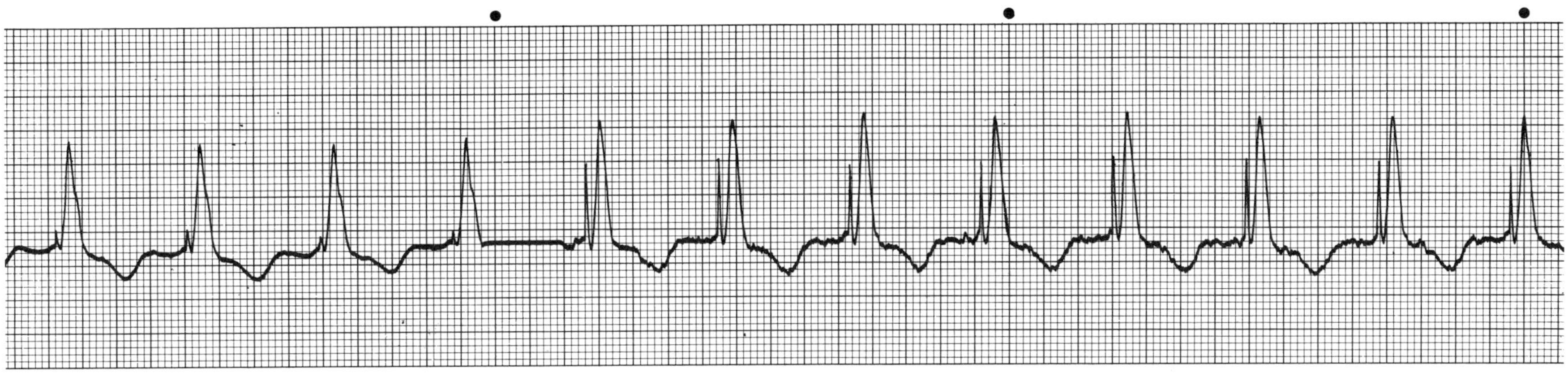

Question: This tracing was recorded from a cat that was recovering from cardiac arrest. The cardiac arrest occurred just minutes after anesthesia was given for repair of a fractured jaw. The first four complexes are lead I, and the rest of the strip is lead II.

1. What procedure had to be performed to help to reverse the cardiac arrest?
2. What is the rhythm diagnosis?

Case 32

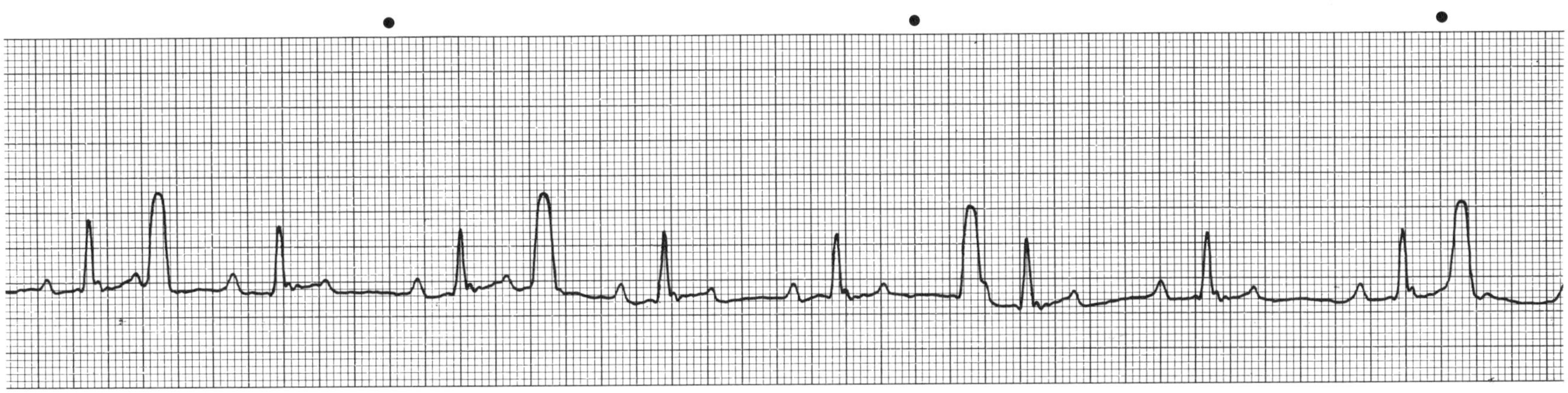

Question: This rhythm strip was recorded from a dog that had experienced 3 seizures over the past 10 days.

1. What is the rhythm diagnosis?

Case 31

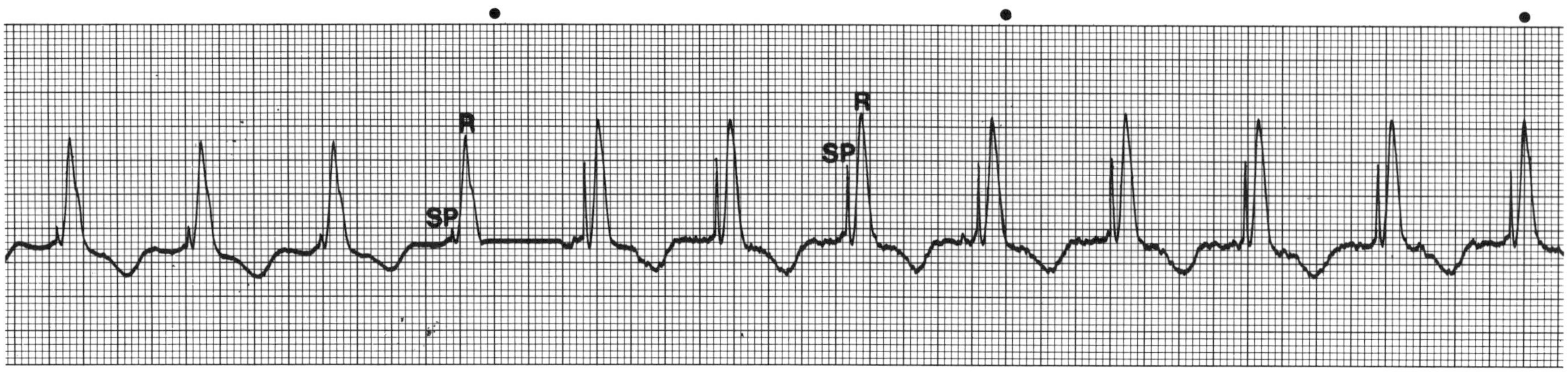

Answer: Fixed-rate, artificial pacemaker rhythm. Left bundle-branch block pattern. Heart rate is 158 beats/min. A transvenous electrode wire has been placed in the right ventricle, resulting in a left bundle-branch block pattern. Each stimulus artifact (SP) is followed by a QRS-T complex. When the pacing lead is placed in the right ventricle, the right ventricular myocardium is depolarized in advance of the left ventricle. The right ventricular pacing results in a QRS complex width that is increased to 0.06 sec and is positive. Electronic pacemakers are used on a temporary or permanent basis for treating symptomatic bradycardia and occasionally are used for controlling a tachycardia resistant to drug therapy. When the condition of this cat has been stabilized, the temporary pacemaker will probably not be needed.

Case 32

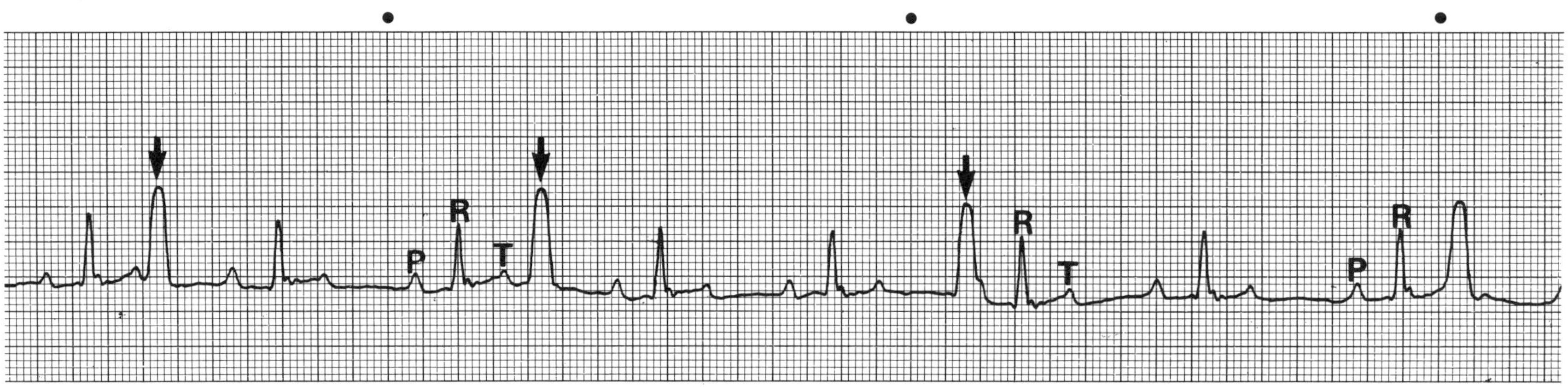

Answer: Normal sinus rhythm and artifact. Heart rate is approximately 110 beats/min. The artifacts (arrows) simulate ventricular ectopic complexes but do not interrupt the normal sinus rhythm. The ECG is a mechanical recording; therefore, several technical or mechanical problems can occur while it is being obtained. The causes of artifact can be placed into two general categories: (1) technical recording problems (fault of the clinician, the machine, or the electrodes and cable) and (2) problems with the animal. Muscle tremor, limb or body motion, poor electrode contact, or surrounding electrical interference can all cause artifactual rhythms. An important method for diagnosing electrocardiographic artifact is the demonstration that normal electrocardiographic activity proceeds despite the artifactual wave forms.

Case 33

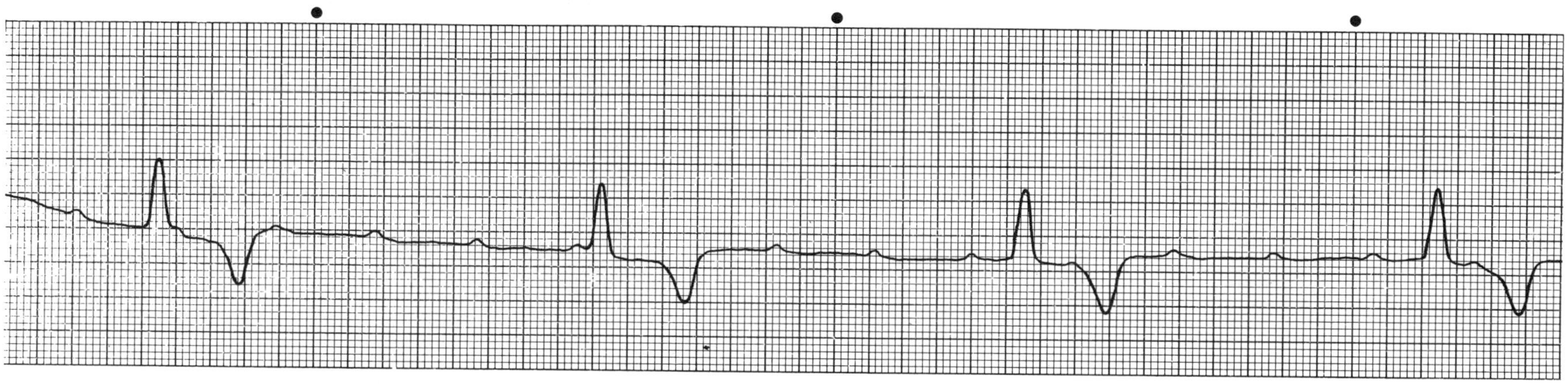

Question: This rhythm strip was recorded from a 12-year-old domestic shorthair cat with a history of lethargy.

1. What is the rhythm diagnosis?
2. What are common causes of this arrhythmia?
3. What is the best therapeutic approach?

Case 34

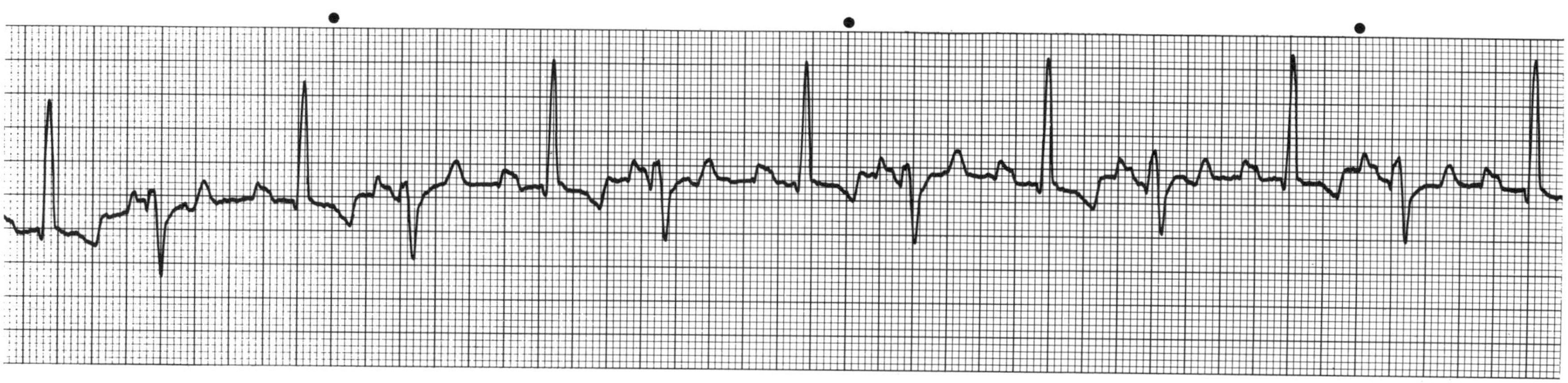

Question: This lead II ECG was recorded from an 8-year-old Collie with a history of coughing at night.

1. What is the rhythm diagnosis?
2. What is the most likely mechanism for this arrhythmia?
3. What is the best therapeutic approach?

Case 33

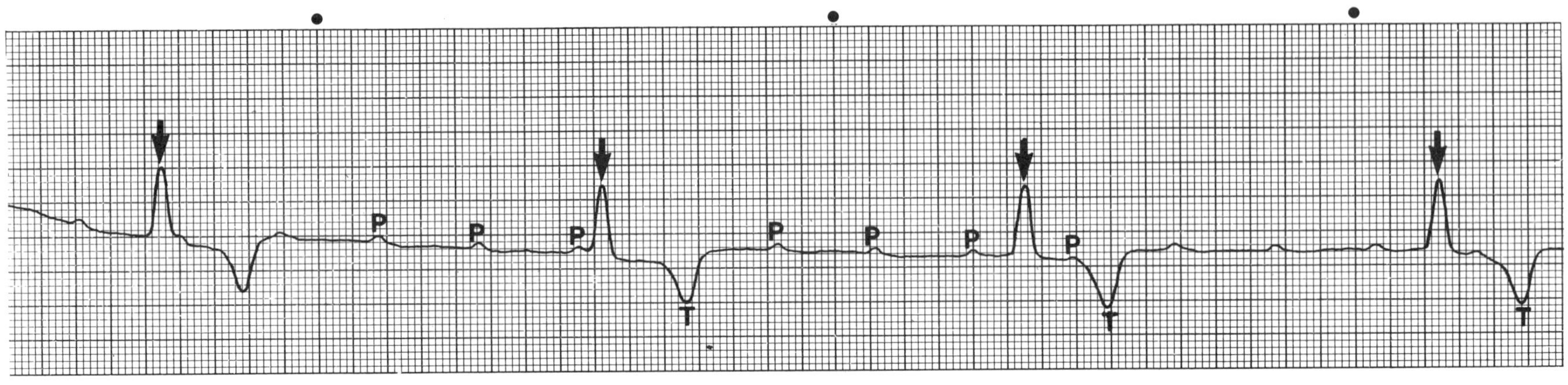

Answer: Complete AV block. Atrial heart rate is 200 beats/min; ventricular heart rate is 48 beats/min. Complete AV block is diagnosed by P waves occurring at a regular interval independent of the slower ventricular escape rhythm (arrows). Complete AV block in old cats is often associated with degeneration or fibrosis of the AV node. Cardiomyopathy, myocarditis, and neoplastic infiltration must also be considered. Complete AV block does not respond to atropine. The ventricular escape rate can sometimes be increased with the use of bronchodilators, such as aminophylline, theophylline, and terbutaline. These drugs increase the rate through direct or indirect stimulation of the adrenergic nervous system. Increases in the heart rate are usually minimal, and pacemaker implantation is sometimes needed to alleviate clinical signs. Arrhythmias related to myocarditis may resolve. Myocarditis is an uncommon cause of AV block in cats.

Case 34

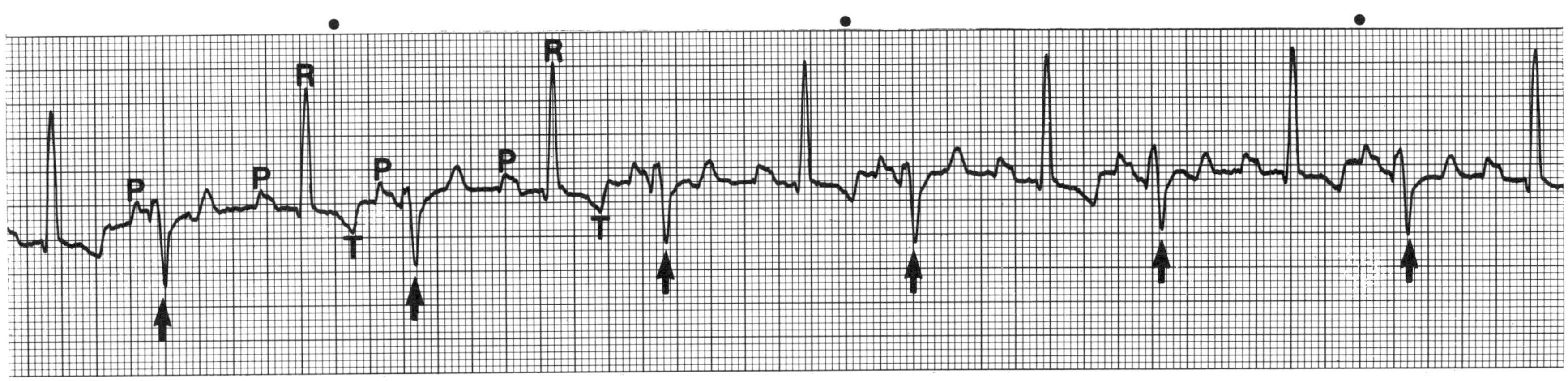

Answer: Sinus rhythm with ventricular bigeminy. Heart rate is 160 beats/min. Ventricular bigeminy is a rhythm characterized by a ventricular premature complex (arrow) alternating with a sinus complex. The regular alternating pattern suggests re-entry as the mechanism for the arrhythmia. The independent P waves happen to precede the ventricular premature complexes. The wide and notched P waves may indicate left atrial enlargement. Thoracic radiographs are indicated to determine if the dog is in congestive heart failure. Furosemide should be prescribed if edema is present. On the basis of the frequency of the ventricular premature complexes and possibility of congestive heart failure, an antiarrhythmic drug should be prescribed. Options include procainamide, quinidine, tocainide, and mexiletine.

Case 35

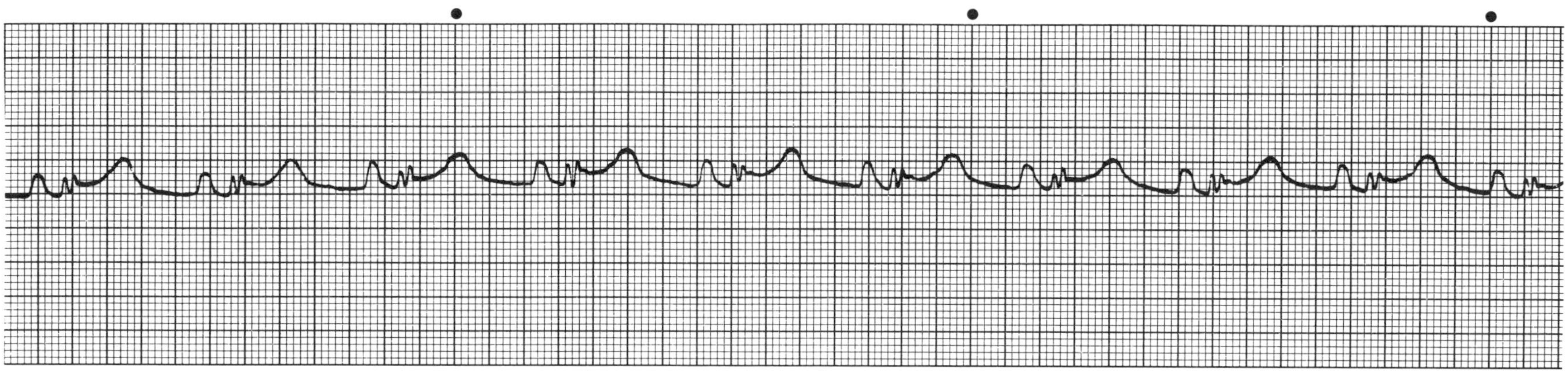

Question: This lead II ECG was obtained from a 13-year-old Irish Setter with cyanosis and muffled heart sounds.

1. What is the rhythm diagnosis?
2. What is the best therapeutic approach?

Case 36

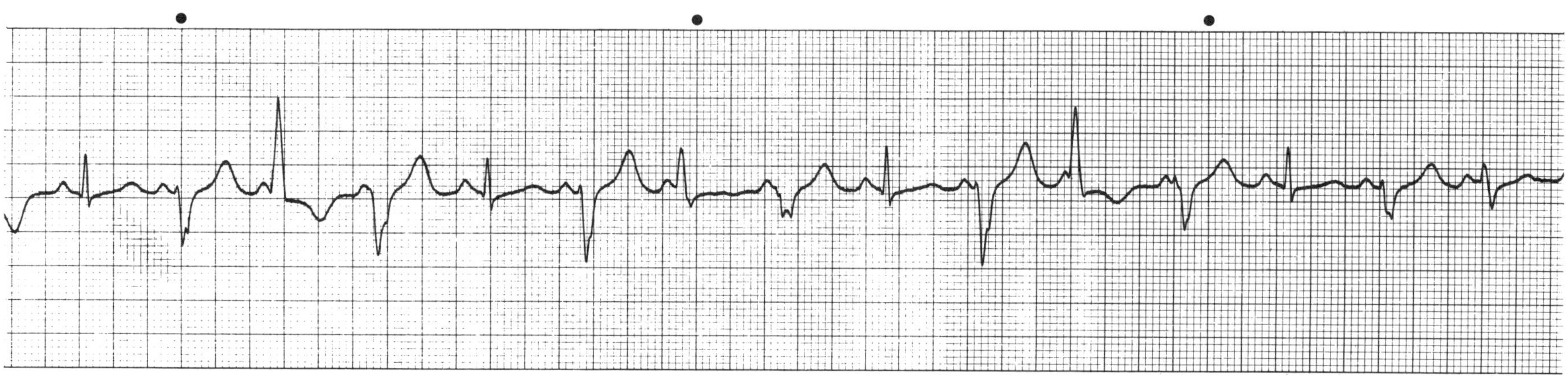

Question: This tracing was recorded from a dyspneic cat with severe pleural effusion. An echocardiographic study documented the dilated form of cardiomyopathy. An abnormality in rhythm was auscultated with a pronounced femoral pulse deficit palpated.

1. What is the rhythm diagnosis?
2. What is the best therapeutic approach?

Case 35

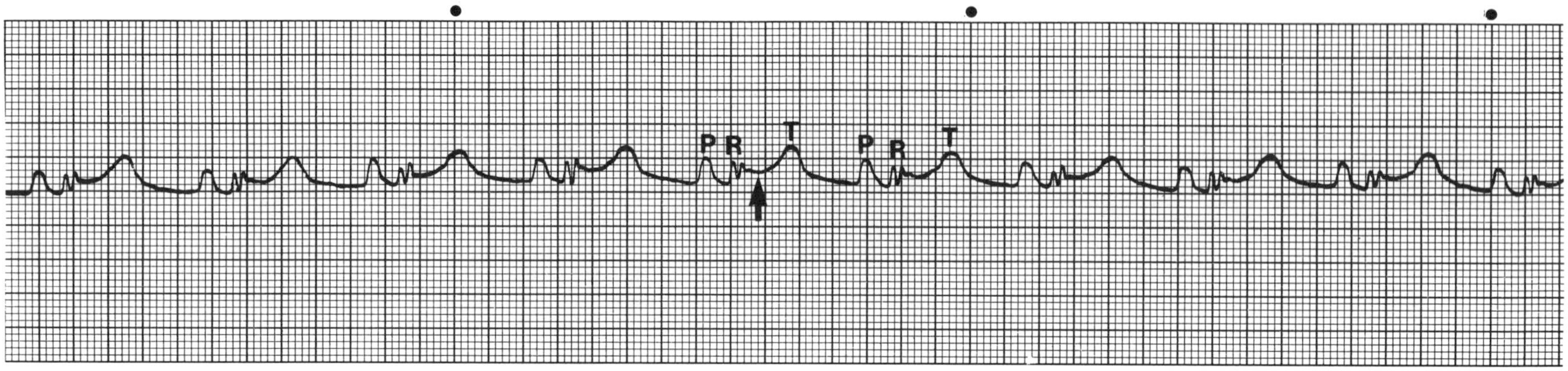

Answer: Sinus rhythm. The heart rate is approximately 120 beats/min. The wide P waves suggest left atrial enlargement. The small QRS complexes and S-T segment elevation (arrow) suggest pericardial effusion. Muffled heart sounds, distended jugular veins, a large, globular-shaped cardiac silhouette, and ascites are typical of chronic pericardial effusion. An echocardiogram is a sensitive and specific test to confirm the diagnosis. Pericardiocentesis is the best therapeutic approach for pericardial effusion. S-T segment elevation suggests pressure or inflammation of the pericardium and is found in animals with pericardial effusion, pericarditis, myocardial hypoxia, and myocardial infarction.

Case 36

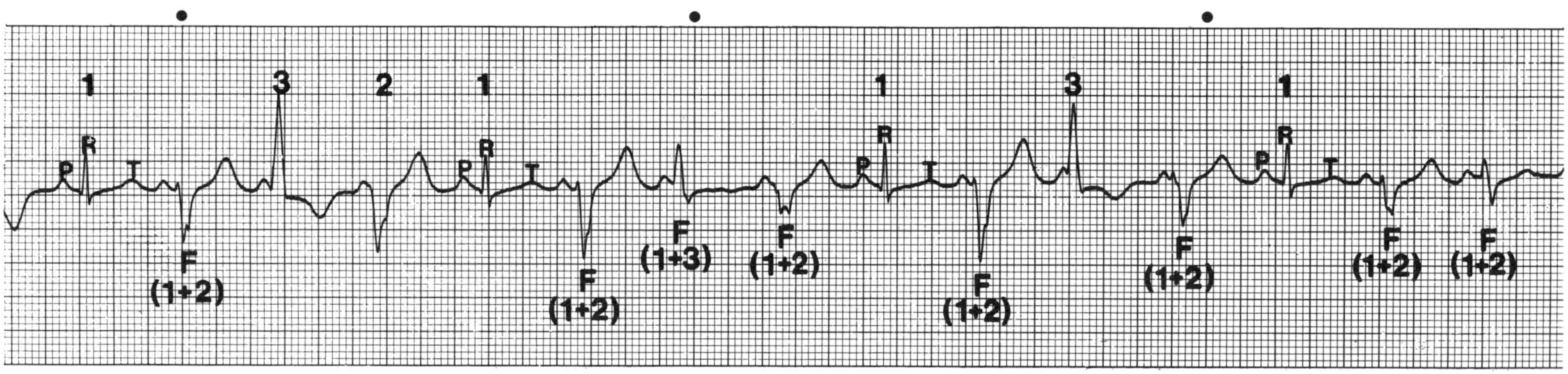

Answer: Multifocal ventricular premature complexes. Heart rate is approximately 200 beats/min. Three different ventricular ectopic foci are probably present in this lead II rhythm strip. The three foci include: (1) a normal sinus complex, (2) a ventricular premature complex (VPC), and (3) another VPC. The simultaneous activation of the ventricles by the sinus complex and one of the other two ventricular foci creates ventricular fusion complexes (F). Some fusion complexes may represent fusion of all three foci. Ventricular fusion complexes have no clinical significance other than to confirm the ectopic nature of the premature complexes. VPCs with different configurations occurring in the same animal are called multifocal or, more appropriately, multiform VPCs. VPCs of uniform configuration are presumed to arise from the same focus. Multiform VPCs may arise either from more than one focus (multifocal) or from a single focus but activating the ventricles along different pathways and causing different QRS complex configurations (unifocal with variable conduction). The term multiform VPCs is preferred because it includes both possible mechanisms. VPCs rarely require aggressive treatment in the cat because they tend to decrease and often disappear spontaneously after the heart failure has been treated. Therapy for heart failure in this cat consisted of furosemide, captopril, and taurine. The prognosis is obviously guarded in this case, given the severity of the presenting signs.

Case 37

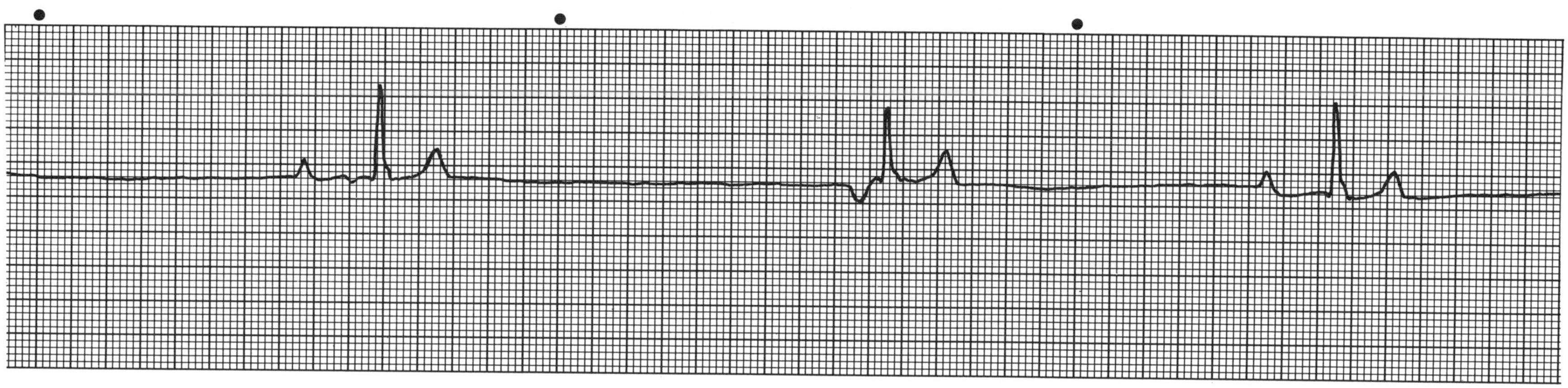

Question: This lead II rhythm strip was recorded from a 14-year-old female Cocker Spaniel with a history of syncope.

1. What is the rhythm diagnosis?
2. What are common causes of this arrhythmia?
3. What is the most likely underlying disorder?
4. What is the best therapeutic approach?

Case 38

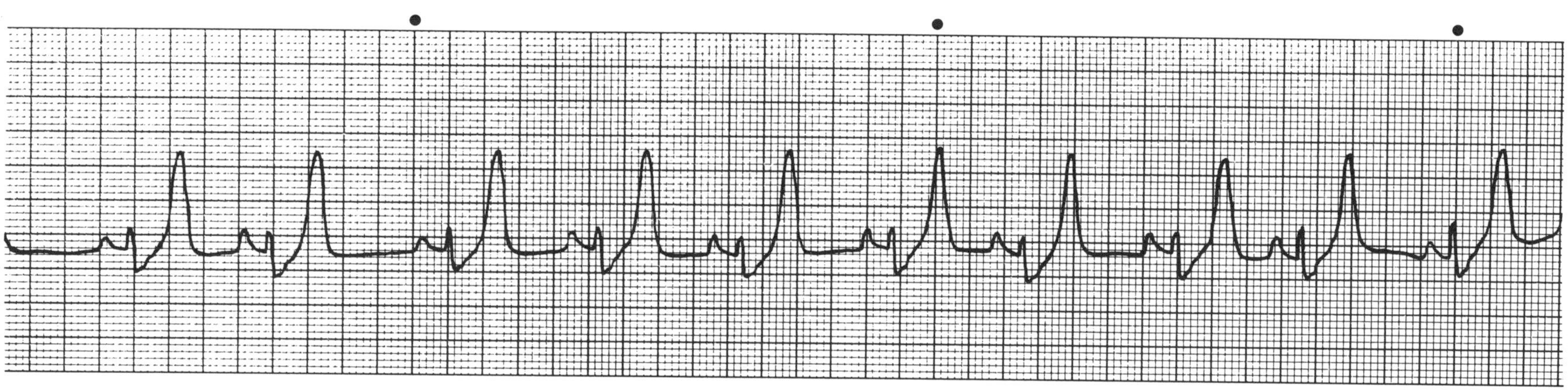

Question: This lead II ECG was obtained from a 6-year-old Beagle with heartworm disease. The clinical signs were severe dyspnea, extreme weakness, and cyanotic mucous membranes.

1. What is the rhythm diagnosis?
2. What is the most likely underlying disorder?
3. What is the best therapeutic approach?

Case 37

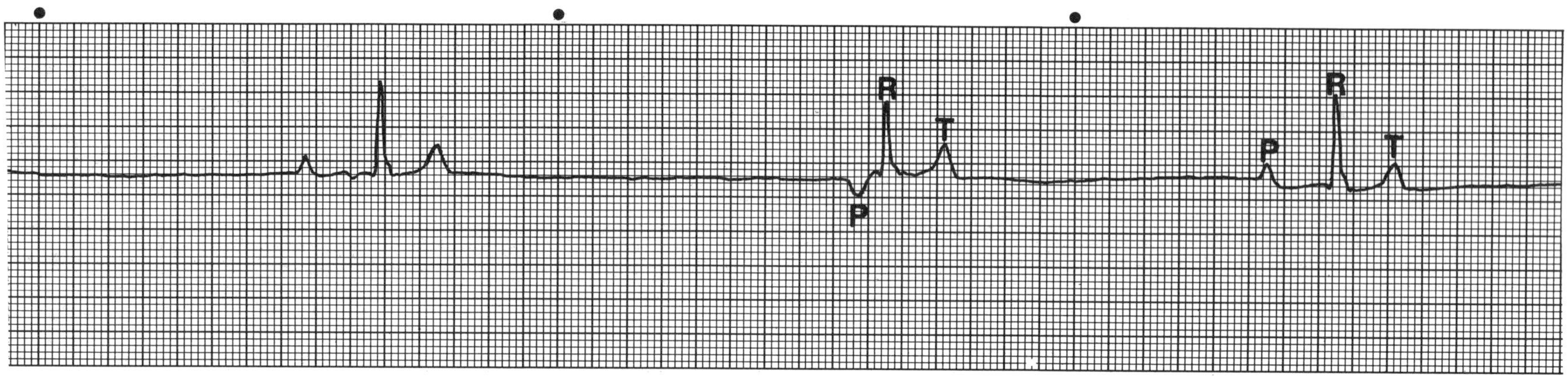

Answer: Sinus bradycardia with first-degree AV block and a junctional escape beat. Heart rate is approximately 40 beats/min. Sinus bradycardia is associated with hypothyroidism, sinus node disease, hypothermia, increased vagal tone, and drug administration (e.g., digoxin, propranolol, diltiazem, and xylazine). Old female Cocker Spaniels are prone to sick sinus syndrome. First-degree AV block can also be associated with increased vagal tone, hypothermia, and drug administration. Degeneration or fibrosis in the AV node of geriatric dogs is a common cause of AV block. Neoplastic infiltration and myocarditis can also affect AV nodal conduction. The junctional escape beat is a normal response to a long sinus pause. The junctional nature of the escape beat is revealed by the negative (retrograde conducted) P wave. P waves are not always seen with junctional escape beats. When they are observed, they can occur before or after the QRS complex and may be positive or negative in polarity. Because of the breed, sex, and age of the dog, the most likely underlying diagnosis is sick sinus syndrome and AV nodal degeneration or fibrosis. For dogs with signs of bradycardia, an oral anticholinergic drug, such as propantheline or isopropamide, and a pacemaker should be prescribed.

Case 38

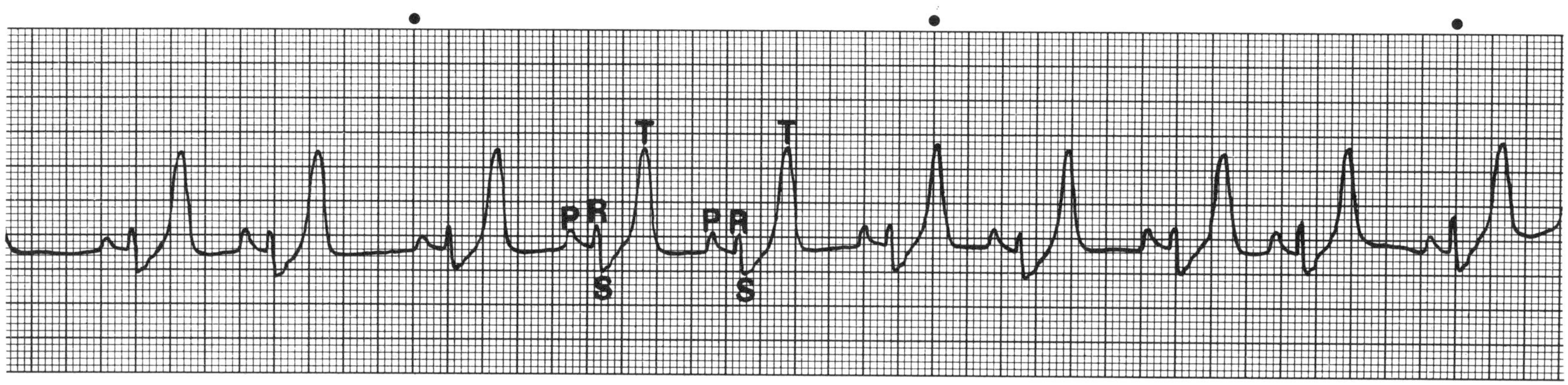

Answer: Sinus rhythm. Heart rate is 140 beats/min. Pulmonary thromboembolism is the most likely underlying disorder. Thoracic radiographs should be taken. Antiarrhythmic drugs are not indicated. Supportive treatment for pulmonary thromboembolism includes cage rest and oxygen, high doses of corticosteroids, fluid support, and aspirin. Severe pulmonary thromboembolism causes acute pulmonary hypertension and right ventricular dilatation. The rapid development of an S wave (when compared with a previous ECG from the same dog) and increased amplitude of the T waves are typical changes that may occur within hours after a pulmonary thromboembolism.

Case 39

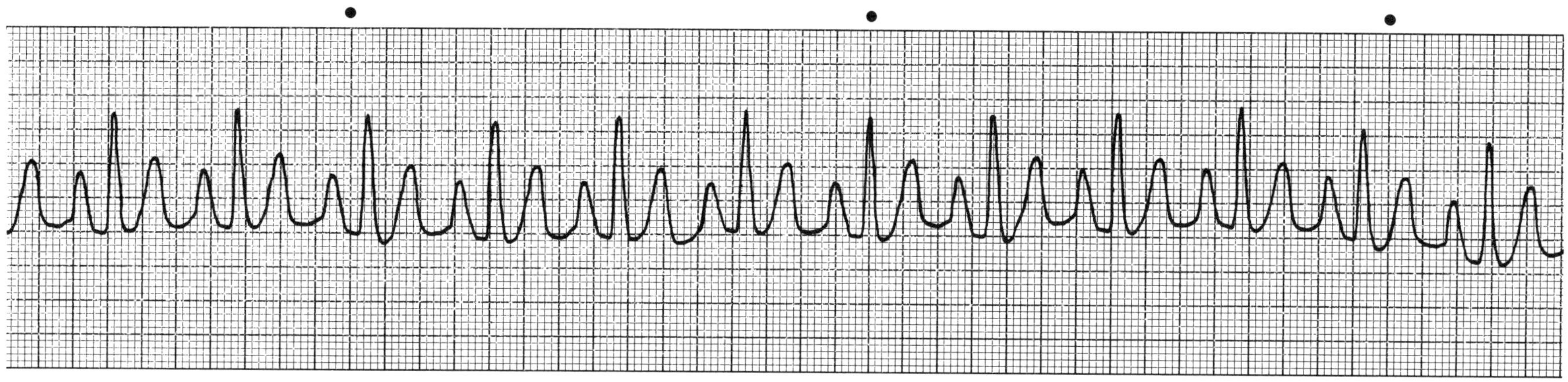

Question: This lead II ECG was obtained from a 7-year-old Pointer with heartworm disease. The dog was examined because of severe dyspnea and cyanosis.

1. What is the rhythm diagnosis?
2. What is the most likely underlying disorder?
3. What is the best therapeutic approach?

Case 40

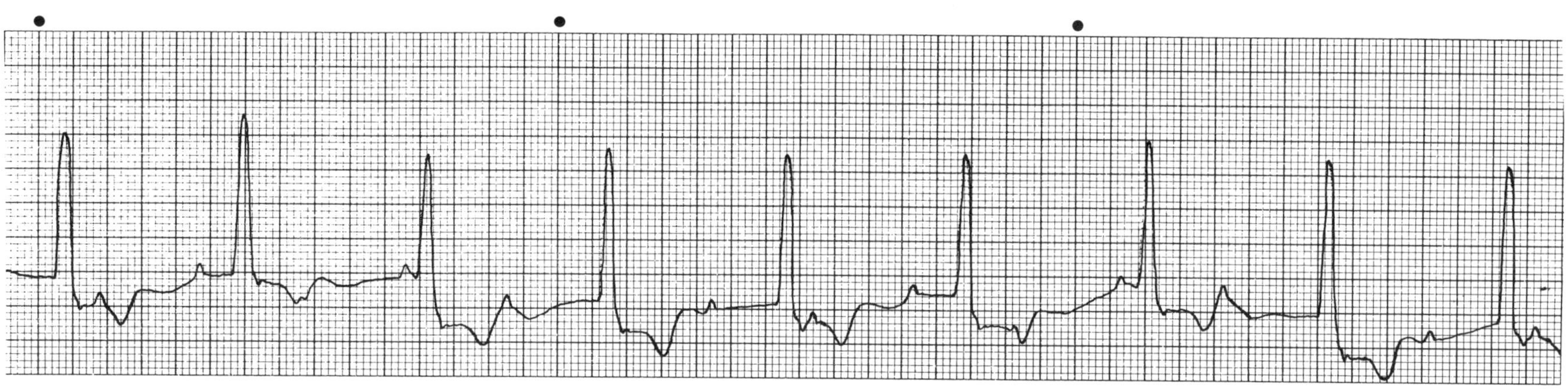

Question: This lead II ECG was obtained from a 16-year-old cat with no clinical signs and a slow heart rate heard on auscultation.

1. What is the rhythm diagnosis?
2. What is the most likely underlying disorder?
3. What is the best therapeutic approach?

Case 39

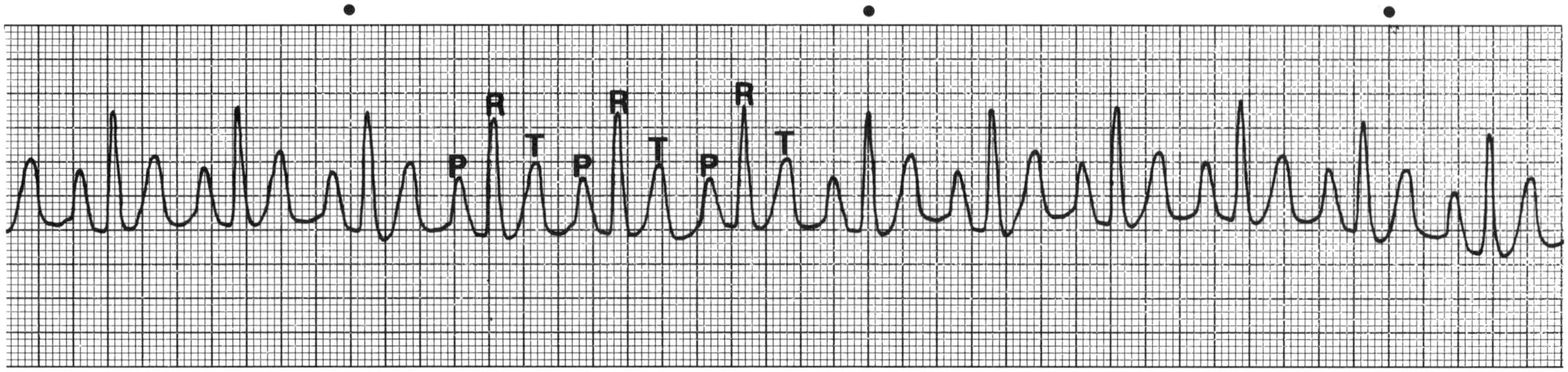

Answer: Sinus rhythm. Heart rate is 165 beats/min. Notice the S-T segment depression and large T waves. Pulmonary thromboembolism is the most likely cause of the acute dyspnea. Treatment for pulmonary thromboembolism includes cage rest and oxygen and corticosteroids. Antithrombotic therapy with either heparin or aspirin may decrease the risk of subsequent emboli. In humans with massive thromboembolism, thrombolytic therapy is often instituted. Thoracic radiographs may support this diagnosis, but can be normal in animals with pulmonary embolism. Pulmonary arteriography is commonly used in humans with suspected pulmonary thromboembolism. In dogs, causes of pulmonary thromboembolism include pancreatitis, glomerulonephritis, chronic renal disease, neoplasia, hyperadrenocorticism, and heartworm disease.

Case 40

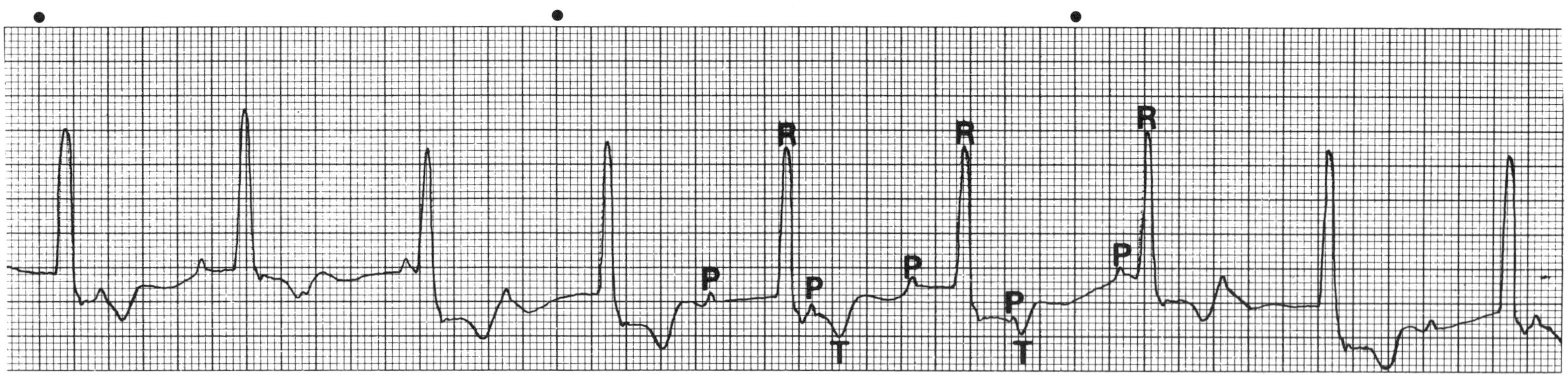

Answer: Sinus rhythm with complete (third-degree) AV block. Atrial heart rate is 200 beats/min.; ventricular heart rate is 115 beats/min. Idiopathic fibrosis of the AV conduction tissue (i.e., His bundle or both bundle branches) is the most likely underlying disorder. Because the cat has no clinical signs, treatment is unnecessary. If clinical signs of weakness or syncope develop, a permanent cardiac pacemaker will have to be considered. An echocardiogram would be recommended. Other possible associated conditions include hyperthyroidism, cardiomyopathy, and chronic renal disease with secondary hypertension. The ventricular rate is slower than the atrial rate. The QRS complexes are wide and tall, thus indicating left ventricular enlargement or escape pacemaker in either the ventricle or the lower AV junction with bundle-branch block.

Case 41

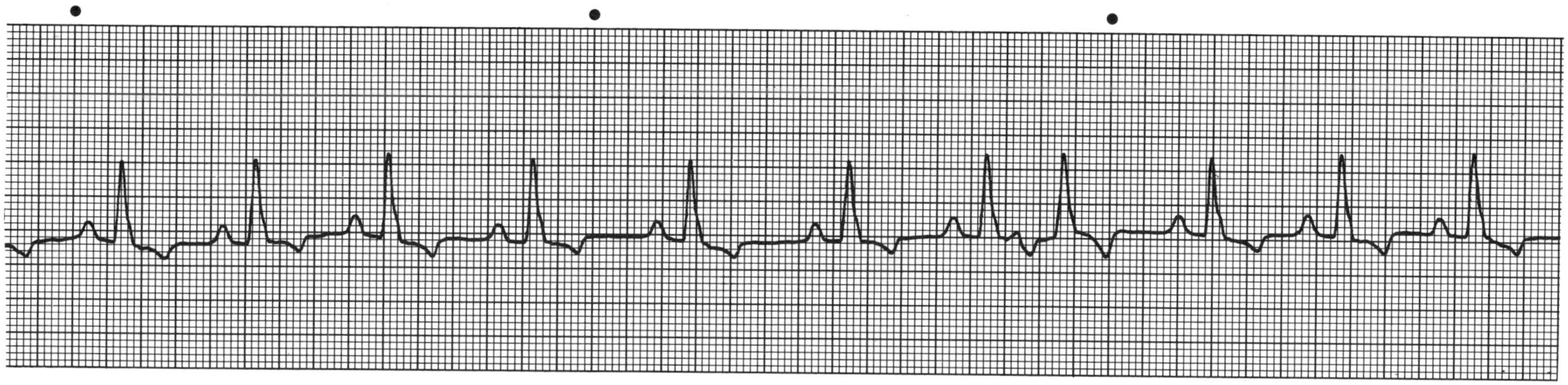

Question: This rhythm strip was recorded from a 5-year-old asymptomatic Terrier.

1. What is the rhythm diagnosis?
2. What are common causes of this arrhythmia?

Case 42

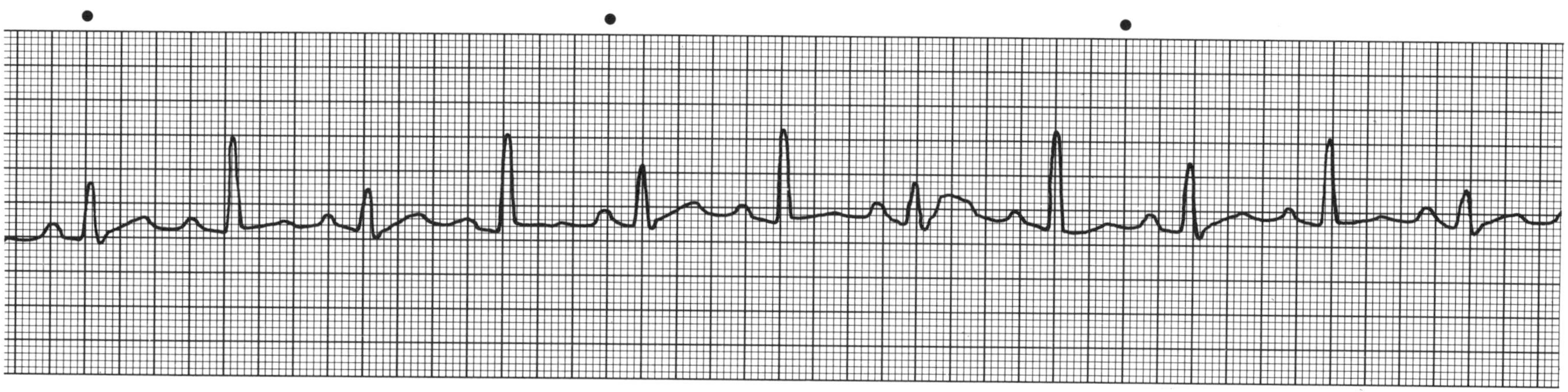

Question: This lead II ECG was obtained from an 11-year-old German Shepherd examined because of severe weakness and difficulty breathing.

1. What is the rhythm diagnosis?
2. What is the most likely underlying disorder?
3. What is the best therapeutic approach?

Case 41

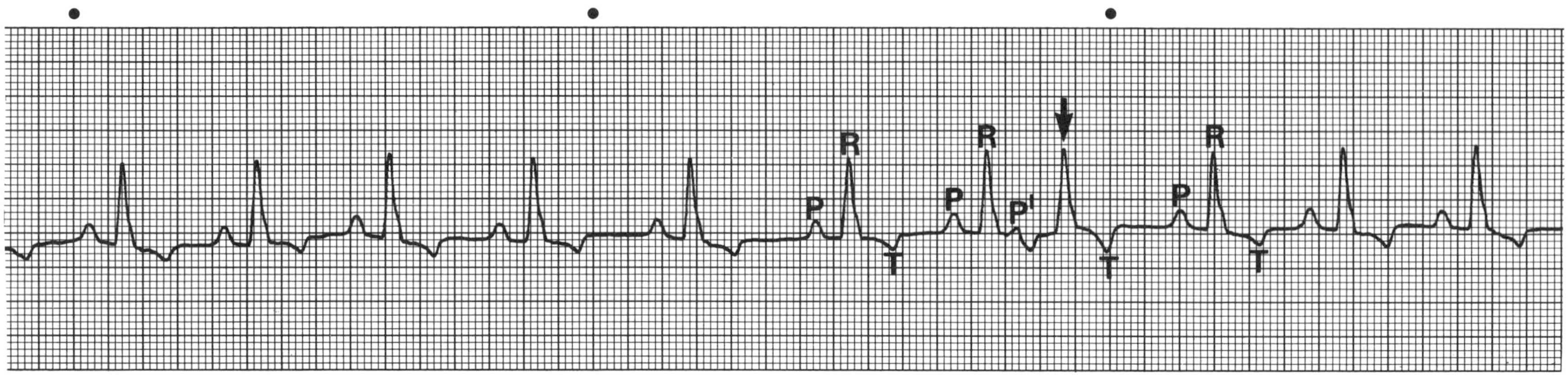

Answer: Sinus arrhythmia with one atrial premature complex (arrow). Heart rate is 160 beats/min. Atrial premature complexes arise from ectopic foci in the atria. They are frequently caused by cardiac disease and may lead to atrial tachycardia, atrial flutter, or atrial fibrillation. The ectopic P′ wave is premature, and its configuration is different from that of the sinus P waves. The QRS complex is premature, and its configuration is usually normal. The P′ and P′-R intervals are usually as long as, or longer than, the sinus P-R interval. The atrial depolarization caused by an atrial premature complex usually depolarizes and resets the SA node. The pause following the atrial premature complex is usually, but not always, less than fully compensatory. The SA node resumes its normal pacemaker activity at a time earlier than what had been expected from the normal R-R interval. As with most premature complexes, the coupling interval (the time between the premature complex and the preceding complex) should be relatively constant. If the coupling intervals are variable, atrial parasystole or multifocal atrial premature complexes may be present. Atrial parasystoles are rare.

Case 42

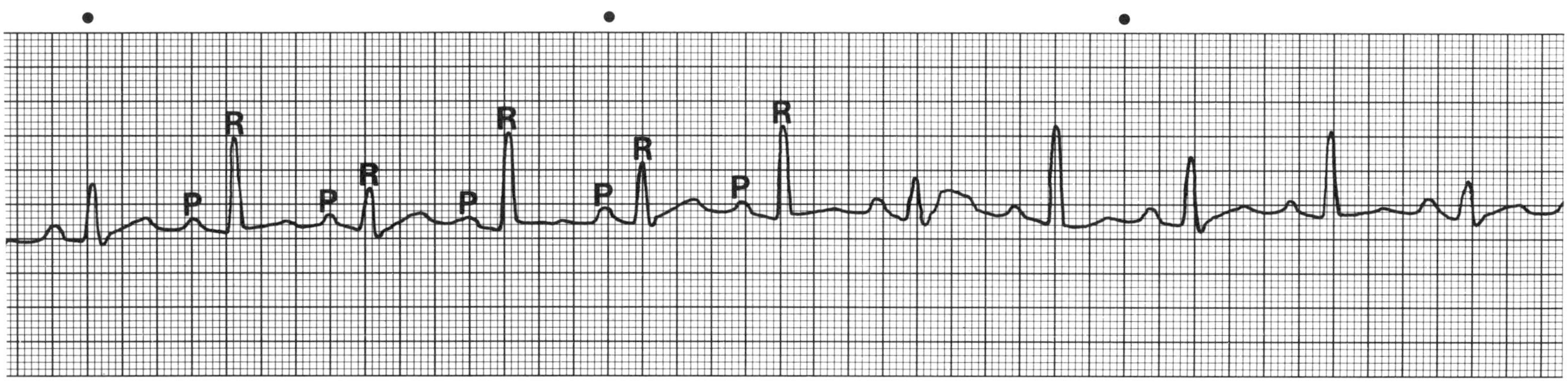

Answer: Sinus rhythm with electrical alternans. Heart rate is 150 beats/min. Electrical alternans is associated with pericardial effusion, alternating bundle-branch block, and supraventricular tachycardia. At least 50 to 75% of animals with pericardial effusion do not have electrical alternans, but rather have small QRS complex amplitudes or S-T segment elevation. Pericardiocentesis and, in selected animals, pericardiectomy are the best therapeutic approaches. Echocardiography is sensitive and specific for detecting pericardial effusion and accompanying right atrial hemangiosarcoma or heart base chemodectoma. Indicators of pericardial effusion that are evident during the physical examination include muffled heart sounds, jugular venous distention or pulsations, and ascites. A large, rounded cardiac silhouette is typically seen on radiographs.

Case 43

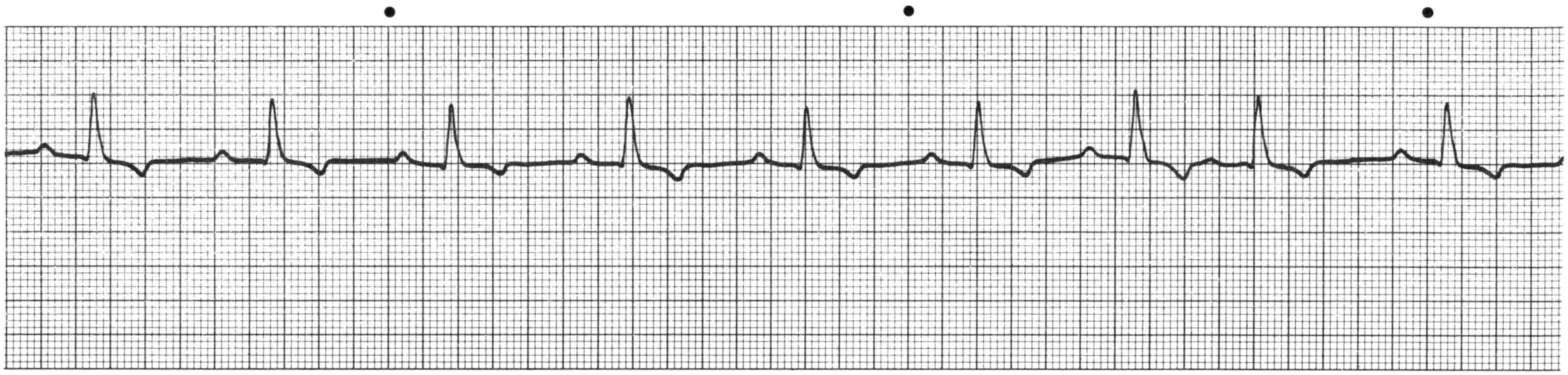

Question: This rhythm strip was recorded from a Burmese cat with dyspnea, hypothermia, and marked lethargy. Thoracic radiographs revealed cardiomegaly and pleural effusion.

1. What is the rhythm diagnosis?
2. What is the most likely underlying disorder?

Case 44

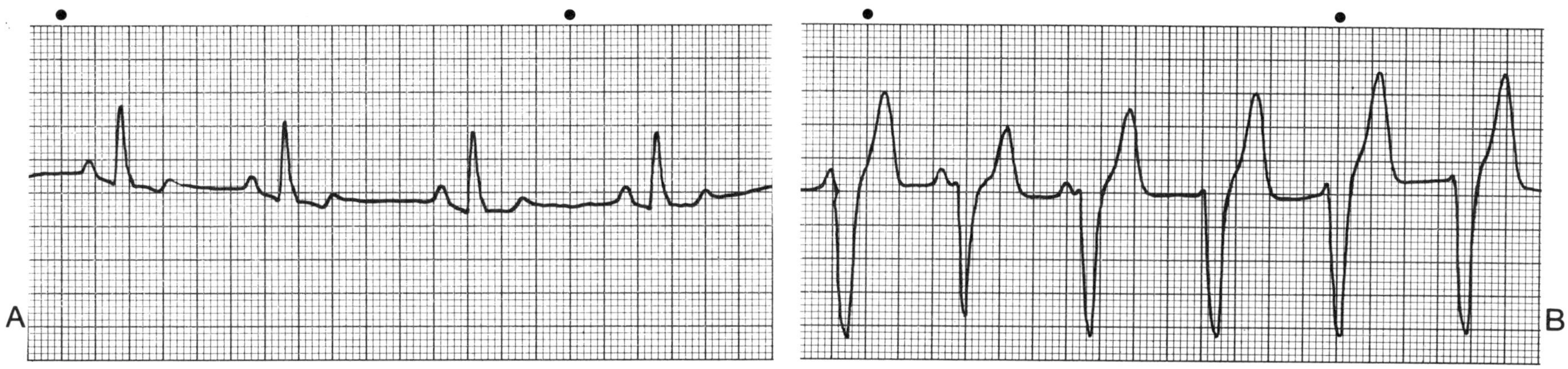

Question: Strip A was recorded from a dog during surgery for a gastric torsion. Strip B was recorded 3 days later.

1. What is the rhythm diagnosis?
2. What is the most likely underlying disorder?
3. What is the best therapeutic approach?

Case 43

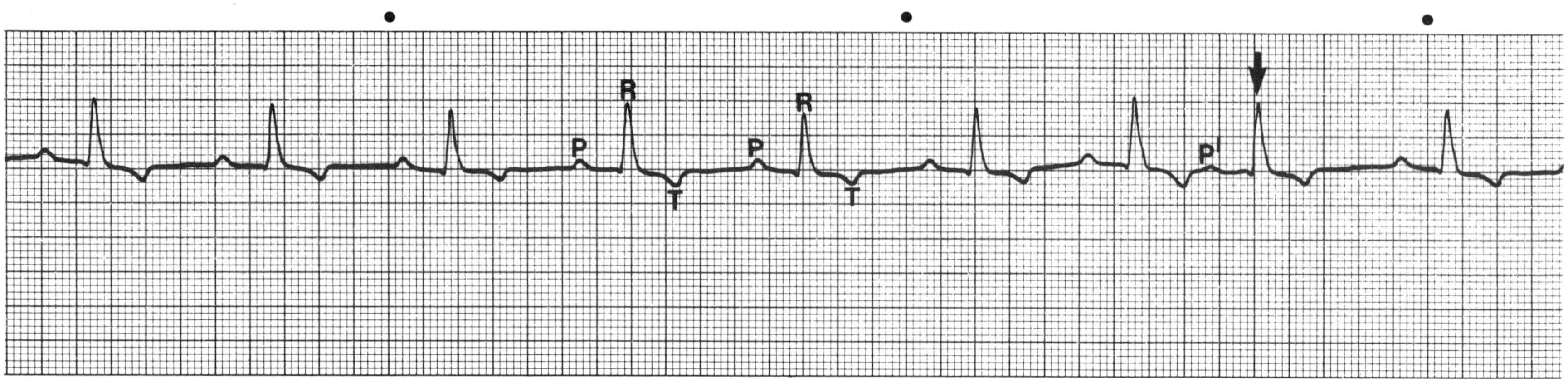

Answer: First-degree AV block (P-R interval 0.13 sec or 6½ boxes; normal not greater than 0.09 sec or 4½ boxes). Sinus bradycardia. Heart rate is approximately 120 beats/min, one atrial premature complex (arrow). When the strip is not read from left to right, the atrial premature complex can be easily missed. The varying QRS complex amplitude is compatible with the pleural effusion. With these electrocardiographic abnormalities and the clinical evaluation, the dilated form of cardiomyopathy should first be considered. A dietary history should be obtained to determine the likelihood of taurine deficiency. Hypokalemia may cause taurine deficiency cardiomyopathy.

Case 44

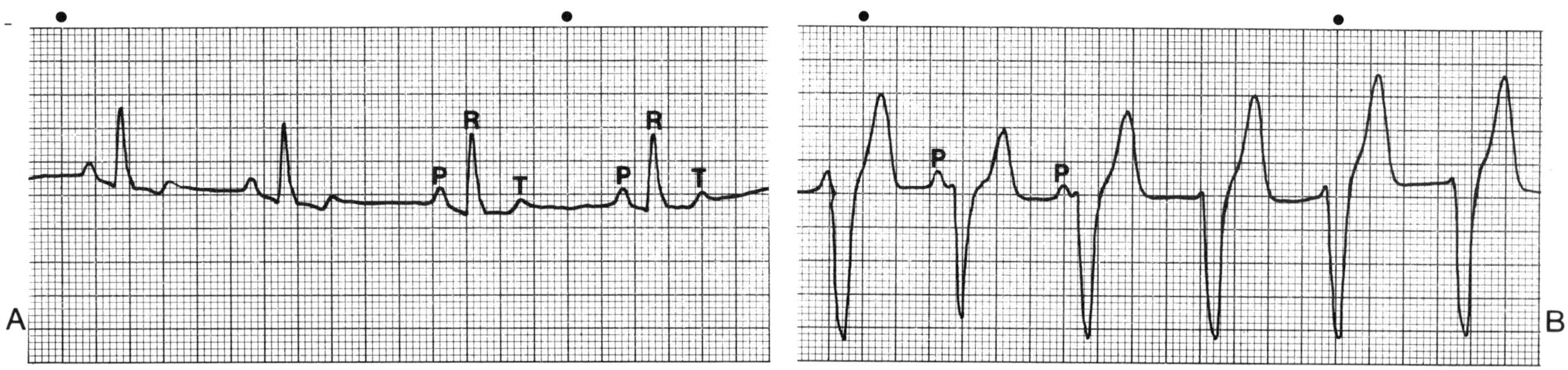

Answer: A. Normal sinus rhythm. Heart rate is 110 beats/min. B. Ventricular tachycardia (no relationship between P waves and bizarre QRS complexes). Heart rate is 165 beats/min. Ventricular ectopic arrhythmias often do not occur until 12 to 36 hours after a myocardial ischemic event (e.g., gastric dilatation-volvulus, myocardial infarction, or traumatic myocarditis). The exact mechanism for these arrhythmias is unknown, but theories include acid-base imbalance, autonomic imbalance, myocardial hypoxia, electrolyte imbalance, or a myocardial depressant factor. The initial therapy for ventricular tachycardia is an intravenous bolus of lidocaine. If such therapy converts the arrhythmia, the animal then is placed on a lidocaine infusion. The infusion rate is adjusted as needed to control the arrhythmia. When the dog can take oral medication, sustained-release forms of procainamide or quinidine should be administered for several weeks.

Case 45

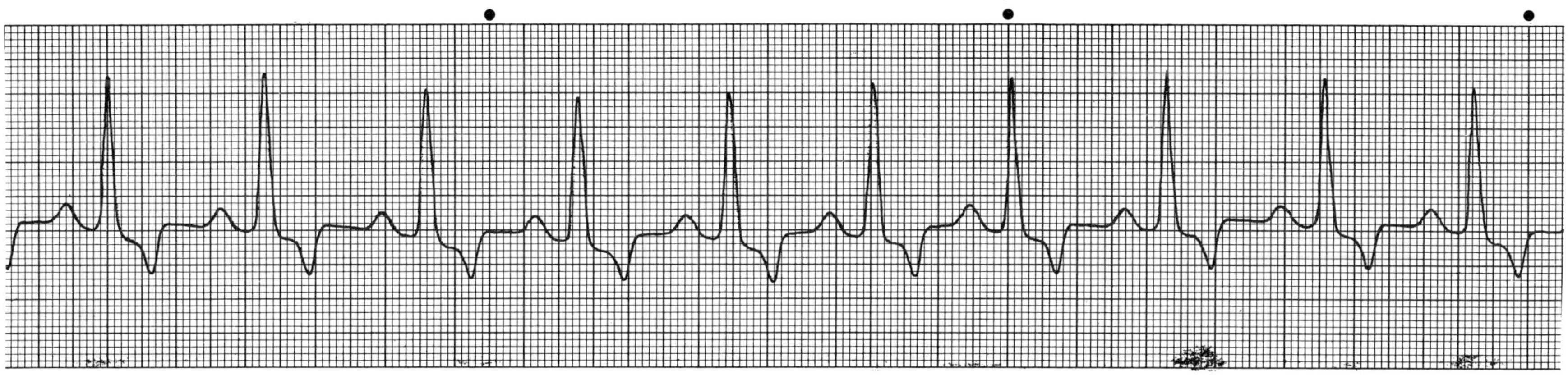

Question: This tracing was recorded from an aged German Shepherd with mitral valvular insufficiency. No clinical signs were present.

1. What is the rhythm diagnosis?
2. What other tests should be performed?

Case 46

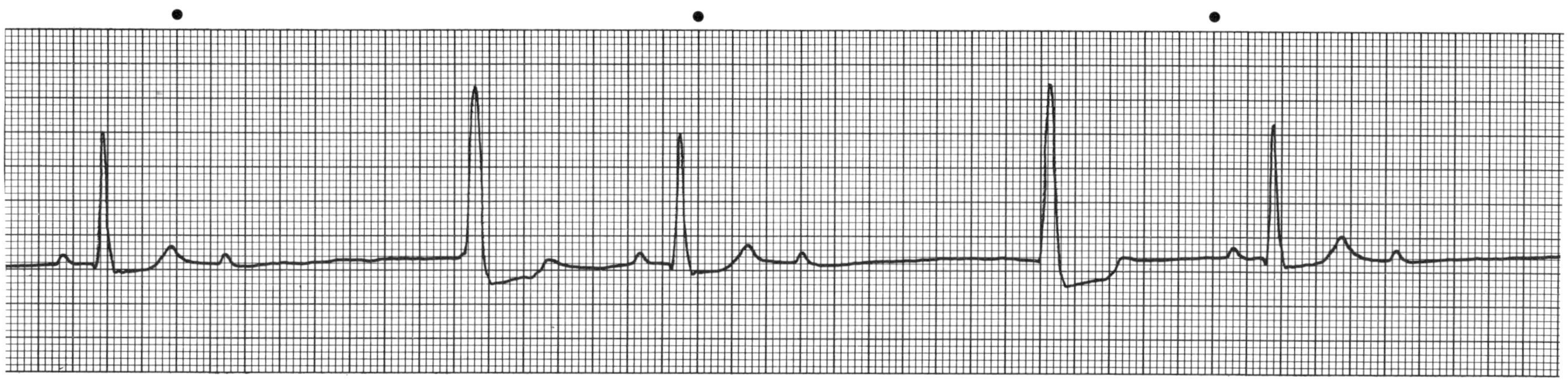

Question: This lead II ECG was obtained from a 9-year-old female Cocker Spaniel examined because of collapsing episodes that had occurred during the past 72 hours. Intermittent pauses were heard on auscultation.

1. What is the rhythm diagnosis?
2. What is the most likely underlying disorder?
3. What is the best therapeutic approach?

Case 45

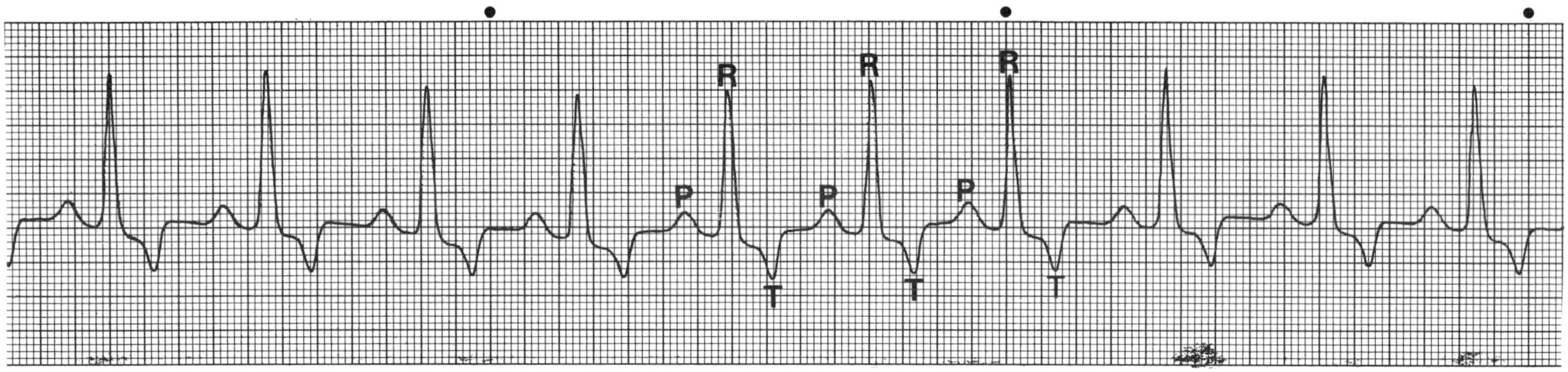

Answer: Normal sinus rhythm. Heart rate is 140 beats/min. Sinus rhythm is the normal mechanism for initiating cardiac systole. The normal cardiac impulse originates in the SA node and spreads to the atrium, the AV node, the His-Purkinje system, and the ventricular myocardium. The normal heart rate can be regular or irregular. A regular sinus rhythm below the normal heart rate range is a sinus bradycardia, and that above the normal heart rate range is a sinus tachycardia. The P-QRS complexes are normal with a constant P-R interval. The wide P waves indicate possible left atrial enlargement. Failure of the rhythm to meet any of the criteria for sinus rhythm indicates a possibility of some abnormality of impulse formation and/or impulse conduction (e.g., an arrhythmia). Because of the possible left atrial enlargement, a chest radiograph should be taken. Atrial arrhythmias may occur with congestive heart failure.

Case 46

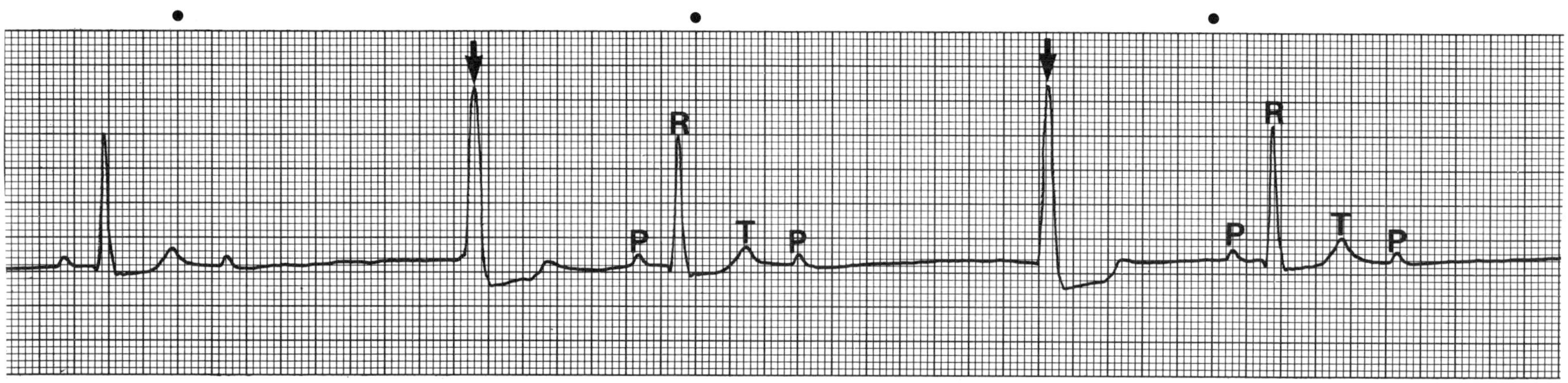

Answer: Sinus bradycardia with intermittent second-degree AV block, periods of sinoatrial block or sinus arrest, and ventricular escape beats. Heart rate is approximately 60 beats/min. Female Cocker Spaniels, as well as Miniature Schnauzers and Dachshunds, are predisposed to sinus node disease (sick sinus syndrome). Atropine sulfate administered intramuscularly or subcutaneously is the initial therapeutic approach. Anticholinergics (e.g., propantheline) can be administered orally for long-term therapy if the response to atropine is favorable. A permanent cardiac pacemaker is required when the response to atropine is poor. Sinus node disease is often accompanied by AV conduction disease; therefore, the second-degree AV block (P wave not followed by a QRS complex) is not unexpected. The ventricular escape (occurs after a pause) complex (arrow) should not be confused with a ventricular premature complex and suppressed with an antiarrhythmic drug. Further increases in the sinus pauses (period before the escape beats) may result in hemodynamic collapse.

Case 47

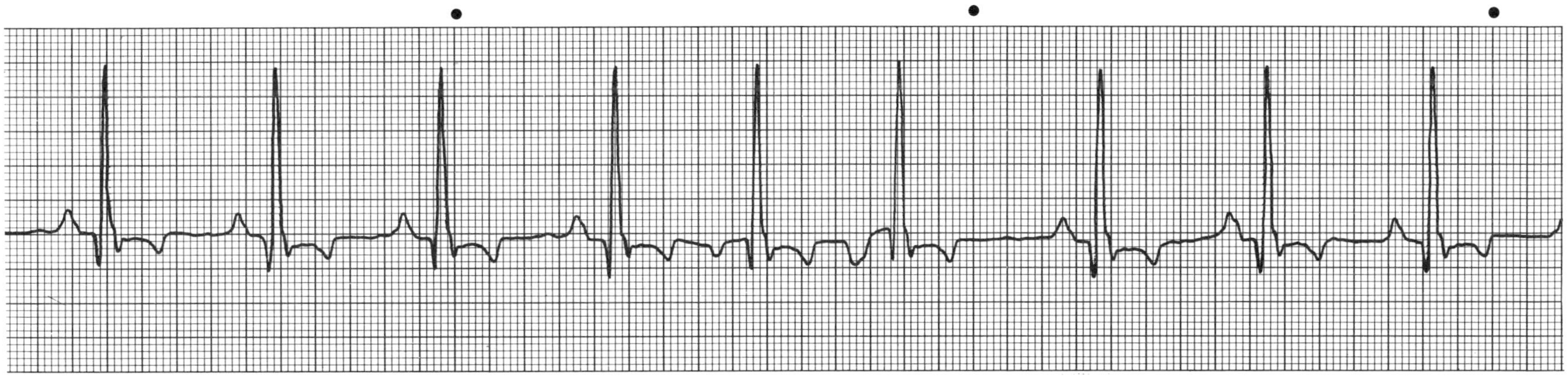

Question: This lead II ECG was obtained from a 2½-year-old male German Shepherd with mitral valvular dysplasia that was diagnosed at 3 months of age.

1. What is the rhythm diagnosis?
2. What is the best therapeutic approach?

Case 48

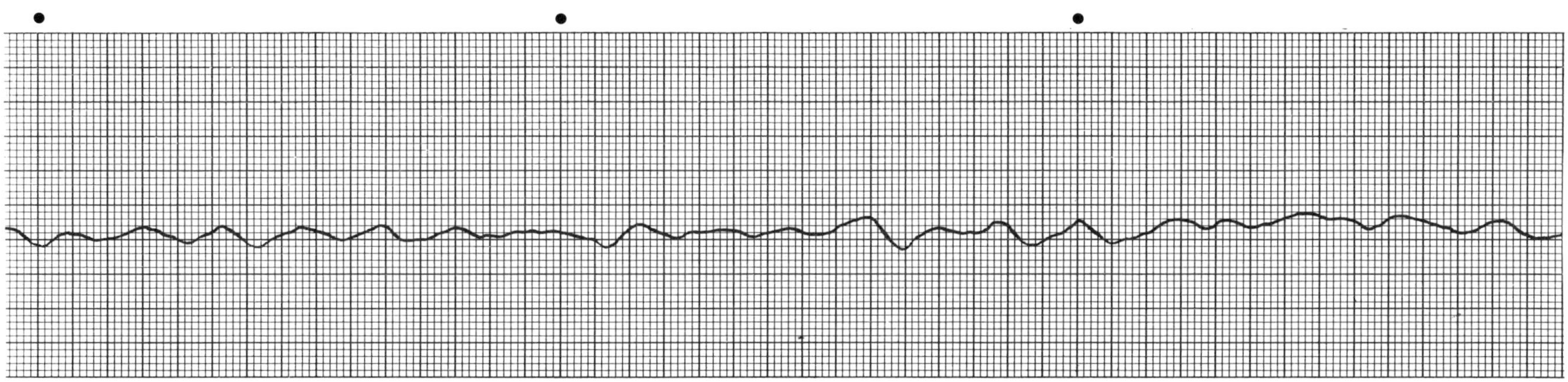

Question: This rhythm strip was recorded from a dog that went into respiratory arrest during induction of anesthesia.

1. What is the rhythm diagnosis?
2. What are common causes of this arrhythmia?
3. What is the best therapeutic approach?
4. What is the prognosis?

Case 47

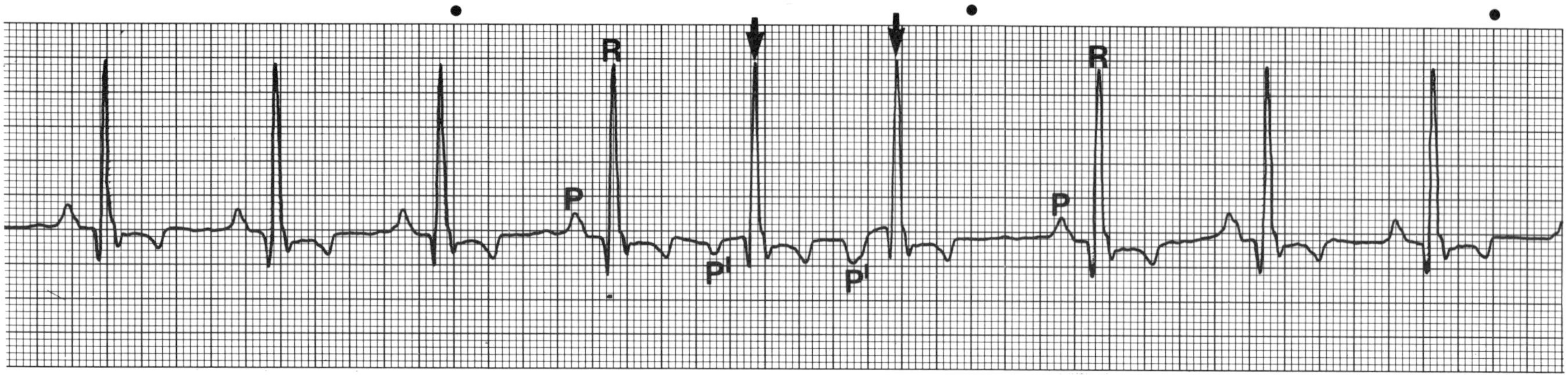

Answer: Sinus rhythm with AV junctional premature complexes. Heart rate is 120 beats/min. If the dog has no clinical signs, antiarrhythmic drugs are not required. Alternatively, if signs of heart failure develop, digoxin is the preferred drug for treating this arrhythmia. The premature QRS complexes (arrows) resemble the sinus beat QRS complexes typical of a supraventricular arrhythmia. The negative P′ waves that precede the premature QRS complexes suggest an AV junctional arrhythmia focus with retrograde conduction from the AV junction to the proximal portion of the atria. Impulses occurring from the left atria, as well as the AV junction, result in negative P′ waves. The negative P′ waves precede, occur simultaneously with, or follow the QRS complexes, depending on the relative speed of conduction retrograde from the arrhythmia focus versus conduction antegrade into the ventricles.

Case 48

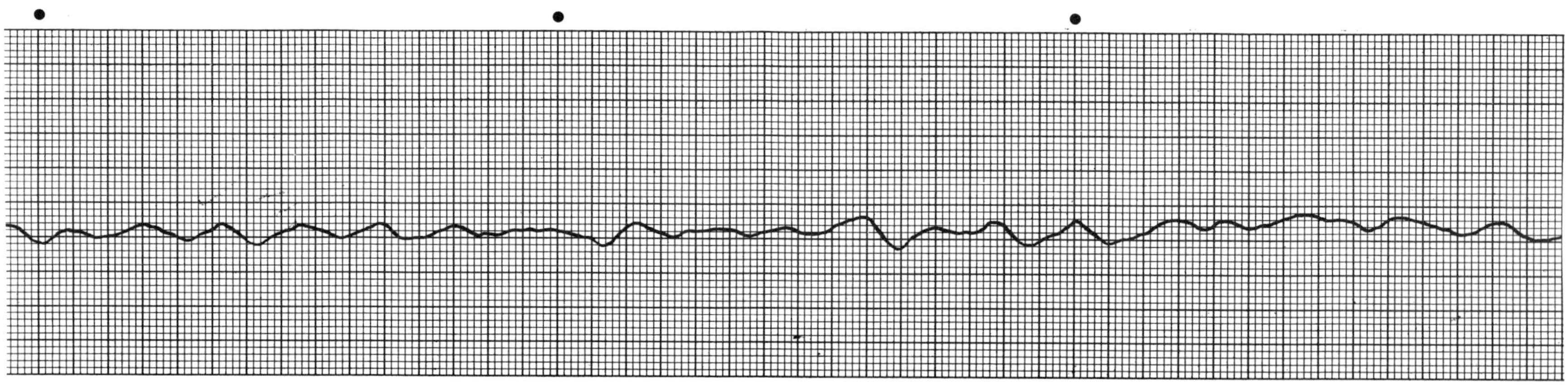

Answer: Ventricular fibrillation (fine). Ventricular fibrillation is characterized by a chaotic, irregular pattern without evidence of recognizable P waves or QRS complexes. The oscillations may be low in amplitude (fine) or large (coarse). Ventricular fibrillation is generally associated with severe cardiac or systemic disorders. Associated conditions include shock, anoxia, myocardial damage, acid-base, electrolyte imbalances (e.g., hyperkalemia, hypokalemia, hypocalcemia, and alkalosis), adverse reactions to drugs (anesthetics and digoxin), myocarditis, and hypothermia. The best therapeutic approach is electrical defibrillation. Drug therapy alone is almost always unsuccessful. The prognosis is guarded to poor with electrical defibrillation and grave without electrical defibrillation.

Case 49

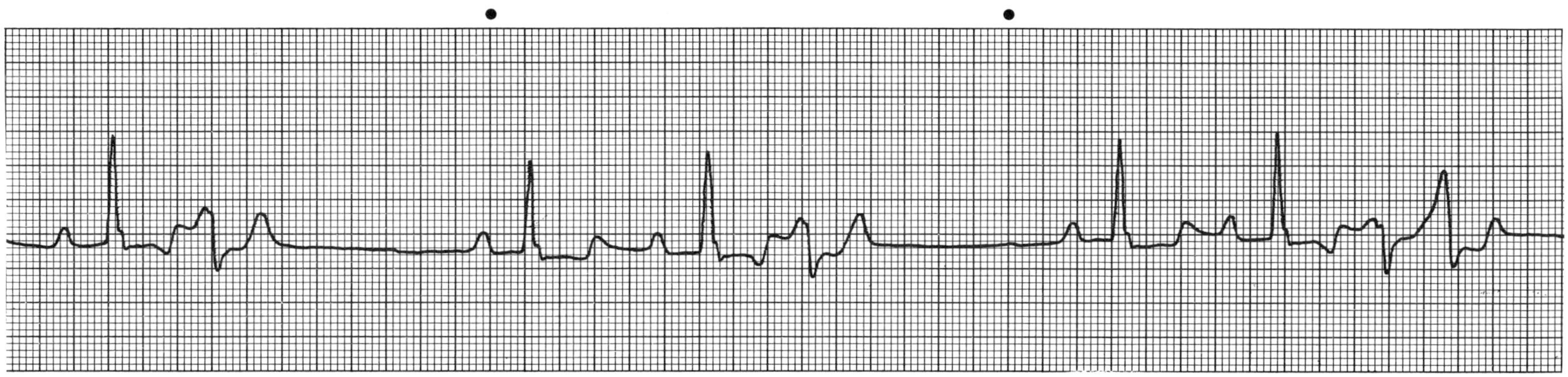

Question: This rhythm strip was recorded from a 6-year-old King Charles Spaniel with congestive heart failure. The dog was being medicated with furosemide and digoxin and was examined because of lethargy.

1. What is the rhythm diagnosis?
2. What is the most likely underlying disorder?
3. What is the best therapeutic approach?

Case 50

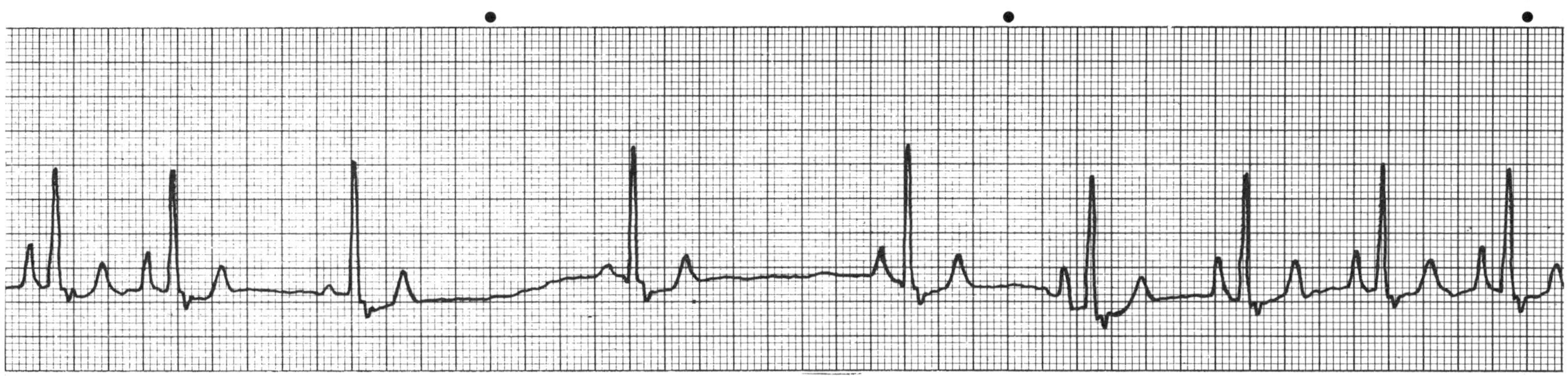

Question: This lead II ECG was obtained from a 10-year-old Yorkshire Terrier examined because of a worsening cough. A grade IV/VI holosystolic murmur, loudest over the left fifth intercostal space, was heard on auscultation.

1. What is the rhythm diagnosis?
2. What is the most likely underlying disorder?
3. What is the best therapeutic approach?

Case 49

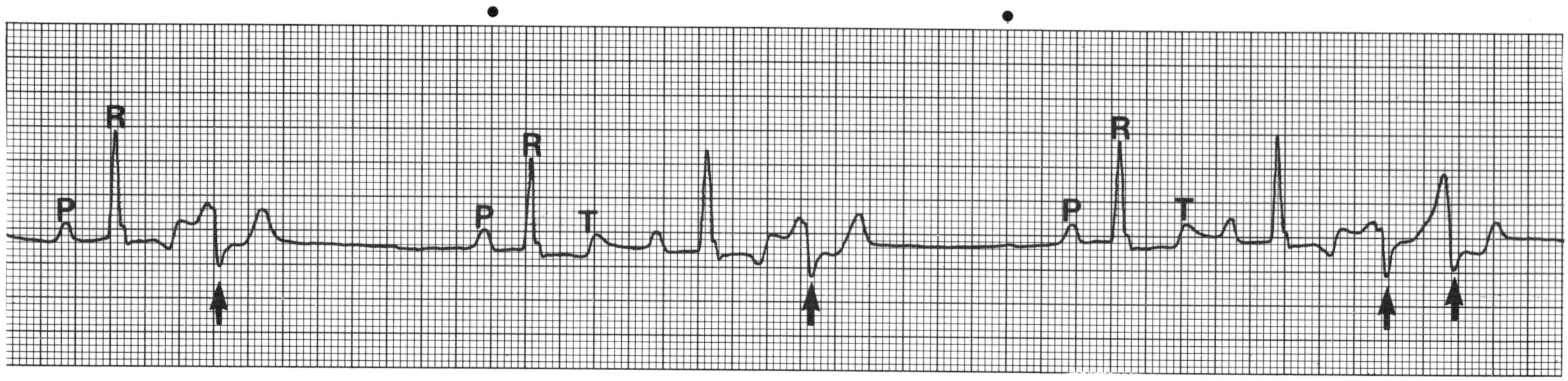

Answer: Sinus rhythm with first-degree AV block and frequent ventricular premature complexes occurring singly and as couplets. Heart rate is approximately 140 beats/min. First-degree AV block is identified by the prolonged P-R interval. Ventricular premature complexes (arrows) occur frequently (approximately 40/min). First-degree AV block and ventricular premature complexes have many causes. Digoxin administration must be considered a primary cause in any animal with this combination of ECG findings, especially if ventricular premature complexes were not present before treatment was initiated. Although this dog was not exhibiting gastrointestinal signs of digoxin toxicity, ECG changes can occur independently of such signs. Digoxin should be discontinued and an ECG re-evaluated in 3 to 5 days. Ideally, serum digoxin concentrations should be obtained to help to confirm the diagnosis and to assess the degree of overdosage. Also, such a determination may assist in establishing the proper dosage to reinstitute after the toxicity resolves. If the formerly used dosage seems appropriate on the basis of the dog's lean body weight, renal and thyroid status, serum electrolytes should be evaluated.

Case 50

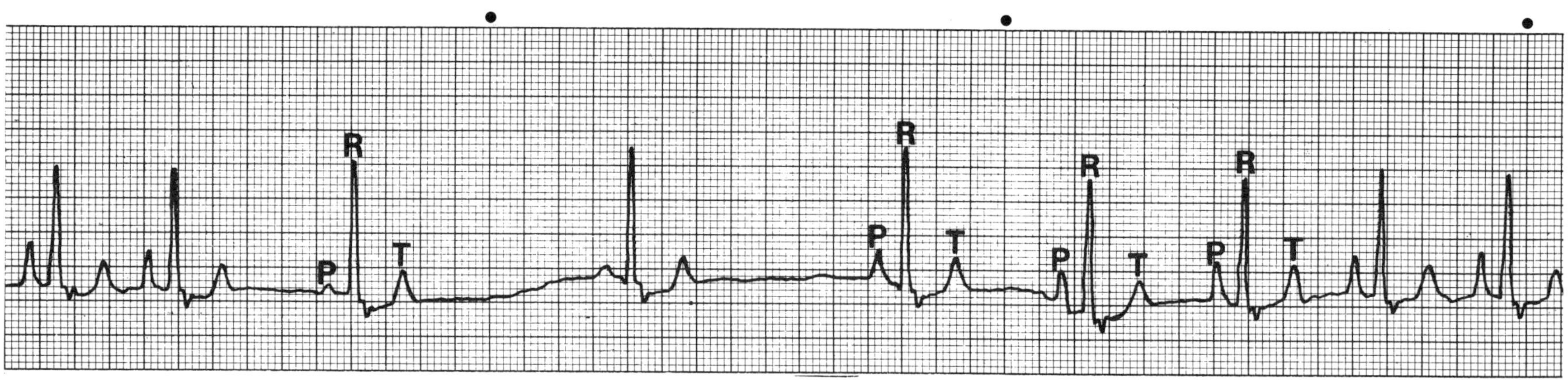

Answer: Sinus arrhythmia with a wandering sinus pacemaker. Heart rate is 110 beats/min. The history and description of the murmur support a diagnosis of degenerative mitral valve disease. The ECG findings, however, suggest tracheobronchial or pulmonary disease. Thoracic radiographs are needed to confirm the diagnosis. Treatment is not required for sinus arrhythmia. Sinus arrhythmia is caused by varying levels of vagal tone to the sinus node and is usually seen in dogs with respiratory disease or in brachycephalic breeds in which vagal tone is increased. The tracheobronchial or pulmonary disorder should be treated. The change in configuration of the P waves (wandering pacemaker) is often found in dogs with sinus arrhythmia and requires no treatment. The high-amplitude P waves (P-pulmonale) are often associated with right atrial enlargement caused by chronic respiratory disease.

Case 51

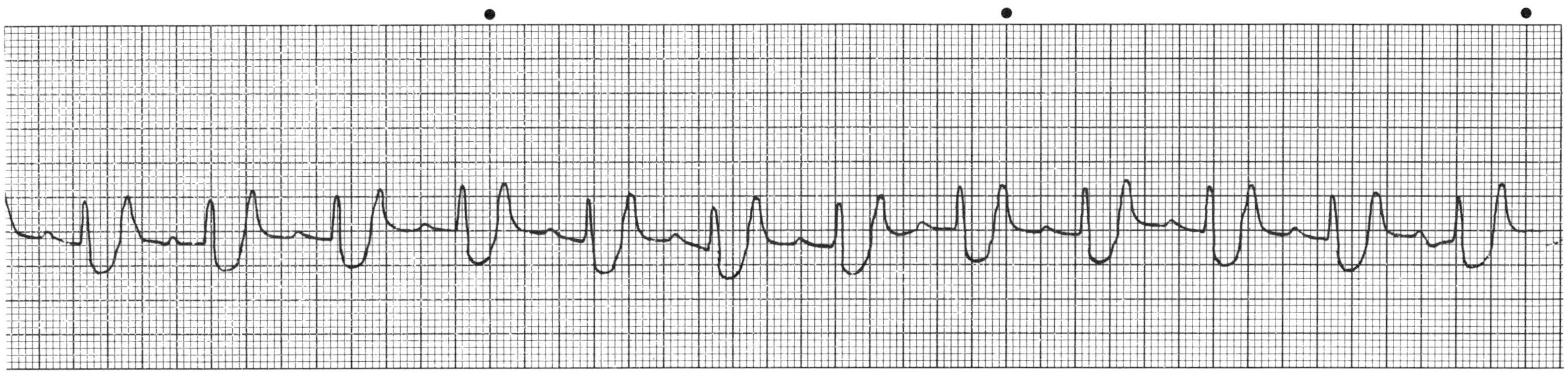

Question: This lead II ECG was obtained from a 10-year-old Miniature Poodle with no clinical signs. A grade IV/VI holosystolic murmur was heard equally in the left and right hemithorax.

1. What is the rhythm diagnosis?
2. What is the most likely underlying disorder?
3. What is the best therapeutic approach?

Case 52

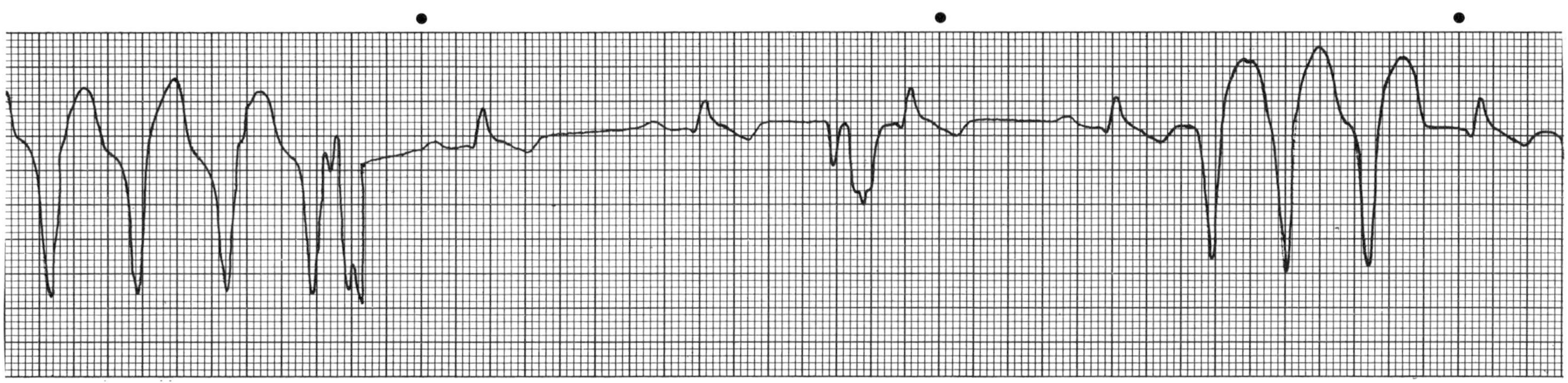

Question: This rhythm strip was recorded from an 8-year-old female Doberman Pinscher with a grade II/VI systolic mitral valvular murmur and a history of exercise intolerance and coughing.

1. What is the rhythm diagnosis?
2. What is the most likely underlying disorder?
3. What is the best therapeutic approach?
4. What is the prognosis?

Case 51

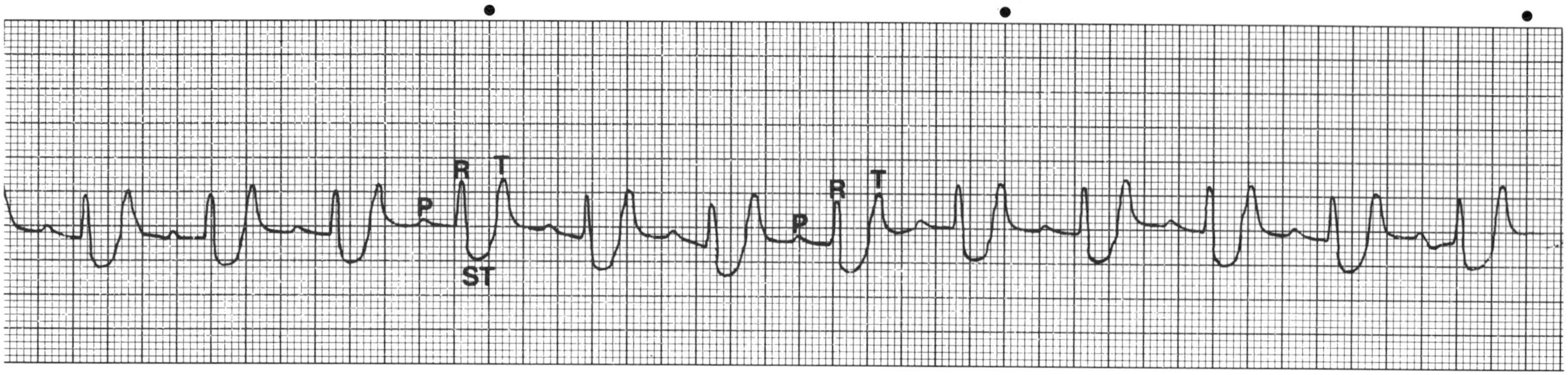

Answer: Sinus rhythm. Heart rate is 165 beats/min. The P waves are of abnormally high amplitude and duration, and large T waves are seen. Mitral and tricuspid valvular insufficiency with corresponding dilated atria account for the size of the P wave. Treatment is not required initially, but monitoring for the development of congestive heart failure is essential. Angiotensin-converting enzyme inhibitor therapy can be considered at this time, although the benefit of its use in animals with asymptomatic heart disease has not been established. The large P waves may be a harbinger of atrial arrhythmias.

Case 52

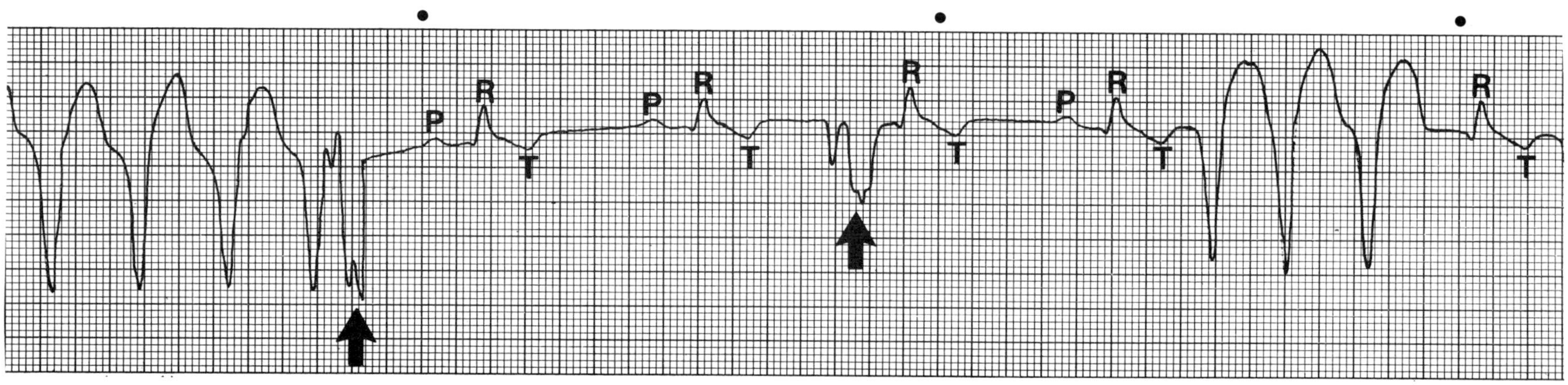

Answer: Sinus rhythm with paroxysmal ventricular tachycardia. Heart rate is variable. Low-amplitude sinus complexes are evident in the center of the strip. Artifact can be seen in two locations (arrows). The artifact can be differentiated from ventricular premature complexes by the absence of T waves. The artifact in the center of the page cannot be a real complex, because it does not interfere with the conduction of the following QRS complex. Paroxysmal ventricular tachycardia in a coughing Doberman Pinscher with a murmur is often associated with dilated cardiomyopathy. The arrhythmia should be controlled with lidocaine while long-term antiarrhythmic therapy with procainamide, quinidine, tocainide, or mexiletine is initiated. If radiographs confirm heart failure, a diuretic and vasodilator should be instituted. Digoxin may eventually be needed for management of myocardial failure. Digoxin should not be prescribed until the ventricular arrhythmia is controlled.

Case 53

A

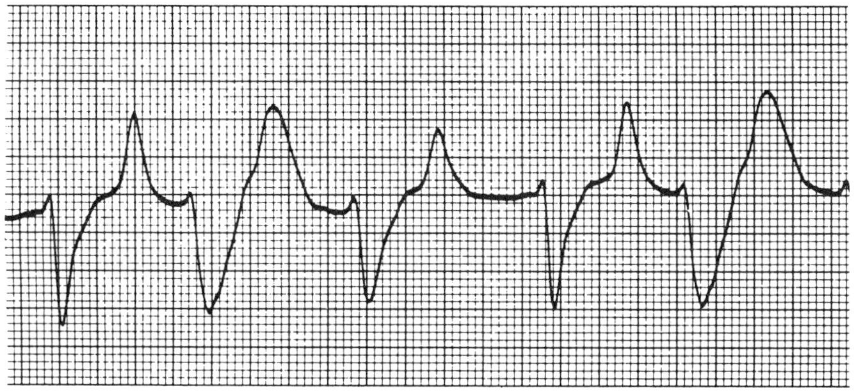

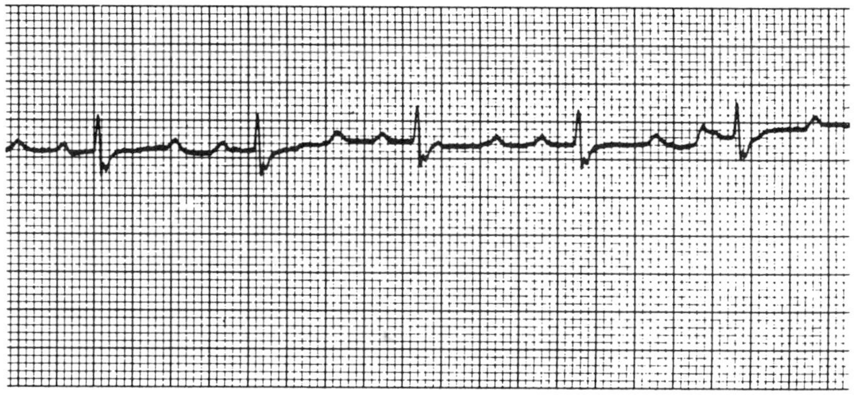

B

Question: Strip A was recorded from a recumbent and vomiting cat with urethral obstruction.

1. What is the rhythm diagnosis?
2. What treatment was given to obtain strip B after a period of 15 minutes?

Case 54

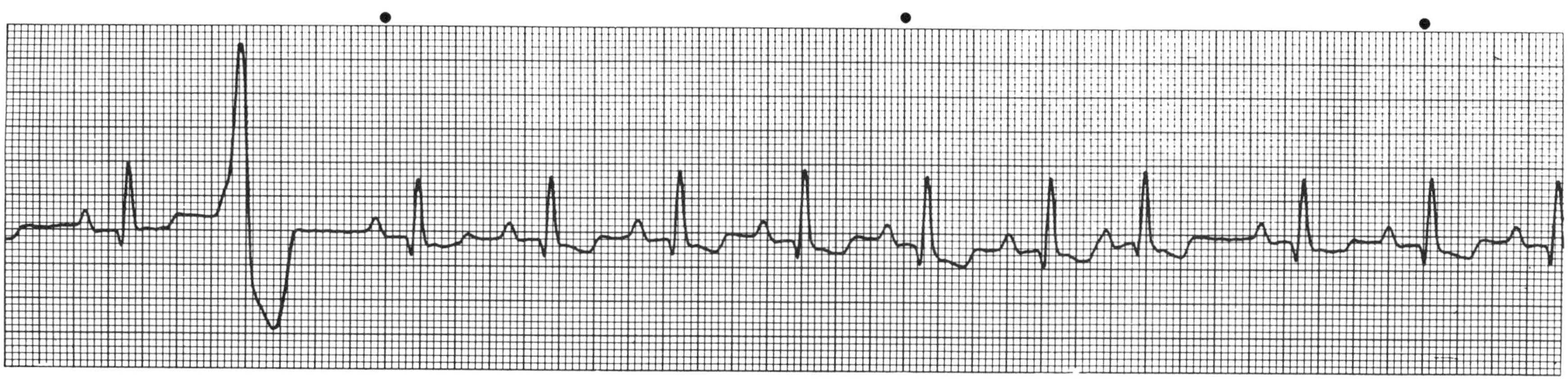

Question: This tracing was recorded from a dog that had been hit by a car 2 days previously.

1. What is the rhythm diagnosis?
2. What has caused the different pauses in this strip?

Case 53

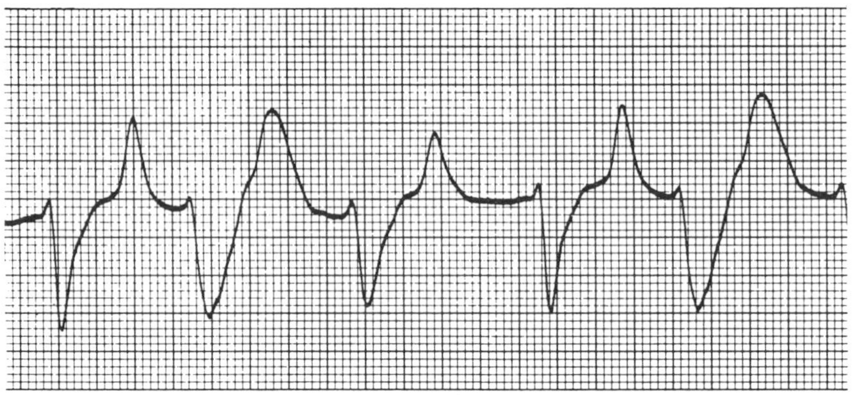

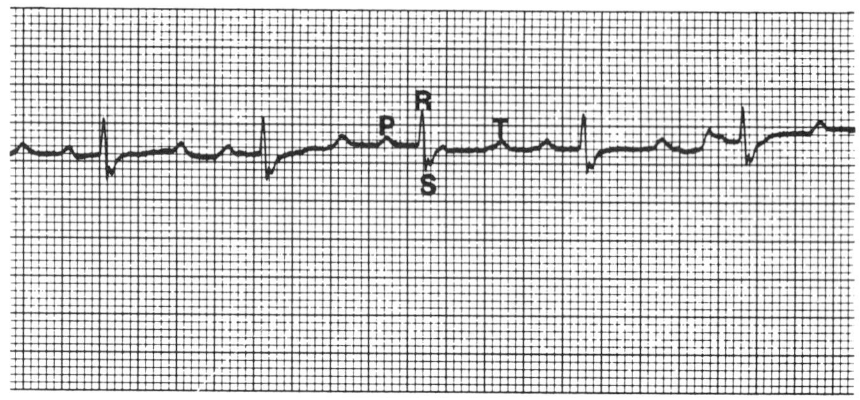

Answer: A. Atrial standstill (no visible P waves) and a sinoventricular rhythm. Heart rate is slow and variable. The wide and bizarre QRS complexes indicate marked conduction delay in the ventricular conduction system. The serum potassium level was 9.0 mEq/L. Ventricular tachycardia should also be considered, but ventricular tachycardia is usually regular with a faster rate (more than 150 beats/min), and P waves are often seen independent of the ventricular complexes. Severe hyperkalemia is not commonly associated with rapid ventricular arrhythmias. To obtain strip B, treatment included relief of urethral obstruction and administration of intravenous 0.9% saline fluid, sodium bicarbonate, and 0.5 unit/kg regular insulin with 2 g dextrose per unit of insulin. Minor changes of hyperkalemia (serum potassium now 6.0 mEq/L) still exist, including a prolonged P-R interval (0.10 sec; normal not greater than 0.09 sec), a wide S wave, and a long Q-T interval.

Case 54

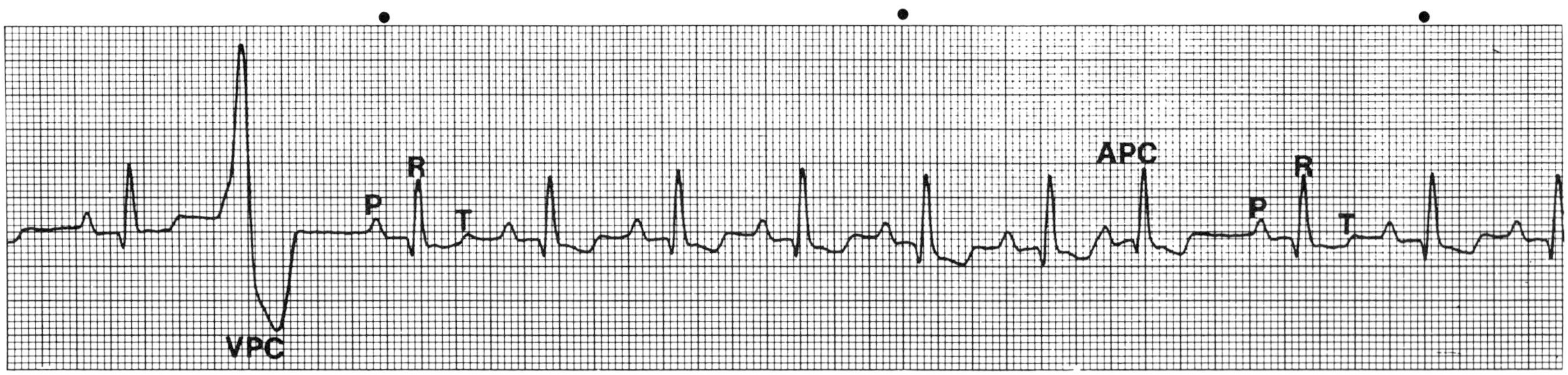

Answer: Sinus rhythm with one ventricular premature complex (VPC) and one atrial premature complex (APC). Heart rate of 165 beats/min. Premature complexes are usually followed by a pause, termed "noncompensatory" (less than two R-R intervals) or "compensatory" (two R-R intervals), according to its duration. With a ventricular premature complex, the ectopic impulse generally cannot penetrate through the AV junction to disturb the normal sinus rhythm. A compensatory pause usually follows a ventricular premature complex, because the next sinus impulse after the ventricular premature complex occurs on time. A noncompensatory pause (or less-than-compensatory pause) occurs with an atrial premature complex. The ectopic atrial impulse discharges the SA node and resets its cycle. Note that the atrial premature complex configuration of the QRS is the same as that of the sinus complexes.

Case 55

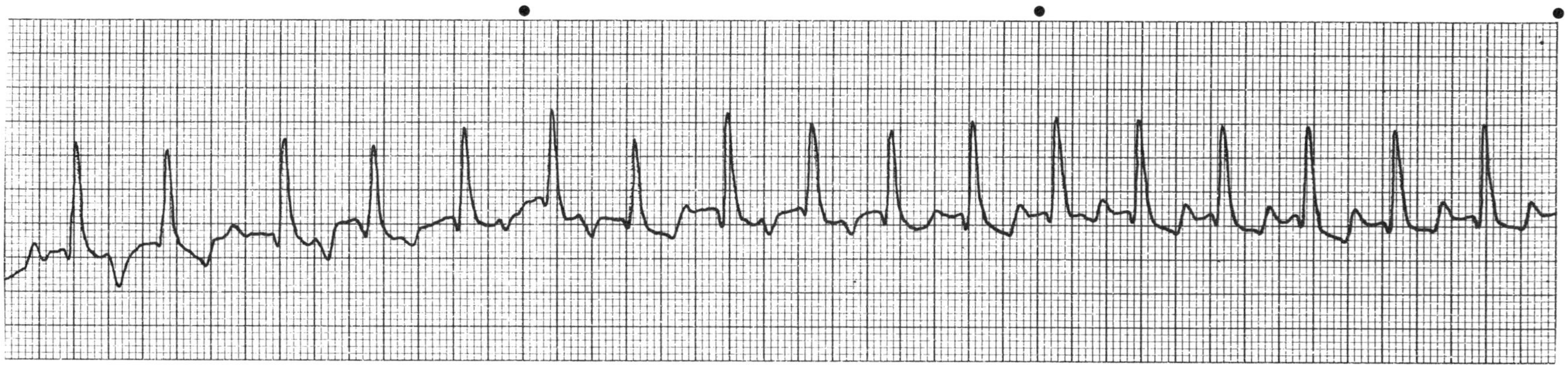

Question: This lead II ECG was obtained from a 6-year-old Boxer with dyspnea and syncopal episodes.

1. What is the rhythm diagnosis?
2. What is the most likely underlying disorder?
3. What is the best therapeutic approach?

Case 56

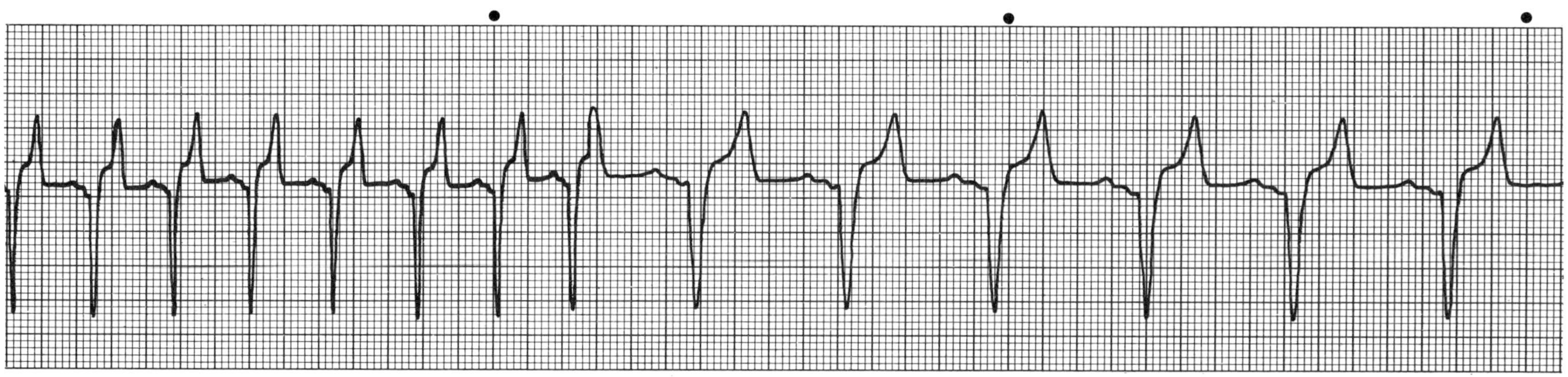

Question: This lead II ECG was obtained from a 9-year-old Beagle as part of a geriatric examination.

1. What is the rhythm diagnosis?
2. What is the best therapeutic approach?

Case 55

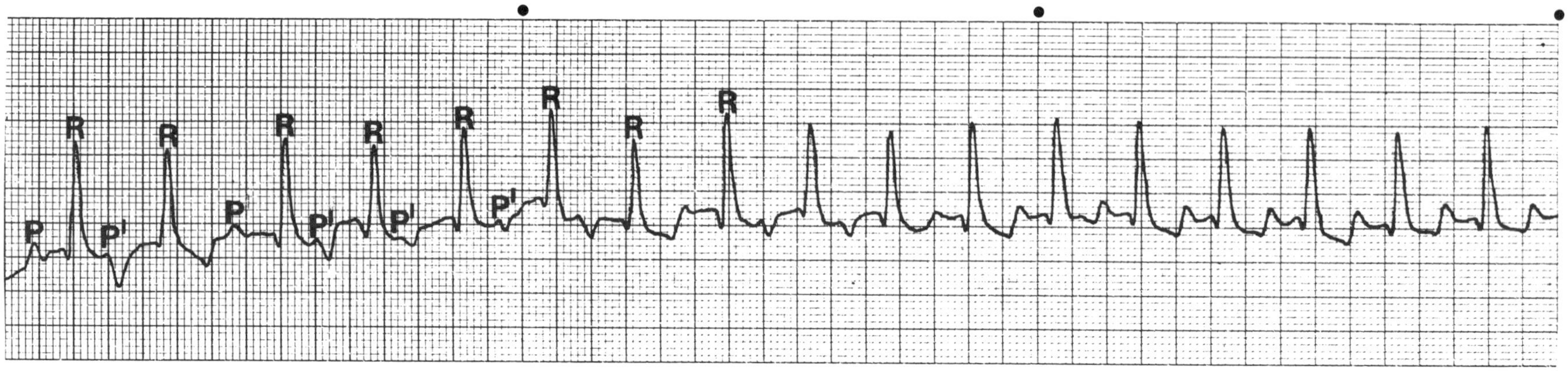

Answer: Sinus rhythm with atrial premature complexes and paroxysmal supraventricular tachycardia. Heart rate during tachycardia is 240 beats/min. Boxer cardiomyopathy is the most likely underlying disorder. Digoxin is the best therapeutic approach for the atrial arrhythmia. If thoracic radiographs confirm congestive heart failure, diuretics and vasodilators should also be administered. The second QRS complex is premature, preceded by a P′ wave, and it resembles the QRS complex of the sinus beats (P-R), a hallmark of atrial premature complexes. The second atrial premature complex (fourth QRS complex preceded by a P′ wave) starts a sustained, supraventricular tachycardia, which continues for the remainder of the strip. Mechanisms that would explain the supraventricular tachycardia, including automaticity or atrial re-entry, cannot be determined without electrophysiologic studies. The slight irregularity of the R-to-R intervals during the supraventricular tachycardia suggests that multiple atrial foci are involved in causing the tachycardia.

Case 56

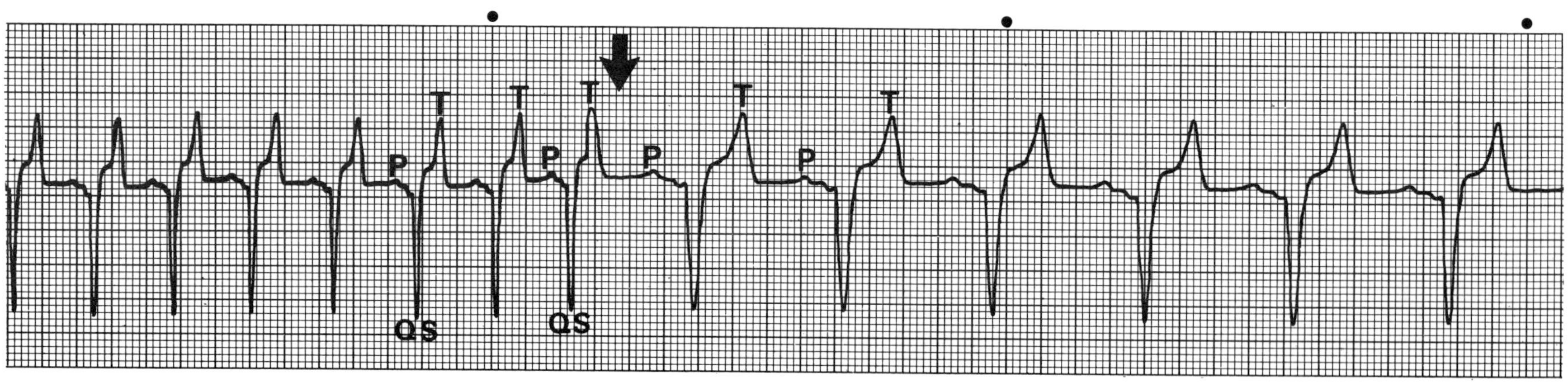

Answer: Sinus rhythm with right bundle-branch block. Heart rate is approximately 120 beats/min. No treatment is required. The apparent change in the heart rate (arrow) is artifactual, because an obvious change in the electrocardiograph paper speed occurs at this point. Notice the change in the P wave and QS complex width. Before the arrow, the paper speed is 25 mm/sec, and after the arrow, the speed is 50 mm/sec. The deep and wide QS wave with a consistent P-R interval is typical of right bundle-branch block. Leads I and III (not shown) also had wide and deep S waves. The change in paper speeds during this lead II rhythm strip, coupled with the negative and wide QRS complexes, could result in a major misdiagnosis of paroxysmal ventricular tachycardia.

Case 57

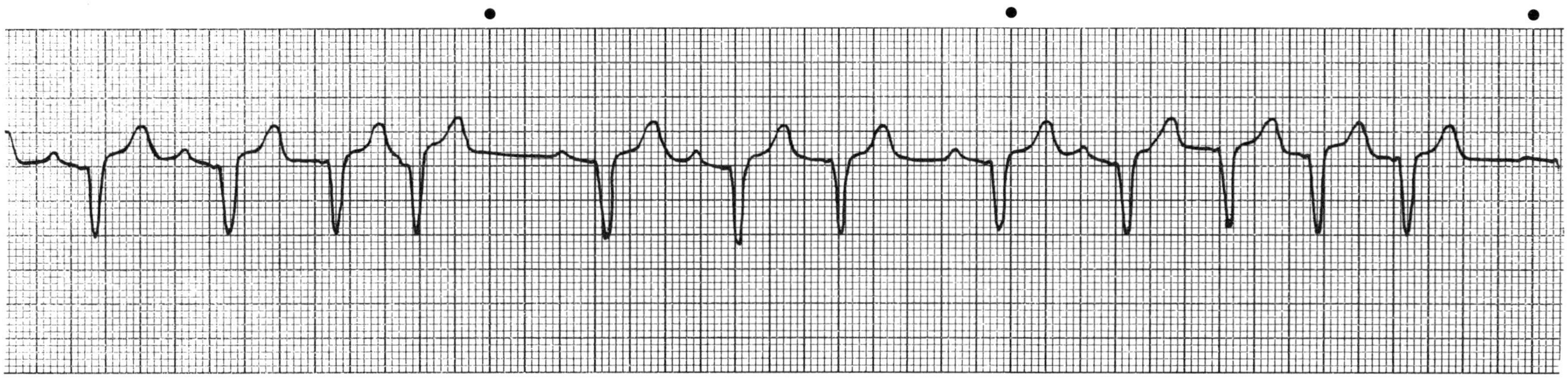

Question: This tracing was recorded from an aged dog with mitral valvular insufficiency and secondary congestive heart failure.

1. What is the rhythm diagnosis?
2. What is the best therapeutic approach?

Case 58

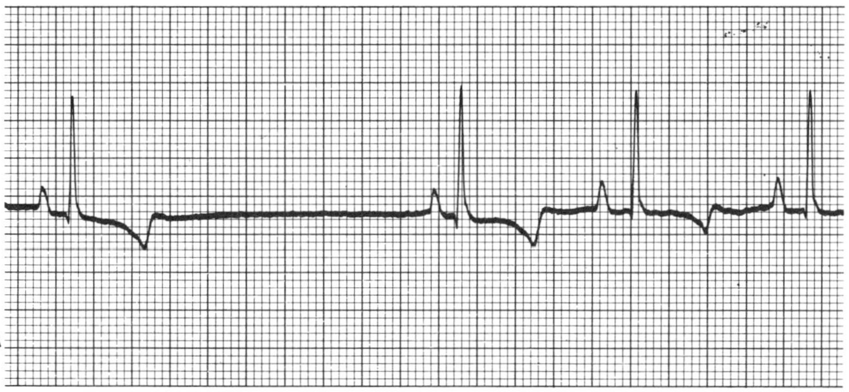

A

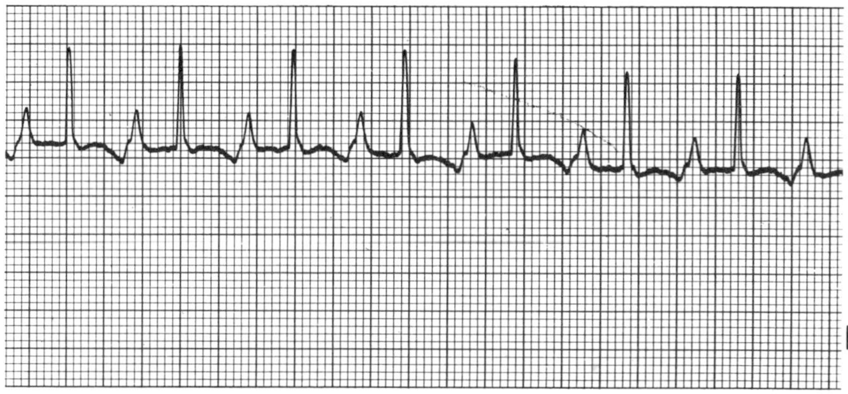

B

Question: This lead II ECG was obtained from a 5-year-old Pug examined because of a worsening cough.

1. What is the rhythm diagnosis in strips A and B?
2. What is the most likely underlying disorder in strip A?
3. What drug probably resulted in the change from the rhythm in strip A to the rhythm in strip B?

Case 57

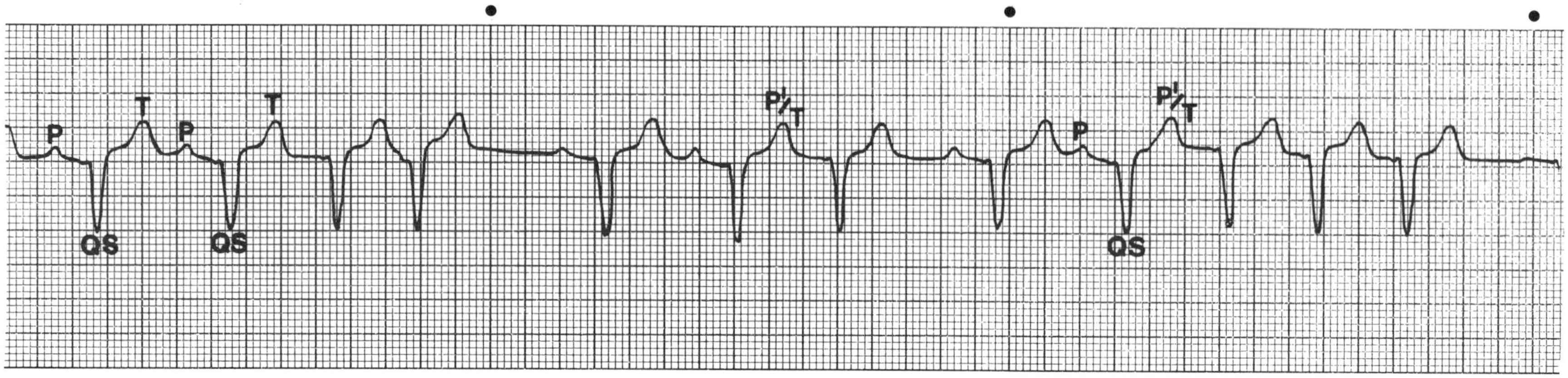

Answer: Numerous atrial premature complexes (complexes 3, 4, 7, 10, 11, and 12). Heart rate is variable. Atrial premature complexes arise from ectopic foci in the atria. They are frequently caused by cardiac disease and may lead to atrial tachycardia, atrial flutter, or atrial fibrillation. The impulses spread through the atria to the AV node, and they may or may not reach the ventricles. The ectopic P′ wave for an atrial premature complex is premature, and its configuration is different from that of the sinus P waves. This P′ wave may be negative, positive, diphasic, or superimposed on the previous T wave (as in this case, P′/T). The QRS complex is premature, and its configuration is usually the same as that of the sinus complexes. The abnormal QRS complexes (QS complexes) here could indicate either heart enlargement and/or an intraventricular conduction defect. Leads I, III, and aVF also had S waves, thus indicating a probable right-sided disorder. Heartworm disease should be ruled out. Digoxin is the treatment of choice for atrial premature complexes in animals with cardiac decompensation. Other drugs should be used to treat the congestive heart failure.

Case 58

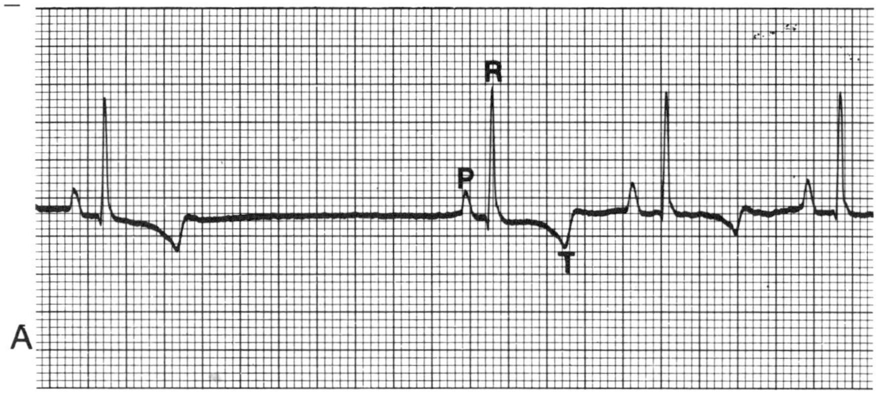

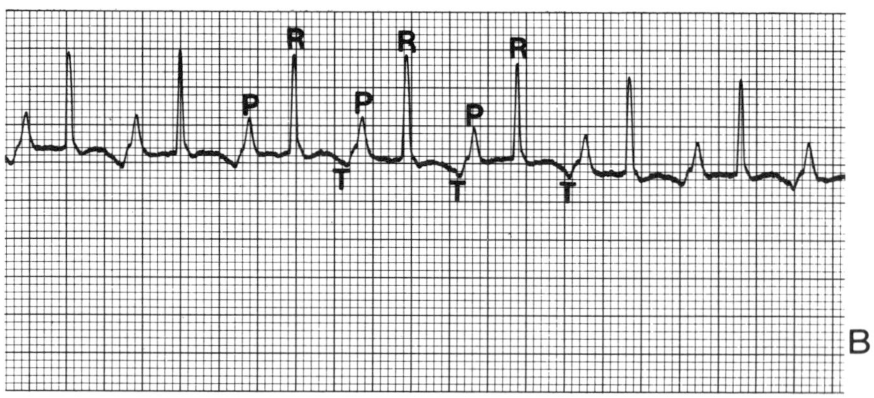

Answer: A. Sinus rhythm with a period of sinoatrial block or sinus arrest. Heart rate is approximately 80 beats/min. B. Sinus tachycardia. Heart rate is 200 beats/min. High levels of vagal tone on expiration probably account for the sinus pause. Atropine was administered and abolished vagal (parasympathetic) tone and unmasked sympathetic tone resulting in the sinus tachycardia. Atropine administered intravenously initially prolongs the P-R interval before an initial increase in heart rate. Bradyarrhythmias are associated with high levels of vagal tone (especially in animals with respiratory disease), hypothyroidism, hypothermia, sinus node disease, and AV conduction system disorders. Parenteral or oral administration of anticholinergics may be useful in abolishing vagal tone, increasing heart rate, and limiting signs of weakness or syncope. A poor response to atropine in an animal with severe clinical signs supports the need for a permanent cardiac pacemaker. A history of coughing suggests the use of bronchodilators to help to reduce the cause of increased vagal tone.

Case 59

A 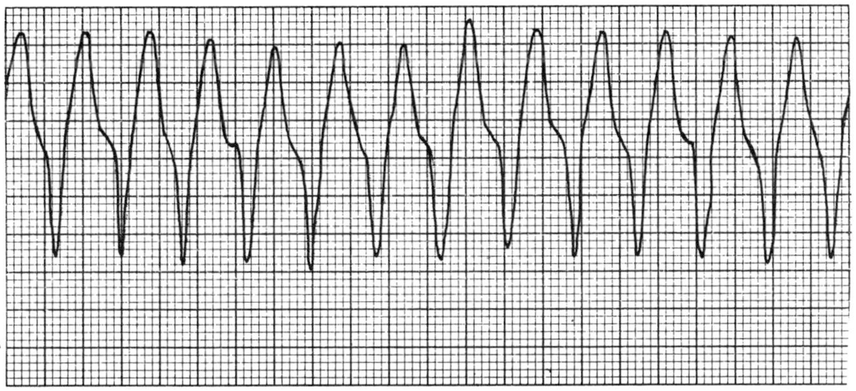

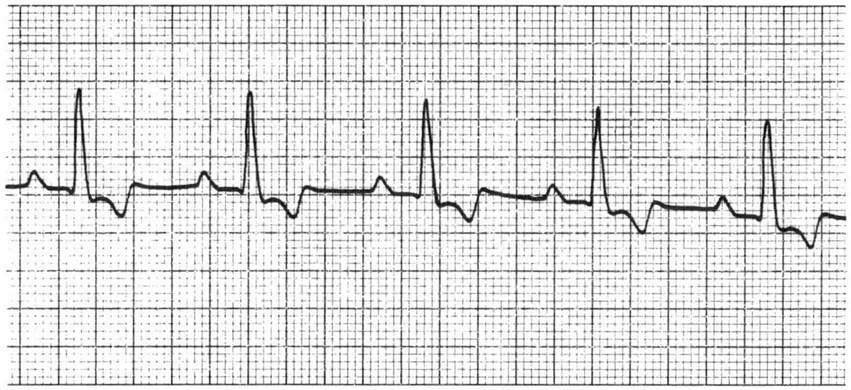 B

Question: This lead II ECG was obtained from a 3-month-old Bulldog puppy examined because of severe dyspnea and collapse.

1. What is the rhythm diagnosis in strip A and in strip B?
2. What is the most likely underlying disorder?
3. What is the best therapeutic approach?

Case 60

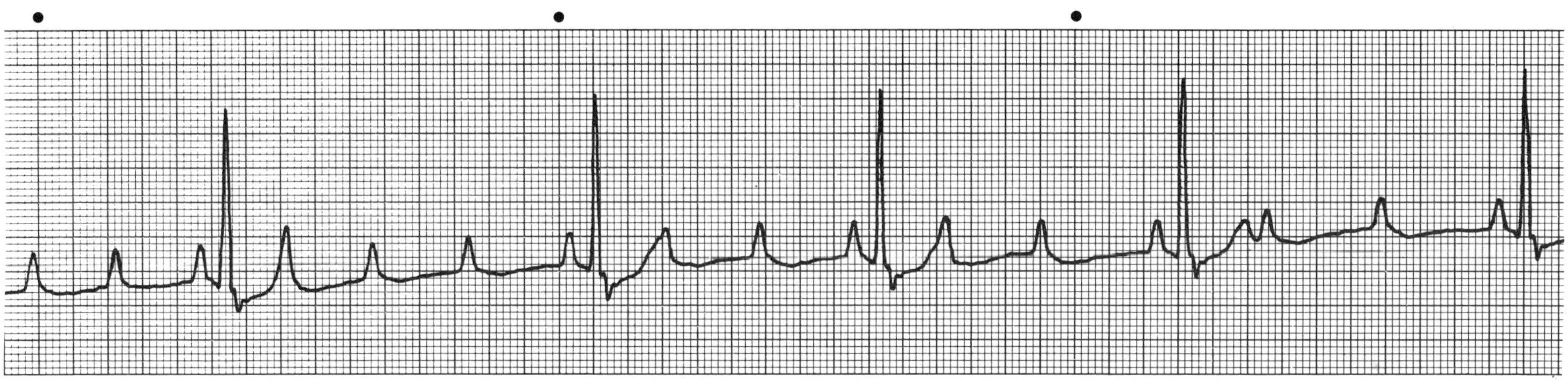

Question: This rhythm strip was recorded from a 12-year-old Pitbull Terrier with a history of exercise intolerance.

1. What is the rhythm diagnosis?
2. What is the best therapeutic approach?

Case 59

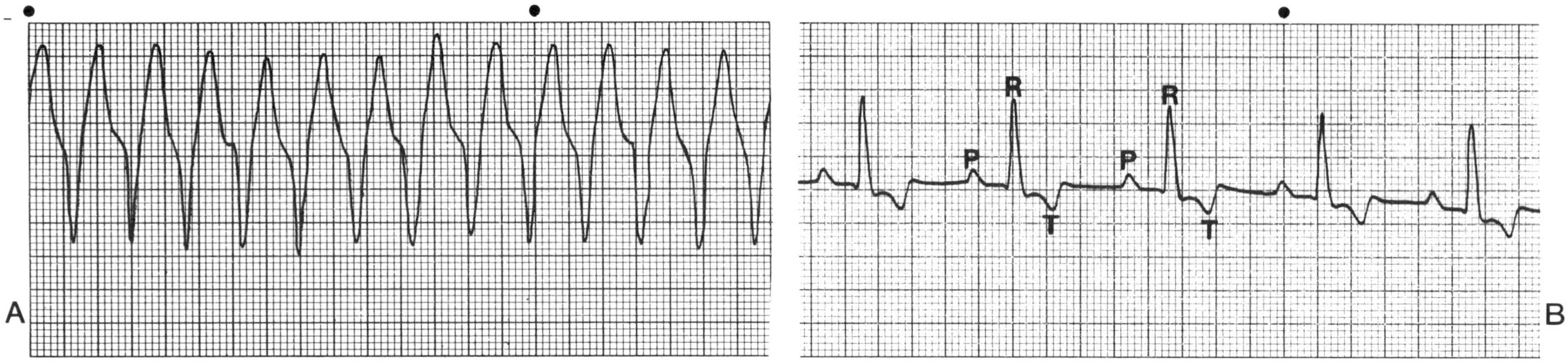

Answer: A. Suspected ventricular tachycardia. Heart rate is 350 beats/min. B. Sinus rhythm. Heart rate is 130 beats/min. The intravenous administration of a bolus of lidocaine followed by observation of the response (B) is the best therapeutic approach. Typically, lidocaine rapidly converts ventricular tachycardia to sinus rhythm. Several boluses of lidocaine are often required (up to 8 mg/kg) within a short period for successful conversion. Notice the sinus beats in B, which appear normal when compared to the wide complex tachycardia in A. The morphology of the sinus beat QRS complexes helps to eliminate the diagnostic possibility of supraventricular tachycardia with pre-existent right bundle-branch block. The rapid rate does not allow observation of the dissociated P waves, another characteristic of ventricular tachycardia. Antiarrhythmic agents, such as procainamide, given orally, with or without propranolol, can now be added for maintenance therapy. The underlying cause should also be treated. The differential diagnosis includes infectious myocarditis, trauma, congenital cardiac defect, and toxicity. A complete cardiovascular data base should be obtained.

Case 60

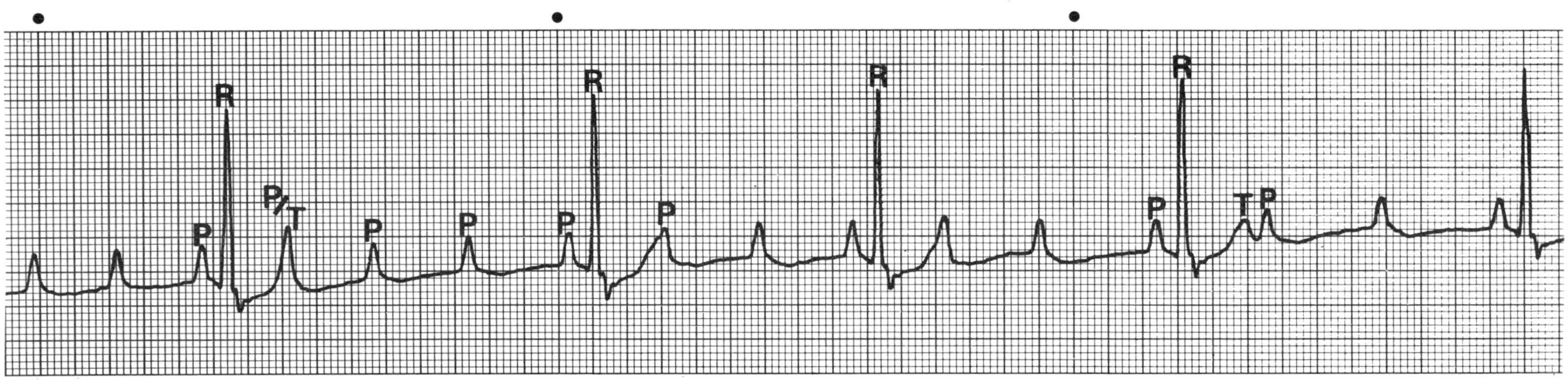

Answer: Advanced second-degree AV block. Atrial rate is 220 beats/min, and ventricular rate is approximately 60 beats/min. Advanced second-degree AV block occurs when more than two consecutive supraventricular impulses are blocked. In this dog, most of the P waves are not conducted. Because the P-R interval in all the ventricular complexes is identical, this condition is advanced second-degree AV block rather than complete AV block. The changing P-P interval is compatible with sinus arrhythmia. An atropine response test would help to determine whether AV nodal conduction can be improved. Atropine should be administered at 0.05 mg/kg intramuscularly, and an ECG should be performed 30 minutes later. If the ventricular rate increases, propantheline bromide or isopropamide iodide should be prescribed. If the animal does not respond to atropine, a trial course of bronchodilator to increase sympathetic tone should be tried. If symptomatic bradycardia persists, a pacemaker should be implanted.

Case 61

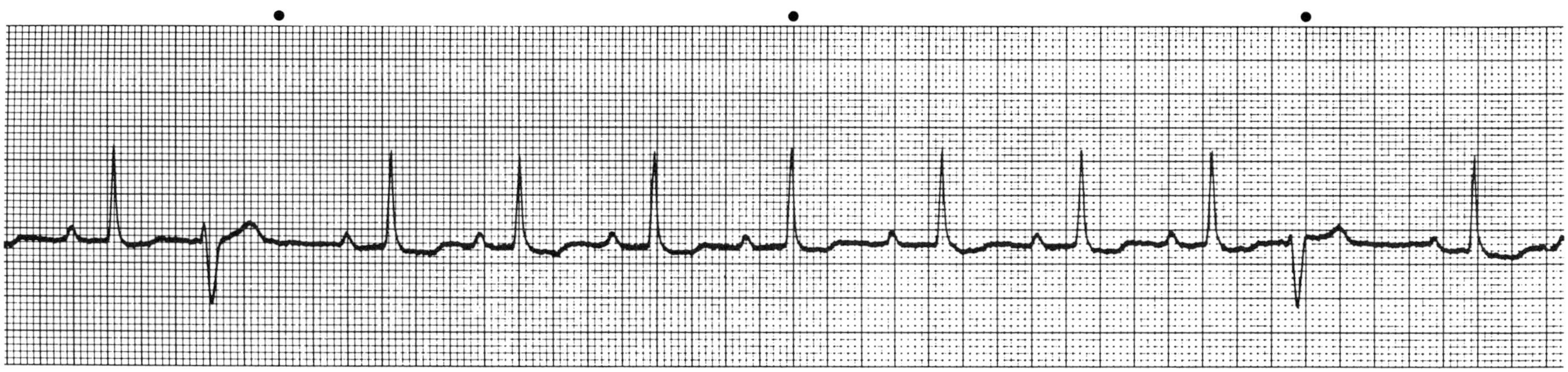

Question: This rhythm strip was obtained from a cat with the dilated form of cardiomyopathy. The cat was being treated with digoxin; its appetite had decreased and it was not active.

1. What is the rhythm diagnosis?
2. What is the best therapeutic approach?

Case 62

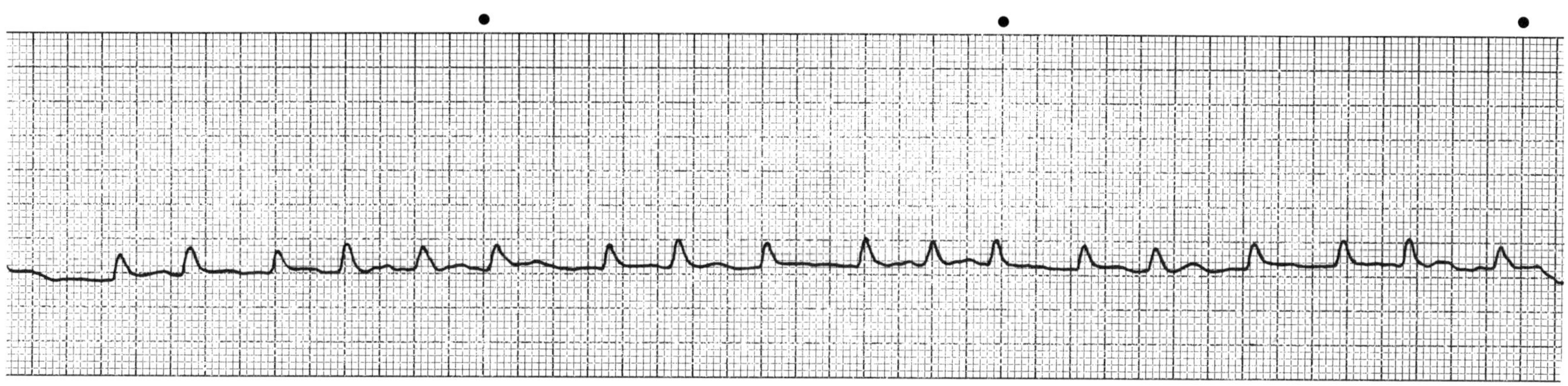

Question: A 5-year-old male domestic shorthair cat was examined because of severe dyspnea. A rapid, irregular heart rhythm was auscultated.

1. What is the rhythm diagnosis?
2. What are common causes of this arrhythmia?
3. What is the best therapeutic approach?

Case 61

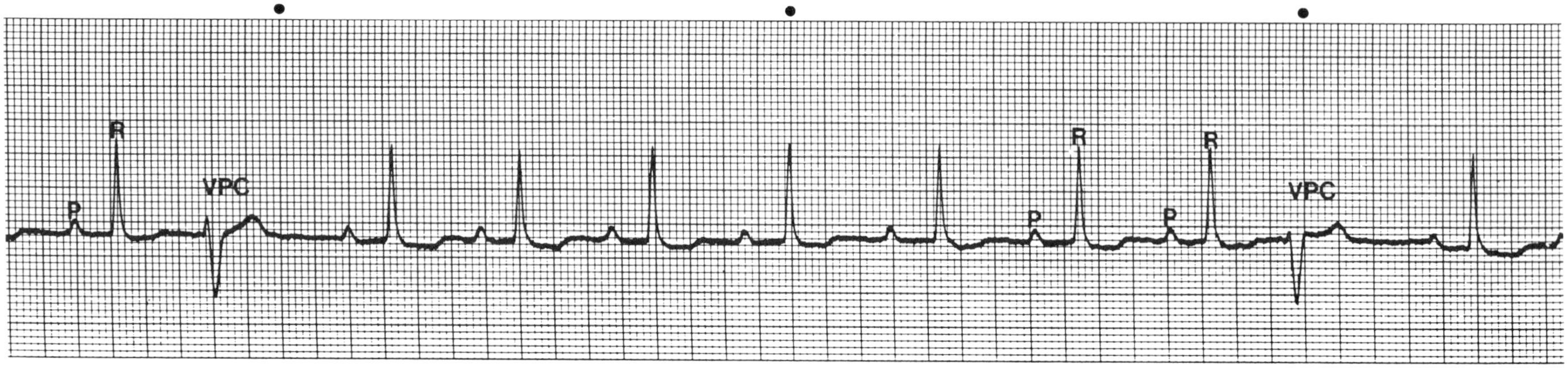

Answer: Sinus rhythm with first-degree AV block and two ventricular premature complexes (VPCs). Heart rate is approximately 150 beats/min. First-degree AV block is present. The P-R interval is prolonged to 0.14 sec or 7 boxes (normal not greater than 0.09 sec or 4½ boxes). The tall R waves of 1.4 mv or 14 boxes (normal not greater than 0.9 mv or 9 boxes) indicate left ventricular enlargement. Digoxin toxicity is the likely diagnosis. The ventricular premature complexes disappeared, the P-R interval returned to normal, and the cat improved clinically after the digoxin was stopped. Vasodilators along with furosemide may be needed to treat any progressive heart failure. Taurine supplementation is advised. Physical examination usually reveals a pulse deficit during a ventricular premature complex, because the cardiac output is temporarily decreased. A reduction in cardiac output is of greater significance when the cat has pre-existing heart disease.

Case 62

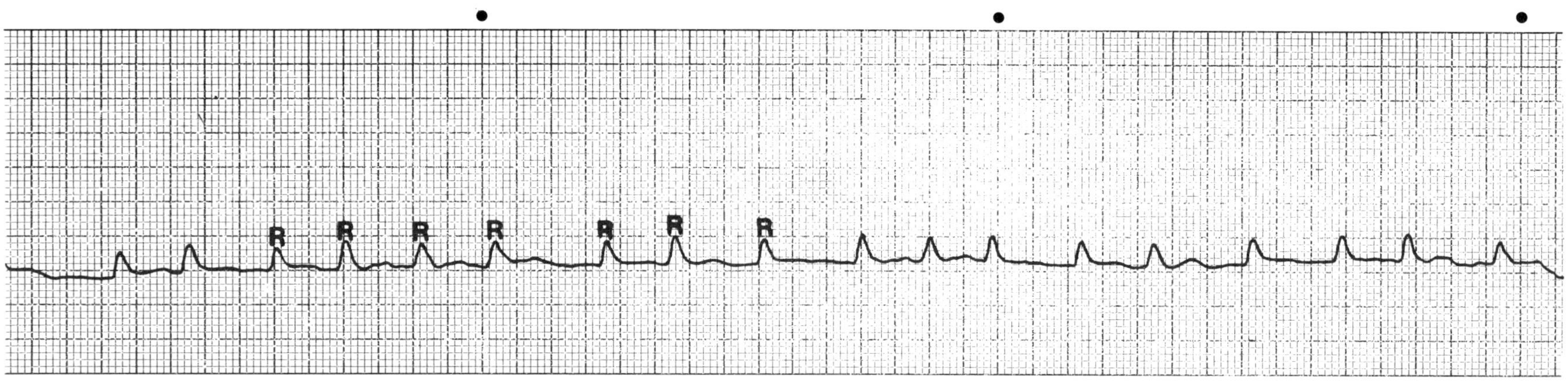

Answer: Atrial fibrillation. Heart rate is 240 beats/min. Hypertrophic cardiomyopathy causes a chronic increase in resistance to left ventricular filling, eventually resulting in severe left atrial enlargement and atrial fibrillation. Diltiazem can be administered to control the ventricular rate. Diltiazem also has a beneficial effect on ventricular diastolic dysfunction, the cause of heart failure in animals with hypertrophic cardiomyopathy. Digoxin or propranolol are alternative or additive medications. The lack of visible P waves and a rapid, irregular ventricular rhythm are the hallmarks of atrial fibrillation. Ineffective atrial contractions may predispose to an atrial, and eventually aortic thrombus. Congenital heart disease, restrictive cardiomyopathy, and hyperthyroidism may also cause atrial fibrillation.

Case 63

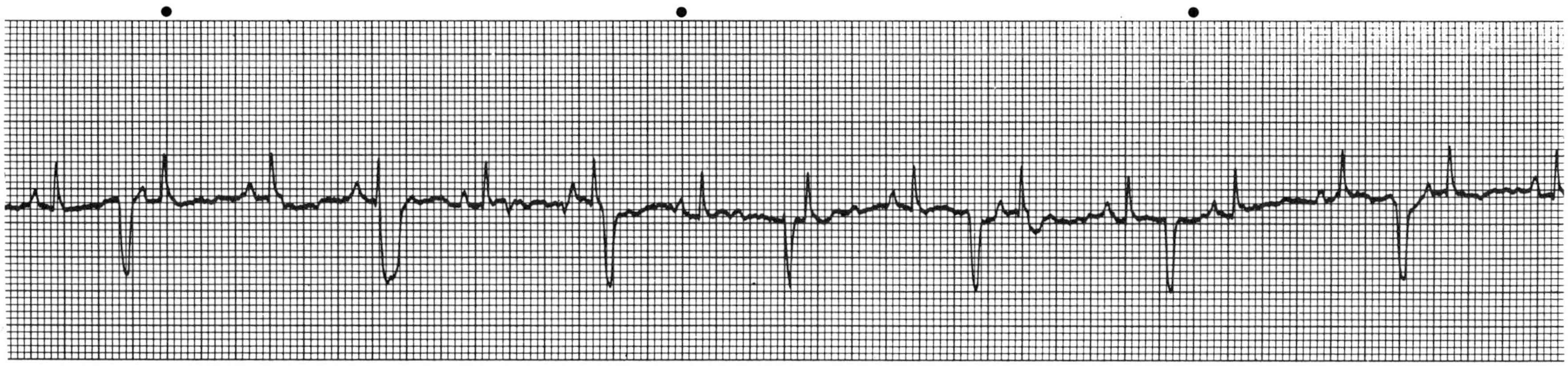

Question: This tracing was recorded from a cat that had fallen seven stories and fractured its humerus.

1. What is the rhythm diagnosis?

Case 64

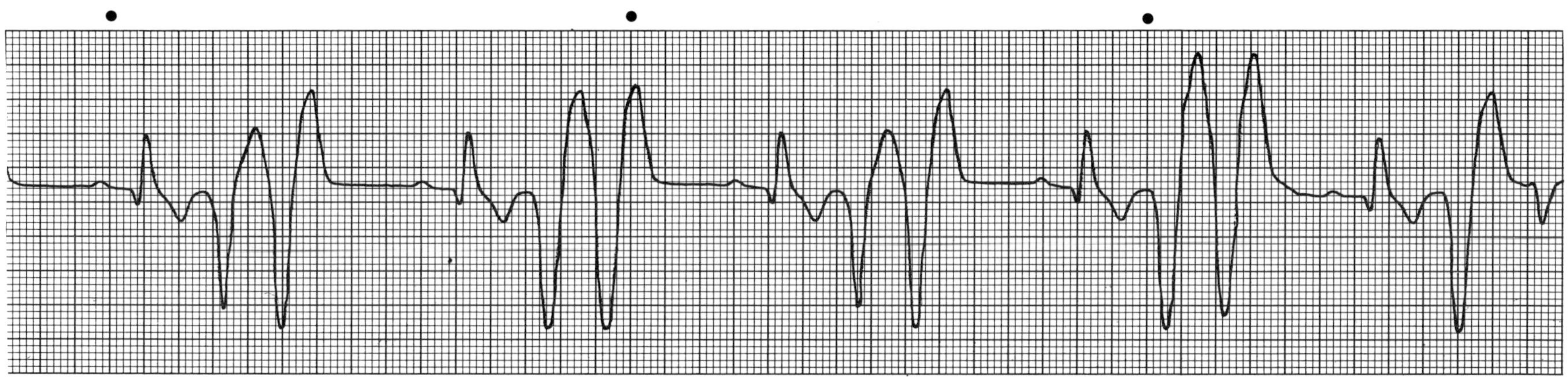

Question: This rhythm strip was recorded from a 5-year-old Viszla with a history of episodic weakness.

1. What is the rhythm diagnosis?
2. What is the likely mechanism for this arrhythmia?
3. What is the best therapeutic approach?

Case 63

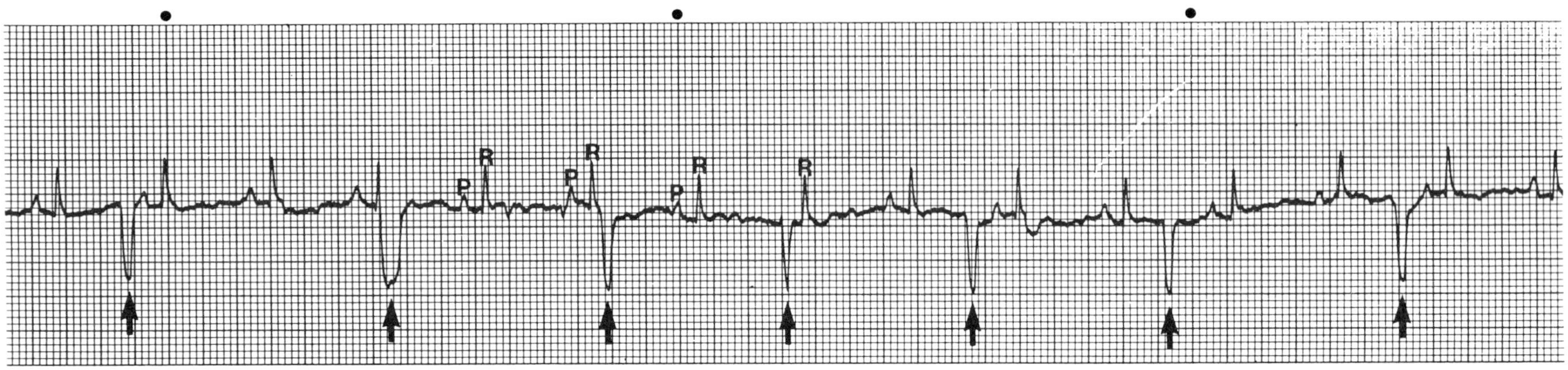

Answer: Normal sinus rhythm with numerous artifacts (arrows). Heart rate is 190 beats/min. Artifacts were created when the cat intermittently jerked its leg. The artifacts happen to fall below, within, and after the QRS-T complexes and resemble ventricular ectopic complexes; some are too close to the sinus complexes to allow double depolarization of the ventricles. Repeat rhythm strips should be evaluated because arrhythmias often occur 48 to 72 hours after the trauma.

Case 64

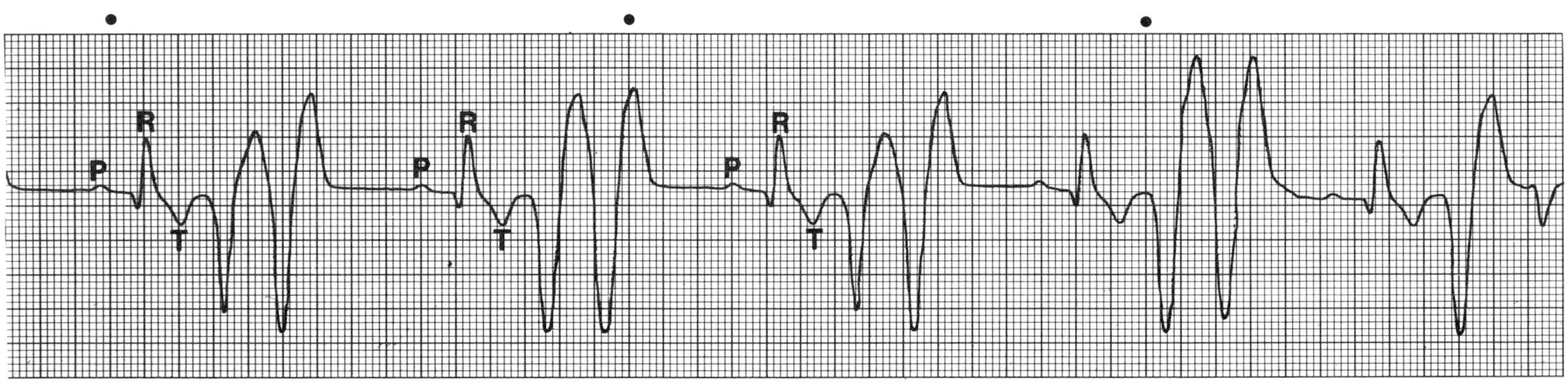

Answer: Sinus rhythm with ventricular trigeminy. Heart rate is 180 beats/min. Two ventricular premature complexes occur for every normal complex. This condition is often termed ventricular trigeminy. It is not possible to determine the mechanism for this arrhythmia without electrophysiologic studies. The ventricular premature complexes certainly could account for the weakness. Thoracic radiographs and an echocardiogram are needed to determine the cause of the ventricular arrhythmia. The dog is hemodynamically compromised. Treatment with boluses of lidocaine should be instituted until the rhythm is stable. After a lidocaine infusion has been started, procainamide, quinidine, tocainide, or mixiletine should be administered for maintenance.

Case 65

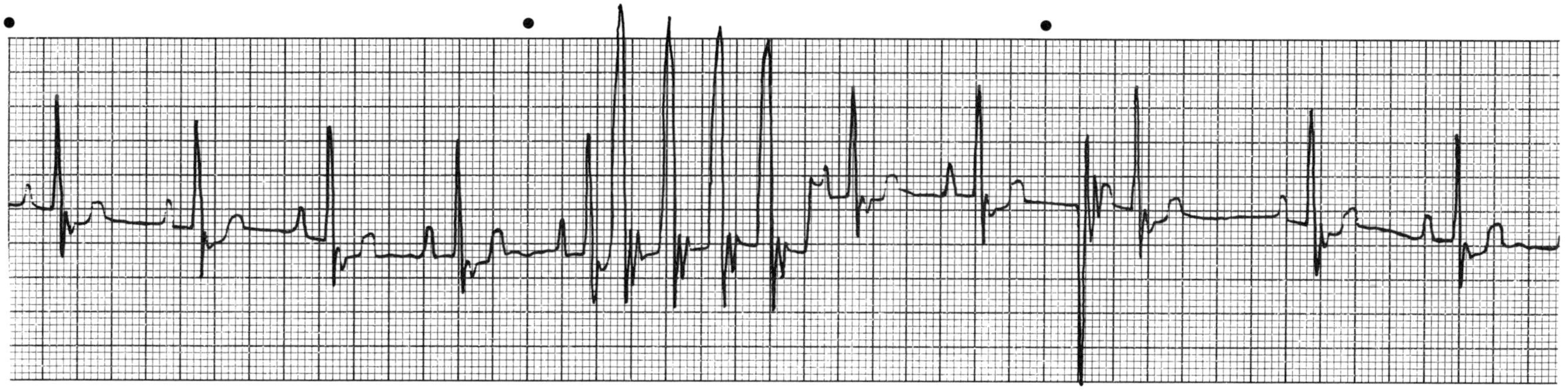

Question: This lead II rhythm strip was recorded from a 6-year-old Dachshund with a cough.

1. What is the rhythm diagnosis?
2. What is the best therapeutic approach?

Case 66

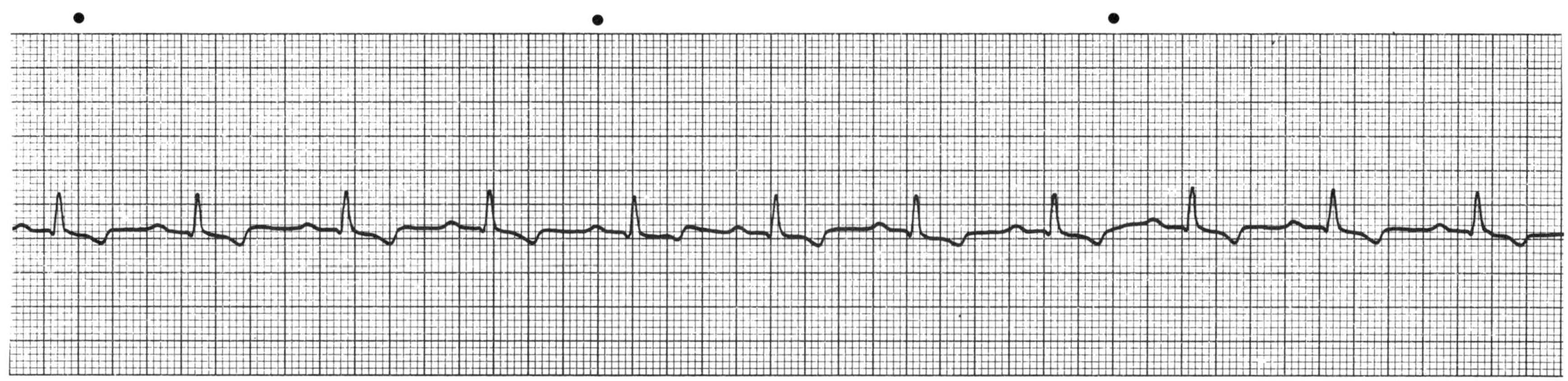

Question: This rhythm strip was obtained from a 17-year-old Burmese cat. The cat was examined because of dental disease and had no other clinical abnormalities. The ECG was done as part of a geriatric work-up.

1. What is the rhythm diagnosis?
2. What is the most likely underlying disorder?
3. What is the best therapeutic approach?

Case 65

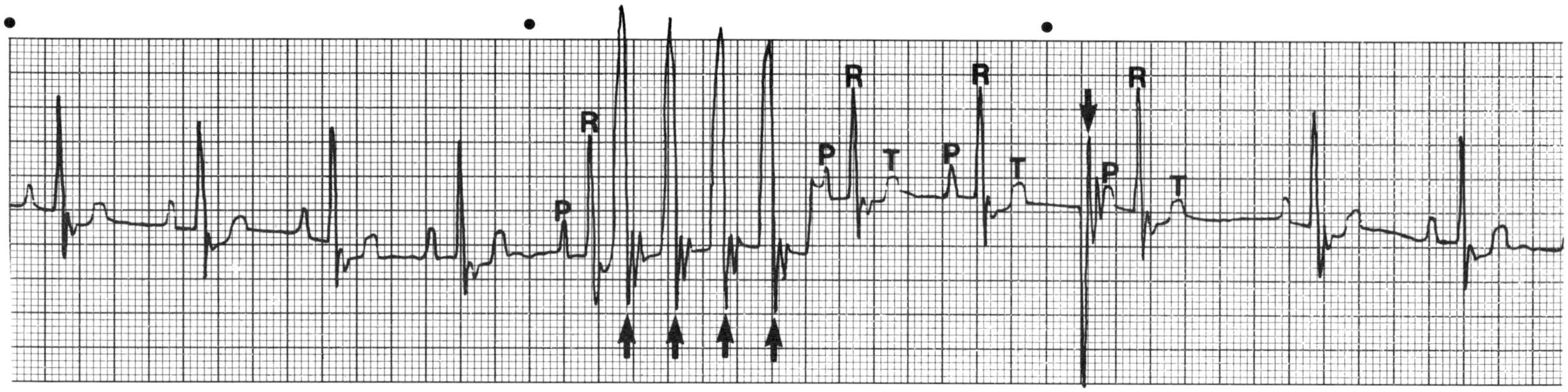

Answer: Sinus arrhythmia. Heart rate is approximately 160 beats/min. Sinus arrhythmia is present. Artifact is marked by arrows. On quick inspection, the artifact might be confused with a serious arrhythmia. Several aspects of the ECG confirm that the abnormal-appearing "complexes" are artifact. None of the artifactual "complexes" has T waves. The first "complex" occurs in the Q-T interval of the sinus complex. This site is an improbable location for ventricular depolarization. The P-R interval following the last artifactual "complex" is normal. If the last artifactual "complex" had been a ventricular ectopic complex, the P-R interval of the following complex probably would have been prolonged because of retrograde depolarization of the AV node. No antiarrhythmic treatment is needed.

Case 66

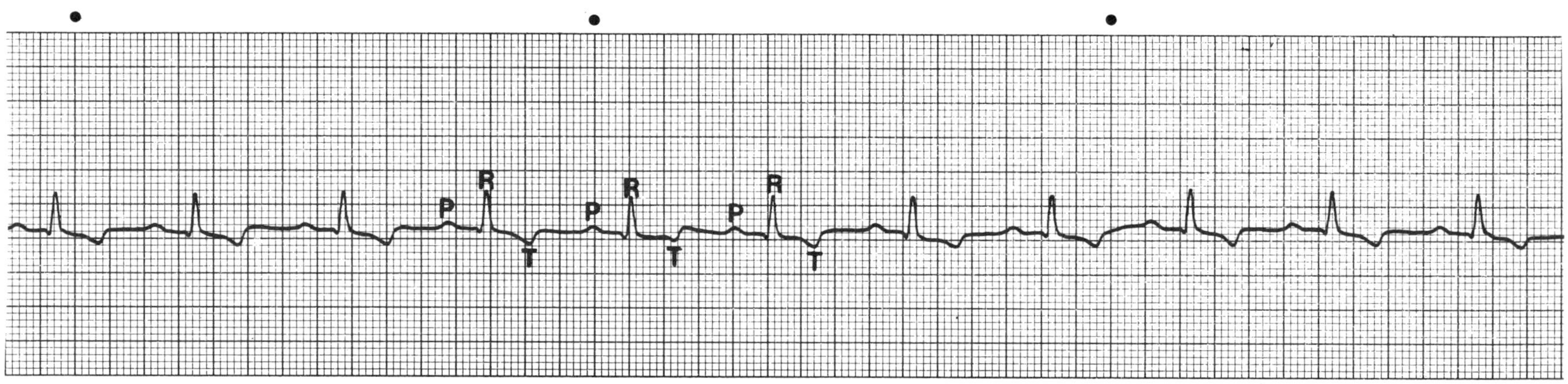

Answer: Sinus rhythm with first-degree AV block. Heart rate is 145 beats/min. The P-R interval is 0.11 sec, which is slightly prolonged for a cat. AV node fibrosis or degeneration is the most likely cause of the conduction disturbance in this geriatric cat. First-degree AV block does not cause clinical signs and requires no treatment. This conduction disturbance does not contraindicate general anesthesia for dentistry in this cat.

Case 67

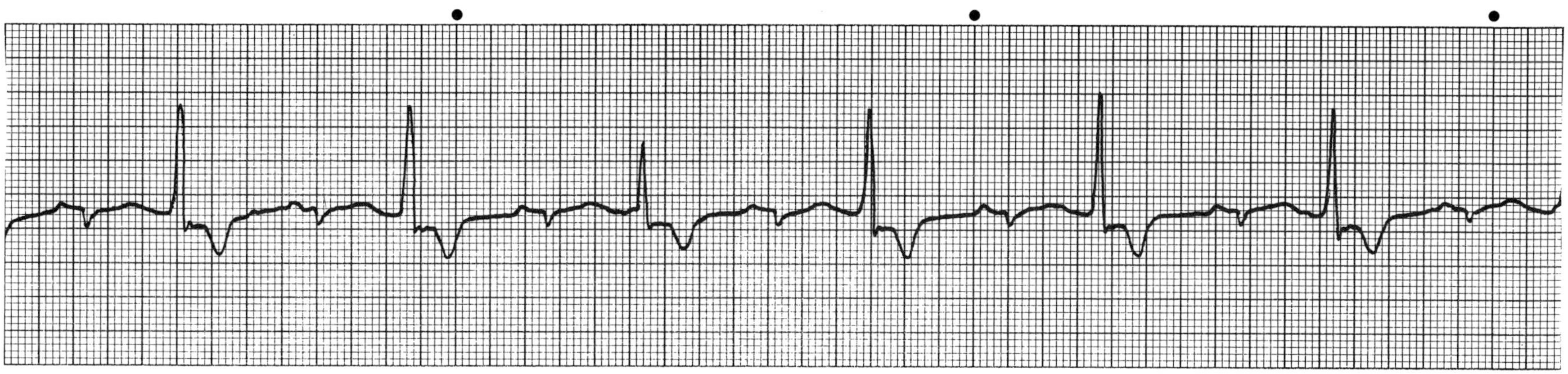

Question: This lead II ECG was obtained from a 13-year-old domestic shorthair cat examined because of severe dyspnea. A gallop rhythm was heard on auscultation.

1. What is the rhythm diagnosis?
2. What is the best therapeutic approach?

Case 68

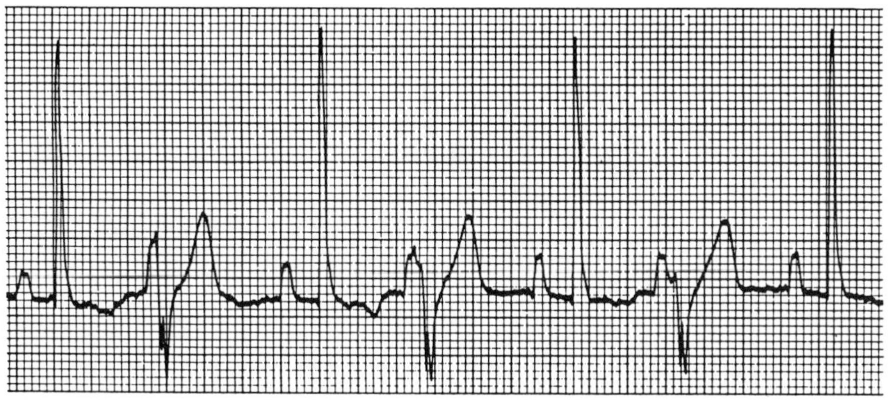

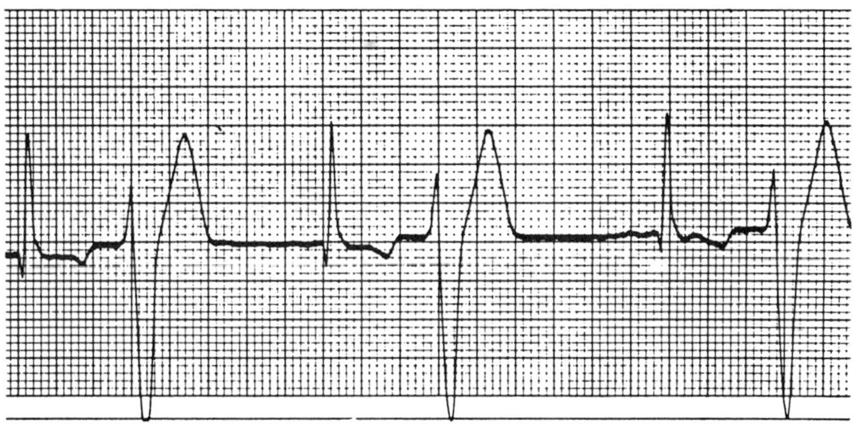

Question: These two strips were recorded from different dogs. Strip A was recorded from a normal dog during anesthesia. Strip B was recorded from a dog with atrial fibrillation; the dog was being treated with digoxin and diuretics for a chronic heart condition.

1. What is the rhythm diagnosis?
2. What two drugs can often cause these undesirable arrhythmias?
3. Will palpation of the femoral pulse reveal any abnormalities?

Case 67

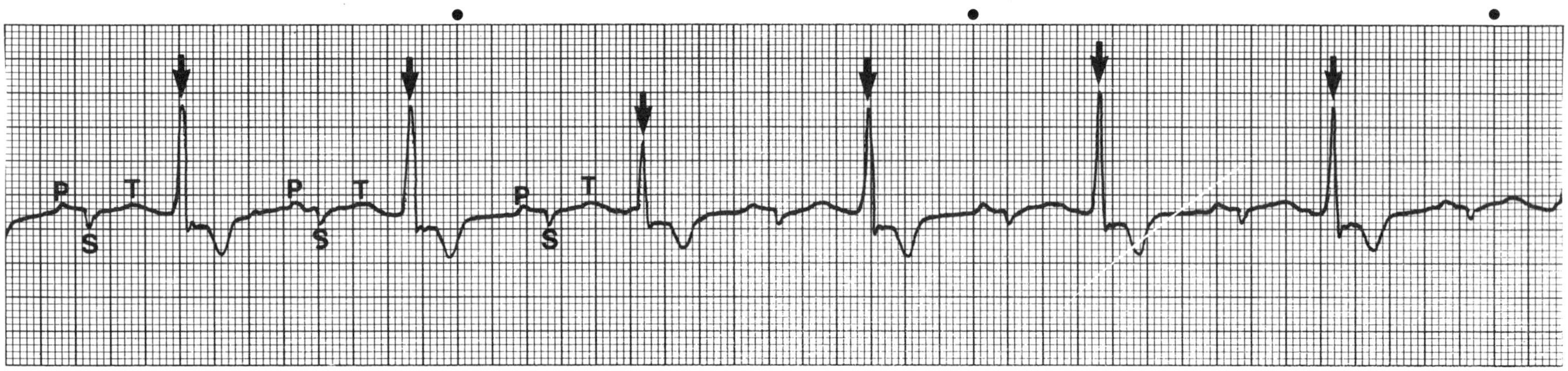

Answer: Sinus rhythm with ventricular premature complexes every other beat (ventricular bigeminy). Heart rate is 180 beats/min. Thoracic radiographs should be assessed before treating the arrhythmia. An echocardiogram would determine whether the cat has cardiomyopathy. Antiarrhythmic medication should be delayed until the underlying disease is identified. Antiarrhythmic medication (e.g., propranolol) may reduce the heart rate and decrease cardiac output. The small P waves and QRS complexes of the sinus beats can be overlooked easily. The high-amplitude, bizarre QRS complexes are ventricular premature complexes (arrows). These complexes are not associated with P waves, a characteristic typical of ventricular arrhythmias. Propranolol can be considered if the ventricular premature complexes persist and the echocardiogram eliminates dilated cardiomyopathy from the differential diagnosis. The underlying condition always should be treated first.

Case 68

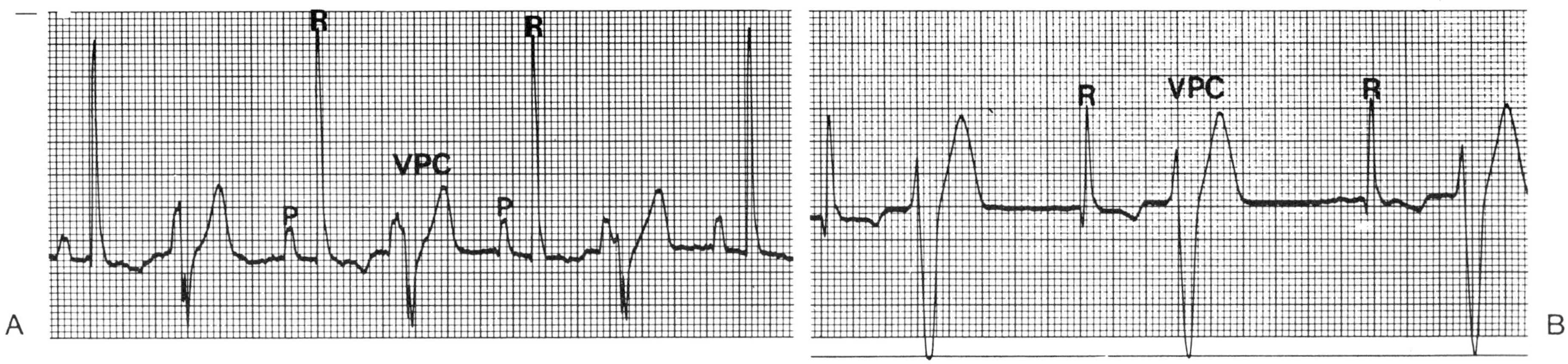

Answer: A and B. Ventricular bigeminy. Heart rate is variable. Strip A has ventricular premature complexes (VPCs) alternating with sinus complexes. Barbiturate anesthetics can often cause this arrhythmia. Strip B is atrial fibrillation and ventricular bigeminy. No P waves are present. The slow, regular ventricular rate (R) indicates a probable block in the AV junction or an AV junctional rhythm. When such a cardiac rhythm disorder is encountered during digoxin therapy, the diagnosis of digoxin toxicity is likely. For both cases, supportive measures are important. Acid base and electrolyte abnormalities should be corrected. Palpation of the femoral pulse in both cases reveals pulsus bigeminus. The premature beat causes the ventricle to contract before the chamber has had time to adequately fill with blood. The blood pressure drops when the premature beat occurs.

Case 69

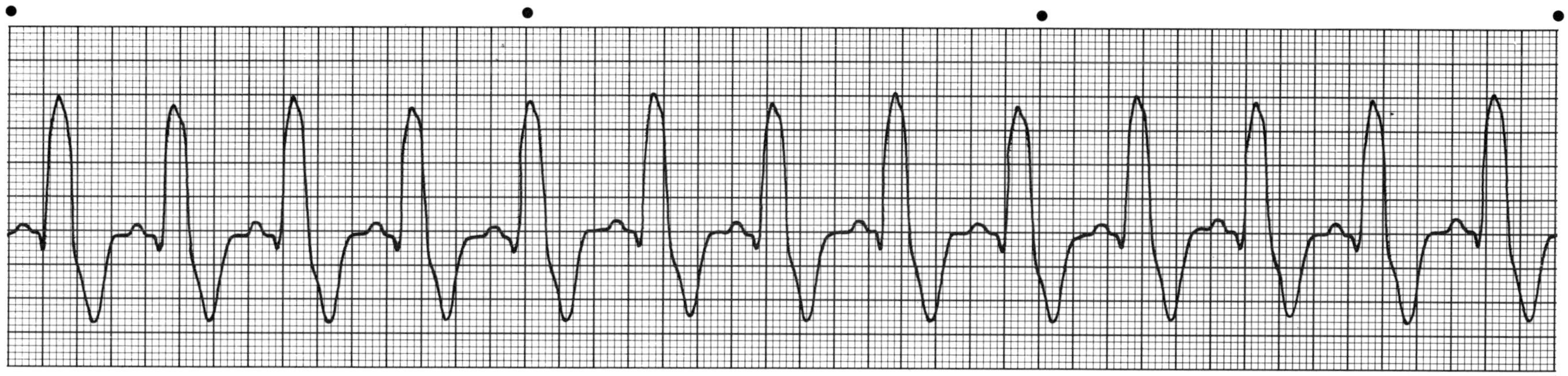

Question: This lead II ECG was obtained from an 8-year-old Boxer that was undergoing chemotherapy for lymphosarcoma.

1. What is the rhythm diagnosis?
2. What is the most likely underlying disorder?
3. What is the best therapeutic approach?

Case 70

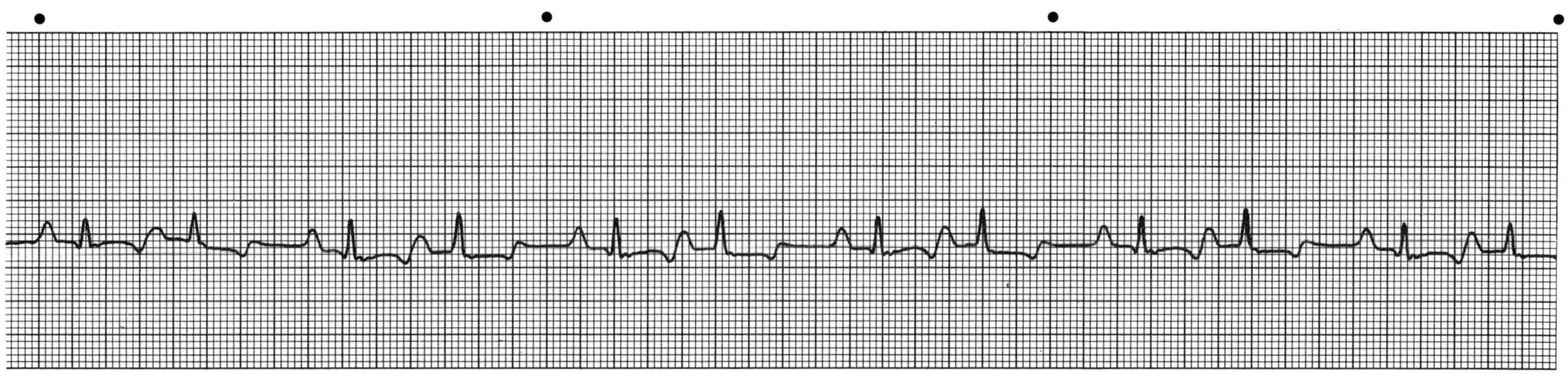

Question: This lead II rhythm strip was recorded from a 6-year-old Chow with a history of coughing at night.

1. What is the rhythm diagnosis?
2. What are common causes of this arrhythmia?
3. What is the most likely underlying disorder?
4. What is the best therapeutic approach?

Case 69

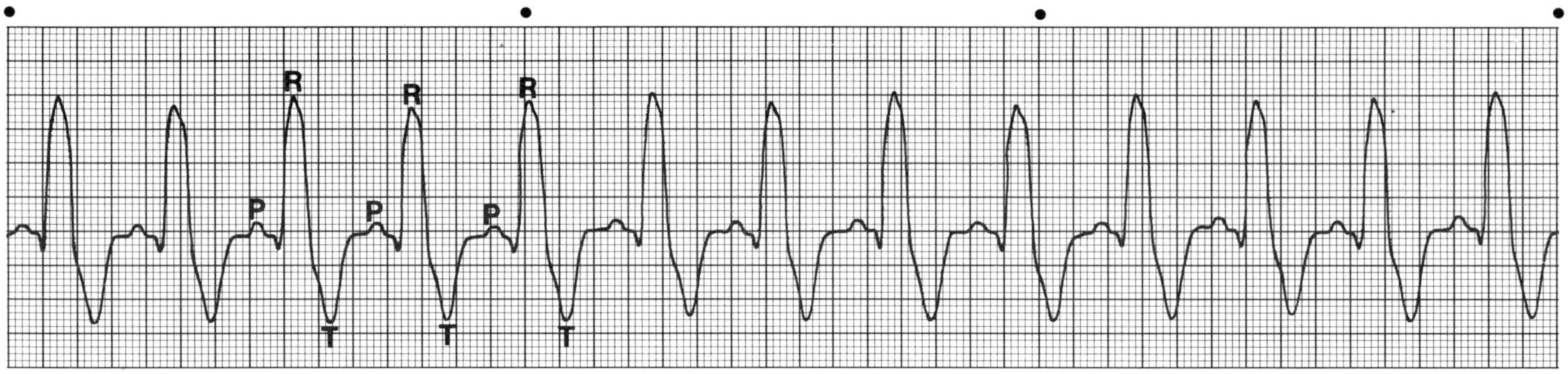

Answer: Sinus rhythm with left bundle-branch block. Heart rate is 175 beats/min. Lymphosarcoma can metastasize to the heart and the intraventricular conduction system. No specific treatment is available or necessary for left bundle-branch block. Serial ECGs should be done to monitor the possible development of complete AV block. Left bundle-branch block is typified by a QRS complex duration of 0.07 sec or greater and a consistent P-R interval. The QRS complexes of left bundle-branch block are positive in leads I, II, III, aVF, CV_6LL, and CV_6LV. The consistent P-R interval quickly differentiates this wide-complex rhythm from ventricular tachycardia.

Case 70

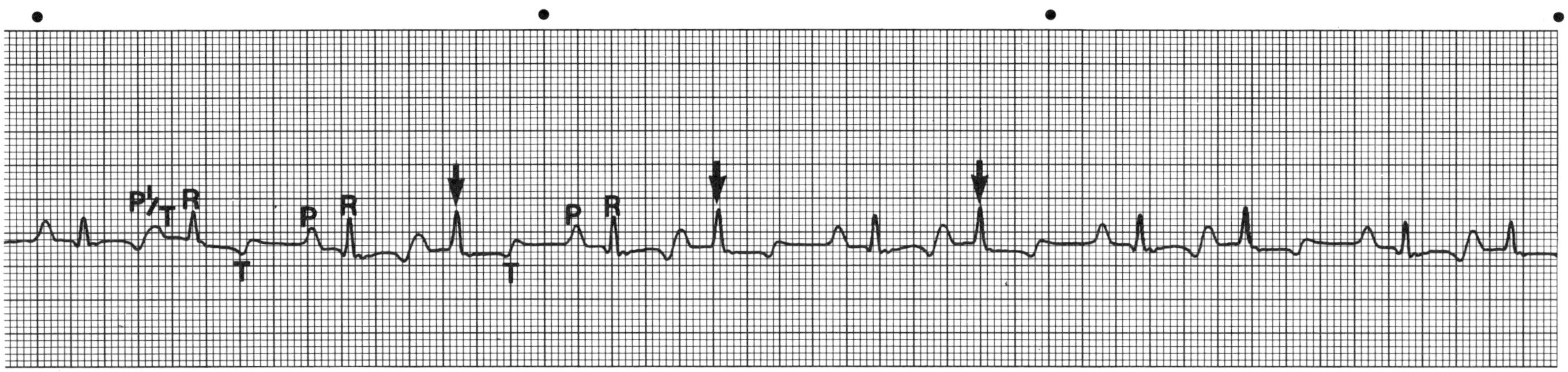

Answer: Sinus rhythm with atrial bigeminy. Heart rate is 160 beats/min. Atrial bigeminy occurs when every other complex is an atrial premature complex (P′/T). The QRS complexes of the atrial premature complexes (arrows) are similar to those of the sinus complexes. The small QRS complexes could be compatible with thoracic effusion or could be a normal variation. Atrial arrhythmias usually accompany atrial distention secondary to valve disease, cardiomyopathy, and pulmonary hypertension. Atrial arrhythmias are also associated with atrial neoplasia, drug administration (e.g., digitalis and general anesthetics), and systemic disturbances (e.g., electrolyte and acid-base imbalances). The arrhythmia, coupled with the history of nocturnal coughing, suggests congestive heart failure. Thoracic radiography should be performed, and echocardiography may be necessary for a definitive cardiac diagnosis. The arrhythmia should be treated with digoxin. Propranolol and diltiazem can also be used for atrial arrhythmias, but are not generally used for initial control in animals with congestive heart failure.

Case 71

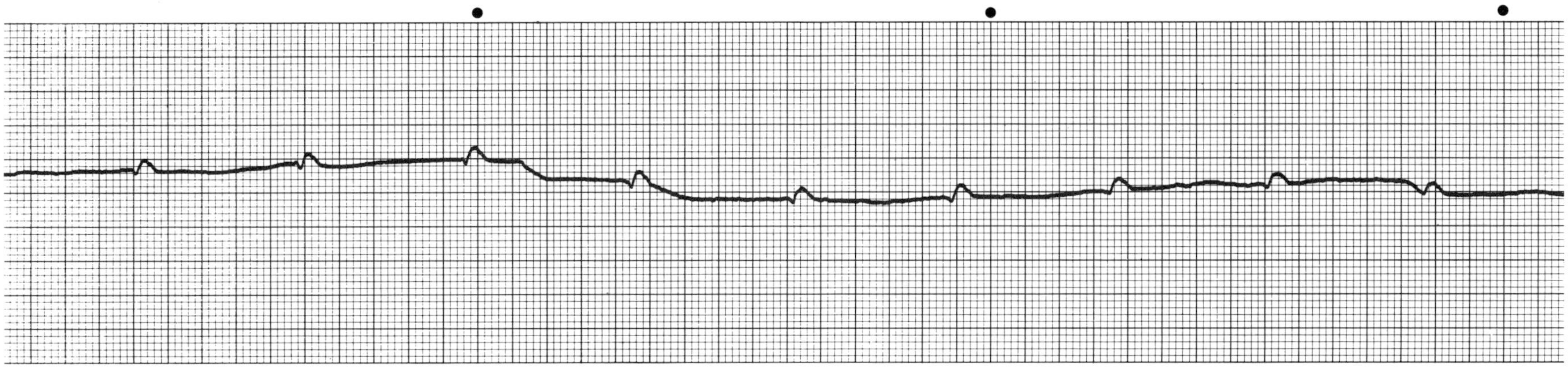

Question: This lead II tracing was recorded from a dog in cardiac arrest. The dog had just been given anesthesia for a routine dental procedure.

1. What is the rhythm diagnosis?
2. What is the best therapeutic approach?

Case 72

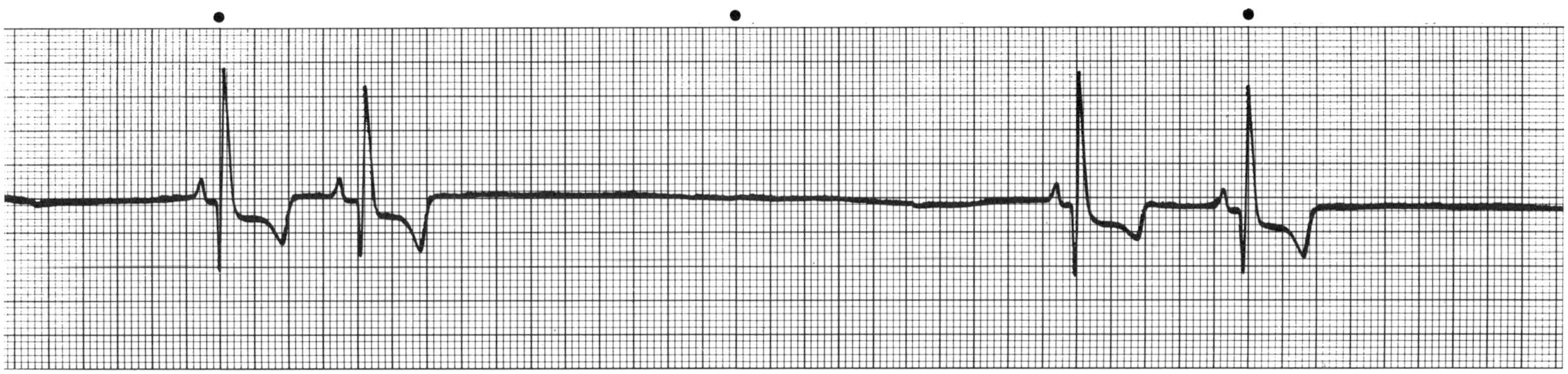

Question: This lead II ECG was obtained from a 10-year-old female Miniature Schnauzer examined because of frequent syncopal episodes that had worsened over a 1-week period.

1. What is the rhythm diagnosis?
2. What is the most likely underlying disorder?
3. What is the best therapeutic approach?

Case 71

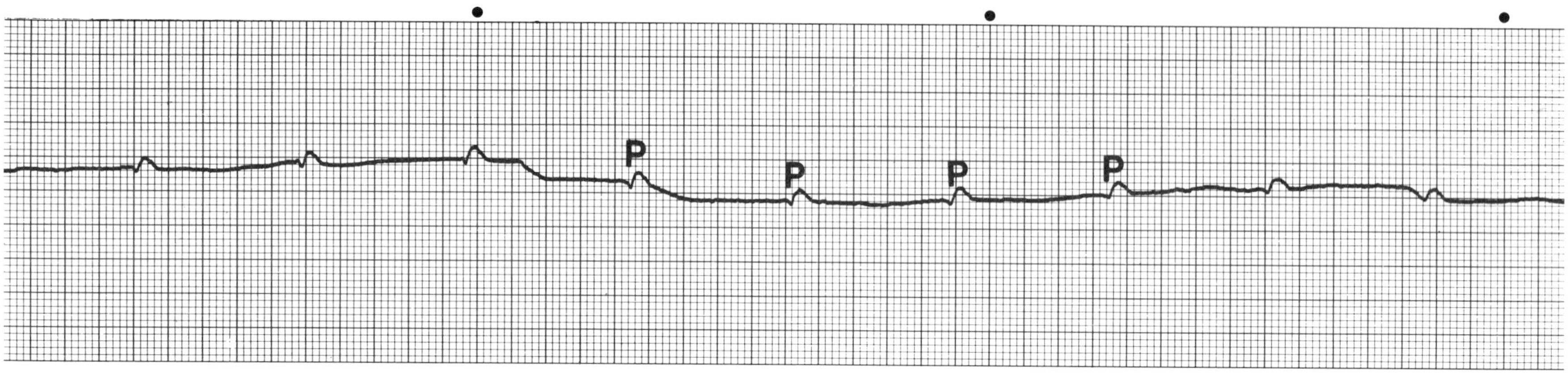

Answer: Ventricular asystole with complete AV block. Atrial heart rate is 125 beats/min. Only P waves (atrial activity) are present. Ventricular activity is absent. Ventricular asystole represents cardiac arrest. The three types of cardiac arrest are ventricular fibrillation, ventricular asystole, and electrical—mechanical dissociation. Ventricular asystole may be caused by severe SA block or by severe third-degree AV block. Cardiac resuscitation should be started immediately. The basic cause of cardiac arrest should be treated, with serum electrolytes and blood gases evaluated. Administer injections of atropine and epinephrine, followed by an intravenous drip of isoproterenol or dobutamine. A transvenous pacemaker may be needed for artificial pacing, but it requires a mechanically responsive myocardium.

Case 72

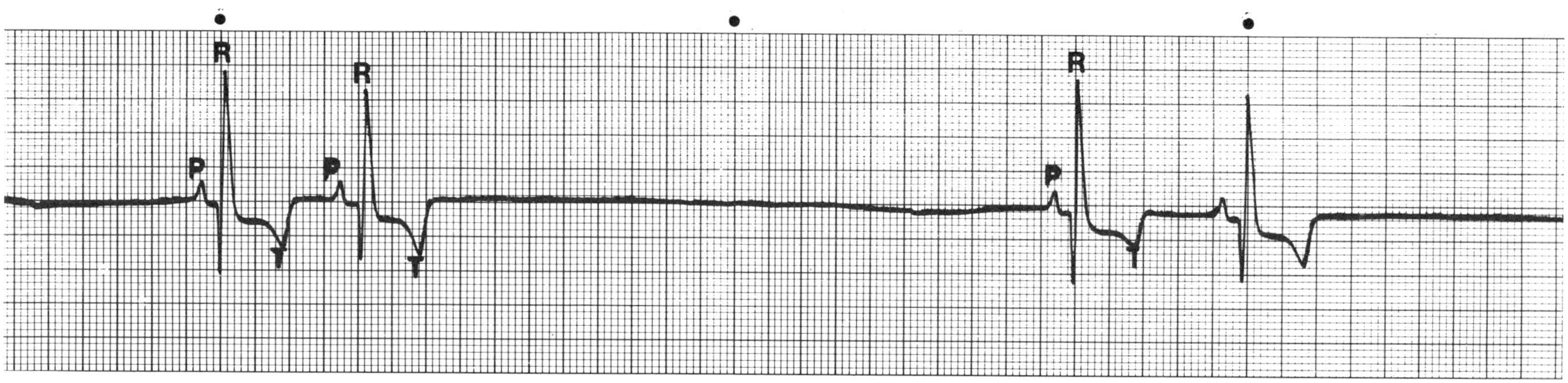

Answer: Sinus rhythm with a prolonged period of sinoatrial block or sinus arrest. Heart rate is irregular. Sinus node disease (sick sinus syndrome) is the probable cause of this arrhythmia. Sinus arrest represents long pauses without P-QRS-T complexes. The pauses are twice or greater-than-twice the normal R-R interval. If pauses are composed of exact series of normal R-R intervals, an SA block is suggested. Hypothyroidism and abnormally high levels of vagal tone are other associated conditions. A poor (blunted) response to atropine supports the diagnosis of sick sinus syndrome. Atropine given parenterally or propantheline given orally may still prevent syncopal episodes. A permanent cardiac pacemaker is required when episodes of syncope or weakness persist. The lack of an AV junctional escape beat at the end of the long pause (a normal physiologic response) supports a finding of disease of the AV conduction system, as well as of the sinus node. The term "sick escape pacemaker syndrome" is sometimes used.

Case 73

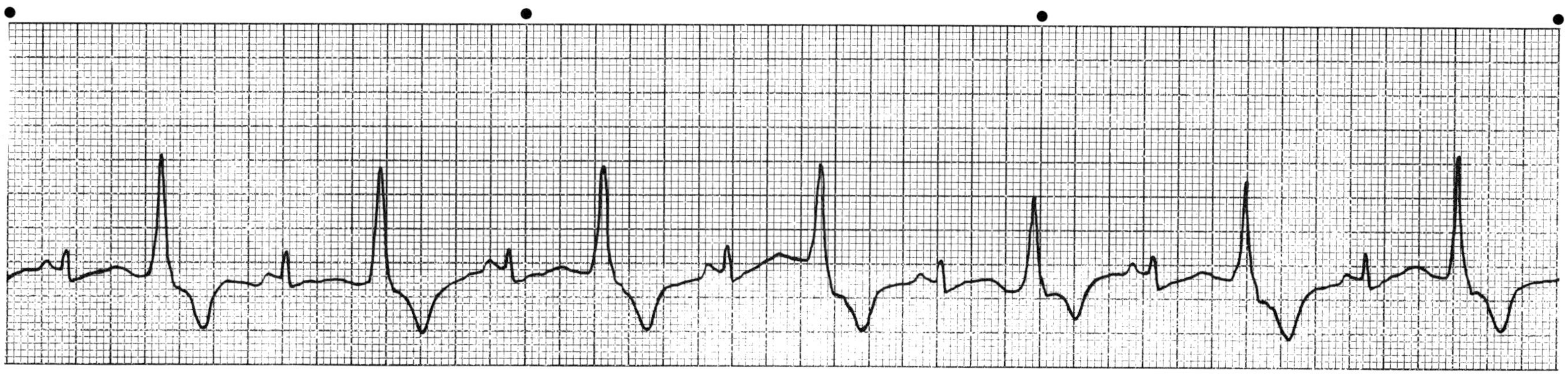

Question: This rhythm strip was recorded from a 3-year-old domestic shorthair cat with a history of dyspnea. Thoracic radiographs revealed cardiomegaly and pulmonary edema.

1. What is the rhythm diagnosis?
2. What is the most likely underlying disorder?
3. What is the best therapeutic approach?

Case 74

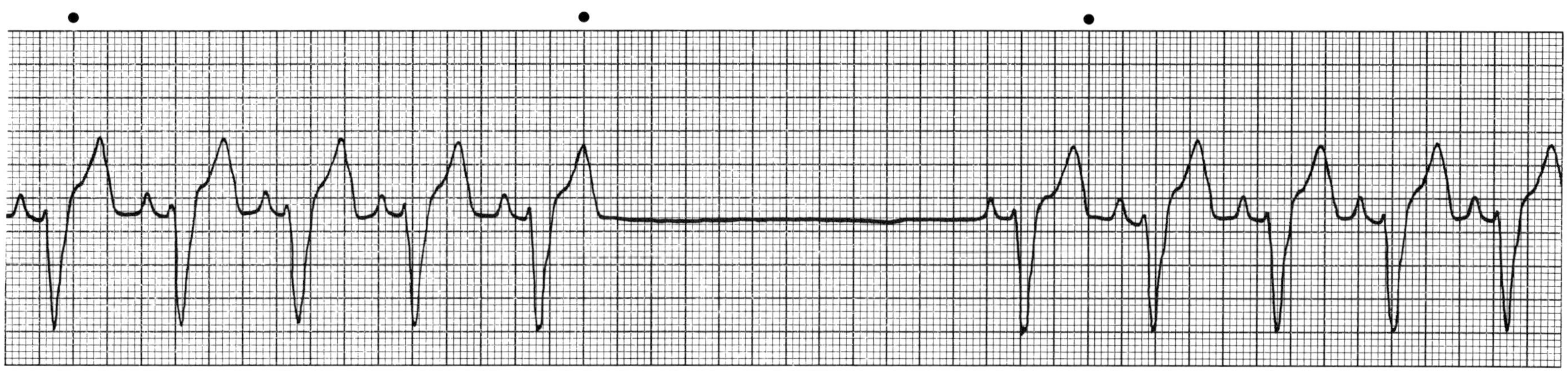

Question: This rhythm strip was recorded from a 10-year-old female Dachshund. The rhythm disturbance was noticed on routine physical examination. The dog had no clinical signs.

1. What is the rhythm diagnosis?
2. What are common causes of this arrhythmia?
3. What is the most likely underlying disorder?
4. What is the best therapeutic approach?

Case 73

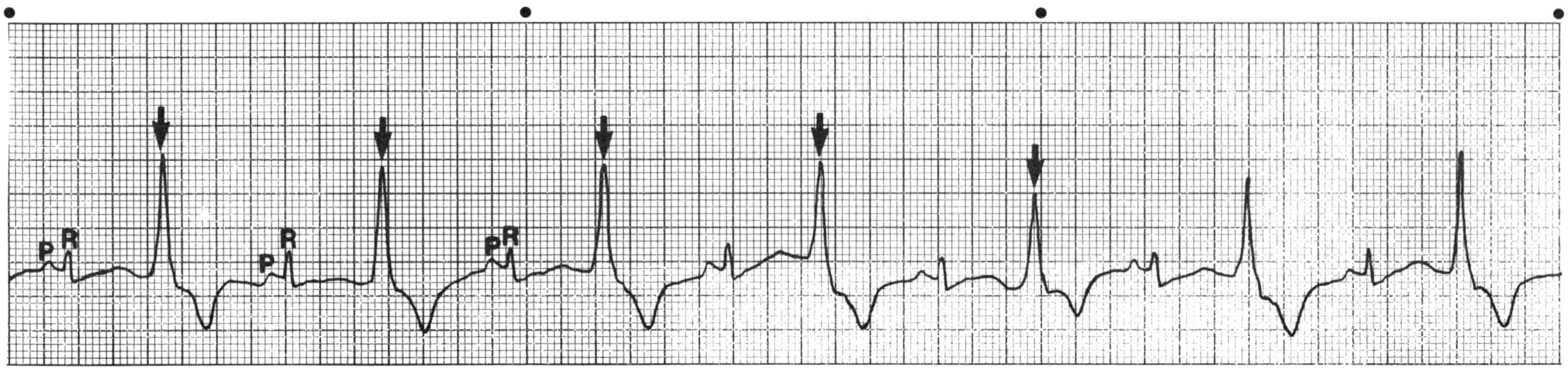

Answer: Sinus rhythm with ventricular bigeminy. Heart rate is 190 beats/min. Every other QRS complex is tall and wide and not associated with a P wave. These configurations are ventricular premature complexes (arrows). The alternating rhythm suggests re-entry as the mechanism for the arrhythmia. The radiographs and history support cardiomyopathy (probably hypertrophic) as the most likely cause of the arrhythmia and clinical signs. Hyperthyroidism could cause the same ECG and radiographic findings, but is extremely unlikely in this instance because of the cat's young age. Echocardiography should be used to establish a definitive diagnosis. Edema should be treated with furosemide. Treatment of the congestive heart failure may resolve the arrhythmia. The arrhythmia can be treated with propranolol and the ECG repeated in 24 hours. If dyspnea worsens after starting the propranolol, the medication should be discontinued. Propranolol can induce bronchoconstriction and aggravate cardiac failure, especially in cats with dilated cardiomyopathy.

Case 74

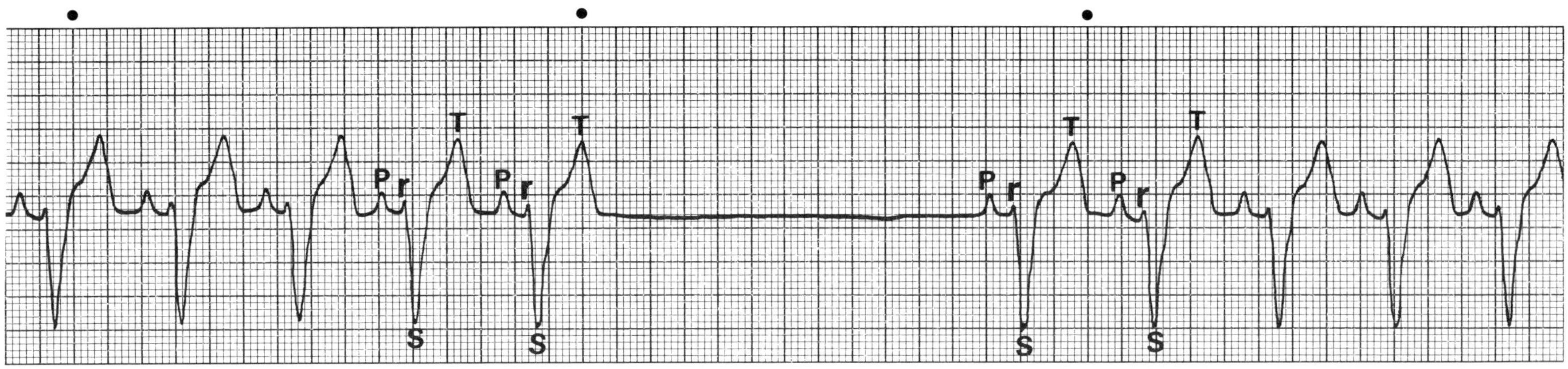

Answer: Sinus rhythm with sinus arrest or sinoatrial block. Heart rate is variable. The QRS complexes are wide and negative and might be confused with ventricular tachycardia. The presence of a consistent P-R interval confirms sinus rhythm. A right bundle-branch block pattern is present. Sinus arrest or sinoatrial block is defined by a sinus pause that is greater than twice the normal R-R interval. Sinus arrest occurs when the electrical discharge from the sinus node is absent. Sinus block occurs when a sinus impulse is generated but then is blocked before leaving the sinoatrial node. After the fifth complex, no P-QRS-T complexes occur for more than 1.4 sec. These findings could indicate sick sinus syndrome, which is prevalent in old female Dachshunds. This dog has no clinical signs and requires no treatment. If weakness is associated with the pauses, an anticholinergic drug should be administered.

Case 75

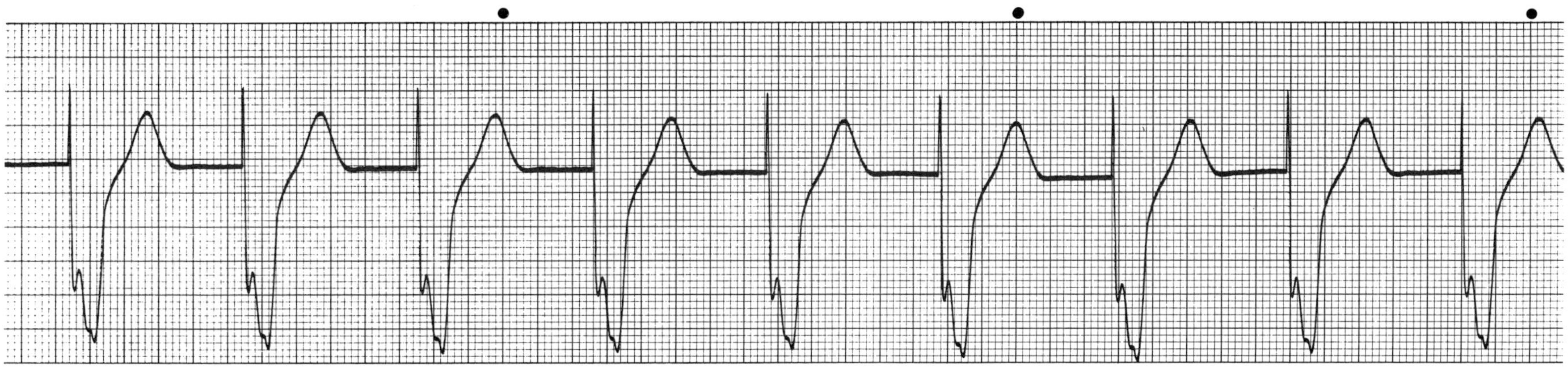

Question: An ECG was recorded from a dog with complete AV block and numerous episodes of fainting. This lead II rhythm strip was recorded 2 weeks after surgery had been performed. No further fainting episodes occurred.

1. What is the rhythm diagnosis?
2. What surgical procedure was performed, and was the procedure successful?

Case 76

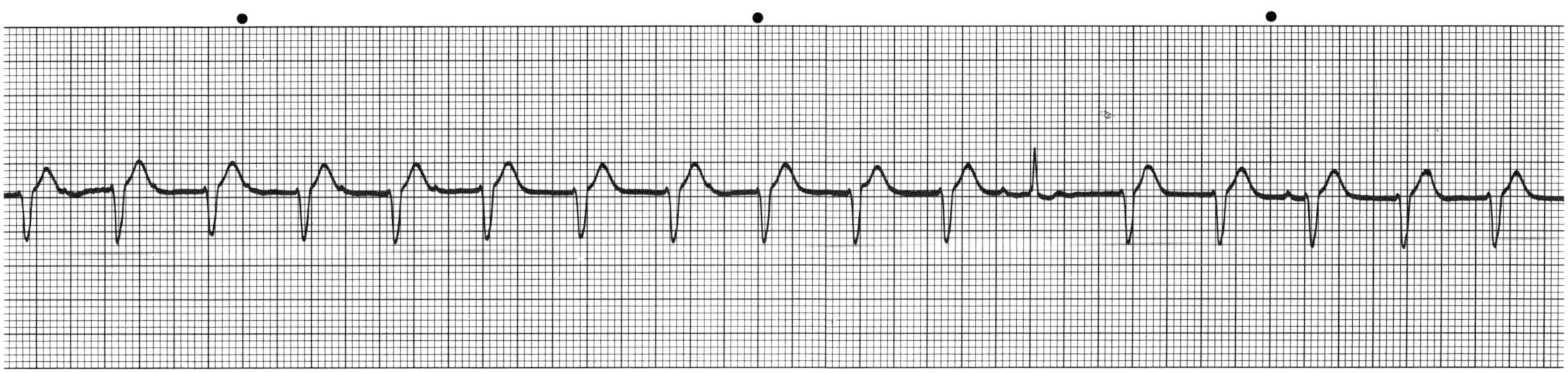

Question: This strip was recorded from a cat with a history of anorexia and lethargy. A femoral pulse deficit was palpated on physical examination. Amplitude scale: 0.5 cm = 1 mv.

1. What is the rhythm diagnosis?
2. What are common causes of this arrhythmia?
3. What is the best therapeutic approach?

Case 75

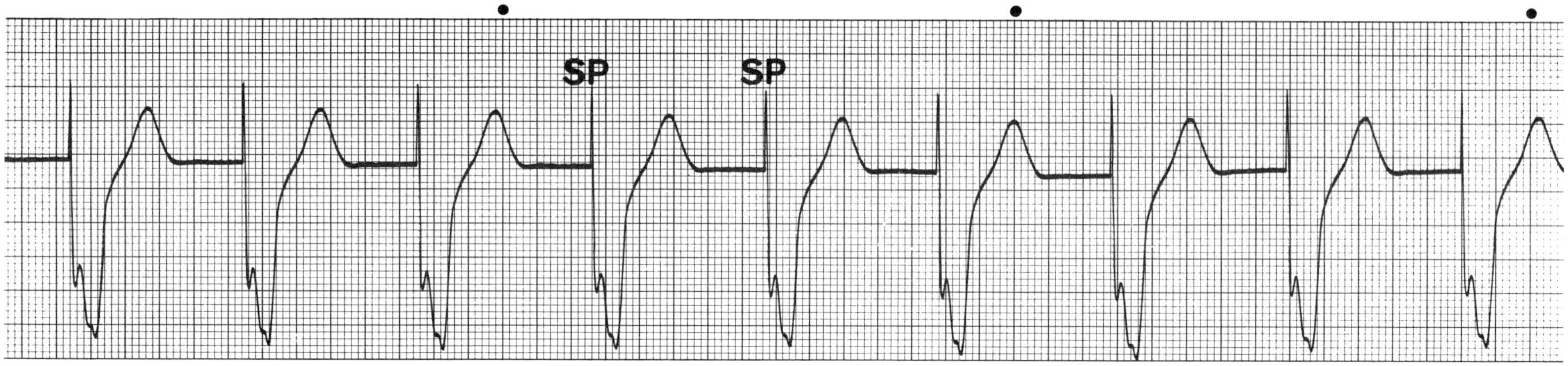

Answer: Fixed-rate artificial pacemaker rhythm with electrode attached to the left ventricle. Heart rate is 120 beats/min. Electronic pacemakers are used on a permanent basis to treat symptomatic bradycardia secondary to complete heart block. The pacemaker pulse rate is regular; a pacemaker spike (SP), or electrical impulse from the artificial pacemaker, is present. Each time the pacemaker gives off an electrical signal, the signal is conducted down the wire to the heart. The pacemaker impulse then spreads into the left and right ventricles, thereby causing the heart to contract. Left ventricle pacing from the attached epicardial electrode implant produces a QRS complex with the configuration of right bundle-branch block. A wide and bizarre QRS complex follows each spike, thereby representing ventricular activation. A thoracic radiograph confirmed the location of the pacemaker generator and lead wire. The pacemaker rate and stimulus artifact should be evaluated on each ECG taken to determine the integrity of the electrode impulse generator. The ECG should be evaluated approximately every 3 months. When the ventricular rate was increased with the pacemaker in this dog, the fainting episodes were eliminated. The QRS complexes are wide and bizarre because the electrical impulse does not travel through the specialized conduction system, but through ordinary muscle, thus spreading to both ventricles with delay. Satisfactory cardiac output is still present.

Case 76

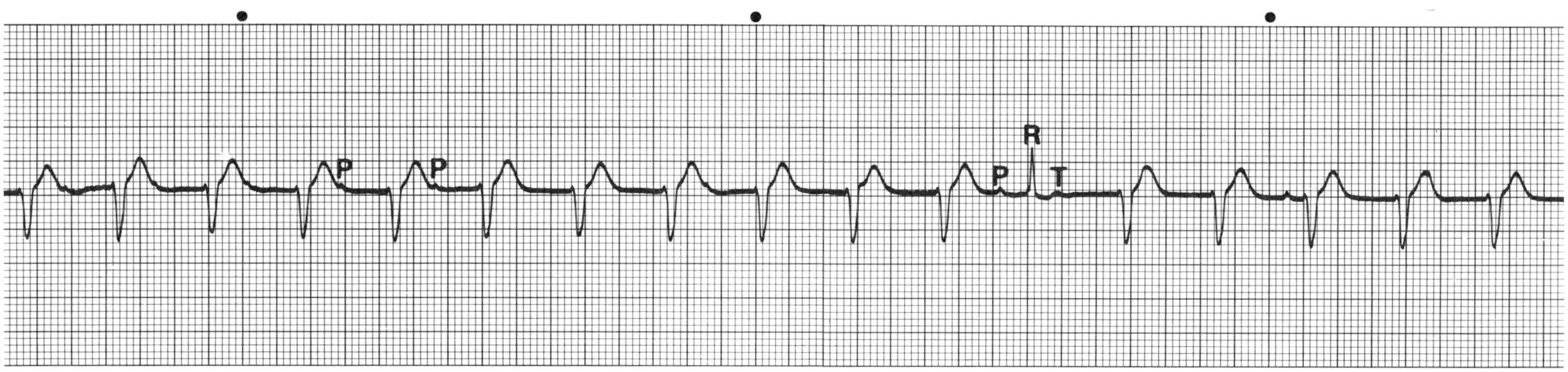

Answer: Paroxysmal ventricular tachycardia. Heart rate is approximately 225 beats/min. Ventricular tachycardia implies a series of repetitive ventricular premature complexes that are usually of sudden onset. The QRS complexes are independent of the P waves. P waves may precede, be hidden within, or follow QRS complexes. The QRS complexes are wide and bizarre. The sixth complex from the end of the strip is a capture complex. A normal sinus impulse has reached the AV junction in a recovered state, thus capturing the ventricles for one complex. Ventricular tachycardia is usually a manifestation of significant heart disease. Associated conditions can include primary cardiac disease, secondary cardiac diseases, and drug therapy. The cardiac conditions include congestive heart failure secondary to cardiomyopathy, myocardial infarction, neoplasia, traumatic myocarditis, hyperthyroidism, and bacterial endomyocarditis. A biochemistry blood profile, complete blood count, determination of serum thyroxine concentrations, and thoracic radiograph complete the initial data base. An echocardiogram may be necessary to determine the underlying condition. The underlying condition should be treated as soon as possible. Supportive measures, including the correction of acid-base and electrolyte abnormalities, are important. Lidocaine should be administered slowly and with extreme caution because cats are particularly susceptible to neurotoxic effects. Propranolol is usually an effective ventricular antiarrhythmic drug in cats.

Case 77

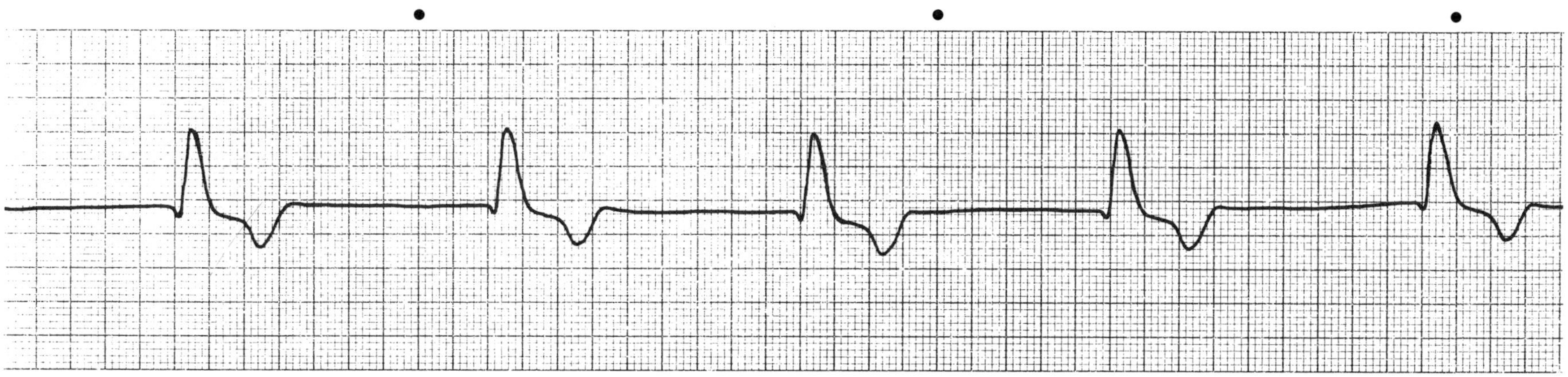

Question: This lead II ECG was obtained from a 2-year-old Miniature Schnauzer examined because of extreme weakness, vomiting, and diarrhea. A slow heart rate was heard on auscultation.

1. What is the rhythm diagnosis?
2. What is the most likely underlying disorder?
3. What is the best therapeutic approach?

Case 78

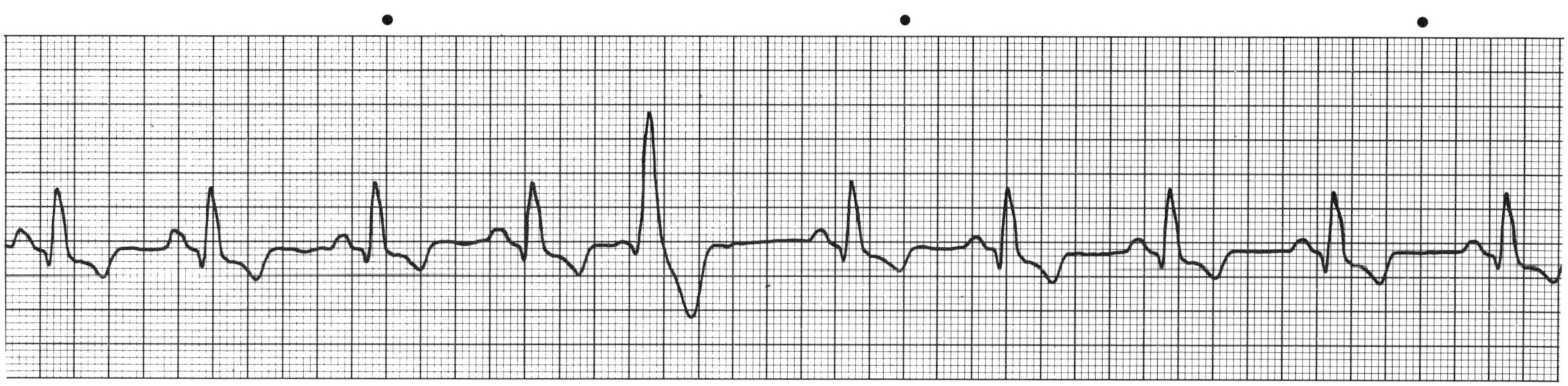

Question: This lead II ECG was obtained from an 8-year-old Doberman Pinscher examined because of exercise intolerance.

1. What is the rhythm diagnosis?
2. What is the most likely underlying disorder?
3. What is the best therapeutic approach?

Case 77

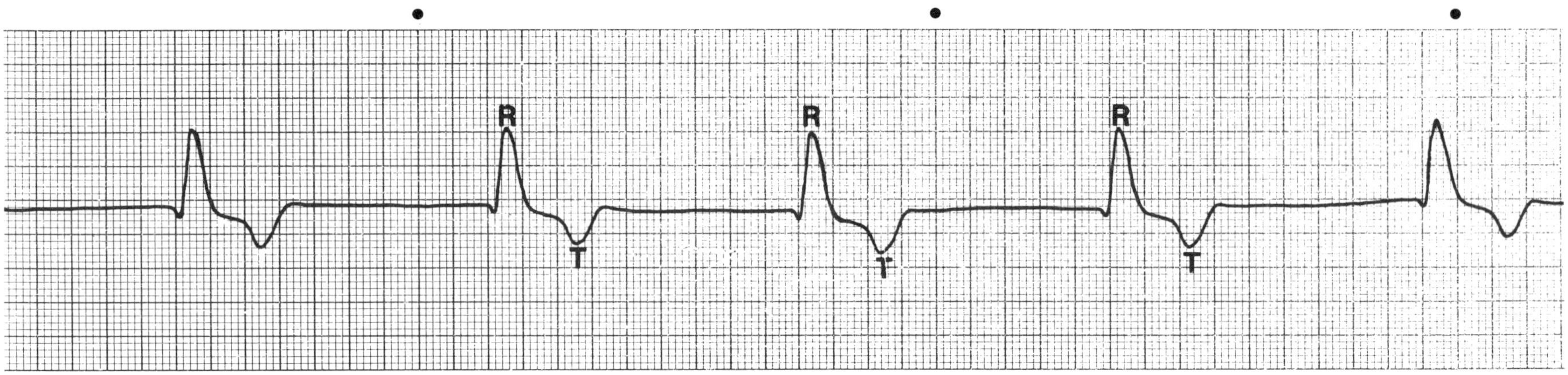

Answer: Atrial standstill. Heart rate is 65 beats/min. Severe hyperkalemia caused by hypoadrenocorticism (Addison's disease), diabetic ketoacidosis, or acute renal failure is the most likely underlying disorder. Treatment for severe hyperkalemia includes intravenous administration of 0.9% sodium chloride, sodium bicarbonate, dextrose, and regular insulin. Calcium gluconate can provide short-term stabilization in life-threatening situations. Sinus rhythm should return within 30 to 60 minutes. Corticosteroids should be administered if hypoadrenocorticism is suspected. Atrial standstill is characterized by no P waves, normal or bizarre QRS complexes, regular rhythm, elevated or depressed S-T segment, and large T waves. Persistent atrial standstill may also be seen in English Springer Spaniels with a form of muscular dystrophy and in cats with dilated cardiomyopathy. Progressive hyperkalemia is typified by tall and broad T waves, flattening and eventual loss of P waves, widening of QRS complexes, and, eventually, ventricular fibrillation or ventricular asystole.

Case 78

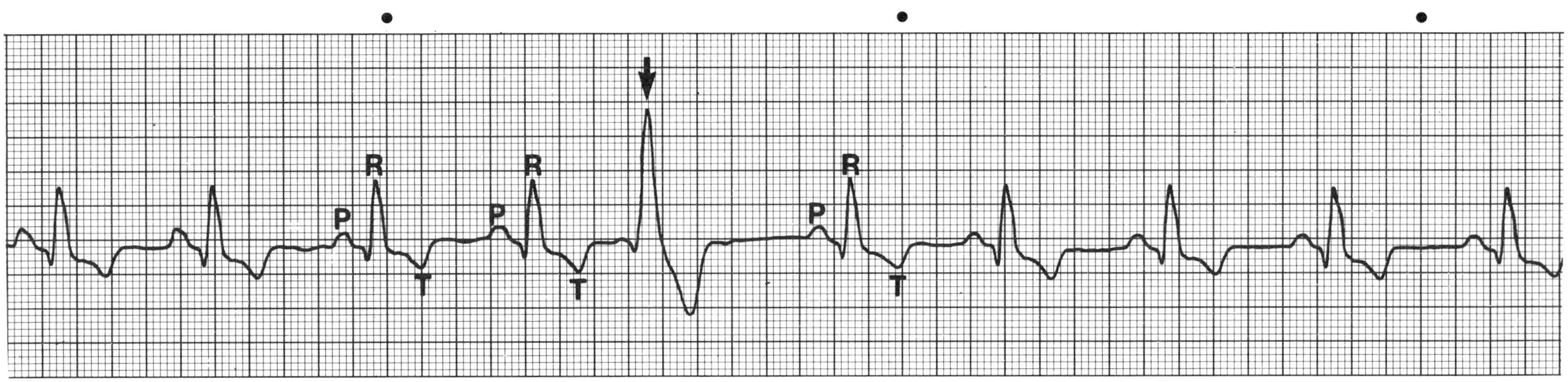

Answer: Sinus rhythm with one ventricular premature complex (arrow). Heart rate is 130 beats/min. Dilated cardiomyopathy and myocarditis are the most likely underlying disorders. Occasional ventricular premature complexes do not require treatment. Treatment should be based on results of a complete diagnostic work-up (i.e., thoracic radiographs, hematologic testing, urinalysis, and, possibly, an echocardiogram). The ventricular premature complex is characterized by a wide and bizarre QRS complex not associated with the preceding P wave. Because the ventricular premature complex deflection is positive, it probably originates in the right ventricle. Accordingly, heartworm disease should also be eliminated from the differential diagnosis.

Case 79

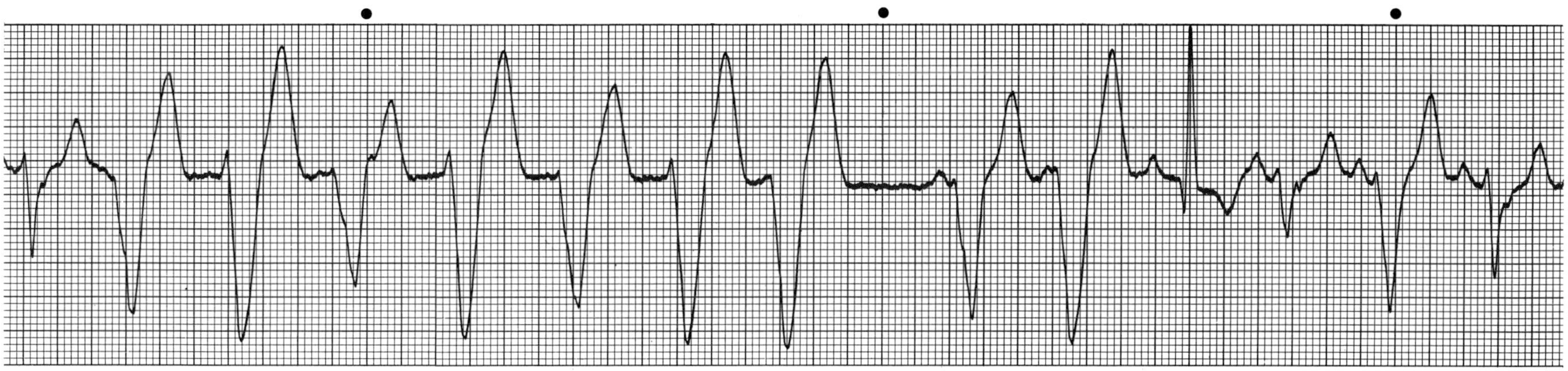

Question: This tracing was recorded from a dog with a gastric dilatation.

1. What is the rhythm diagnosis?
2. What is the best therapeutic approach?

Case 80

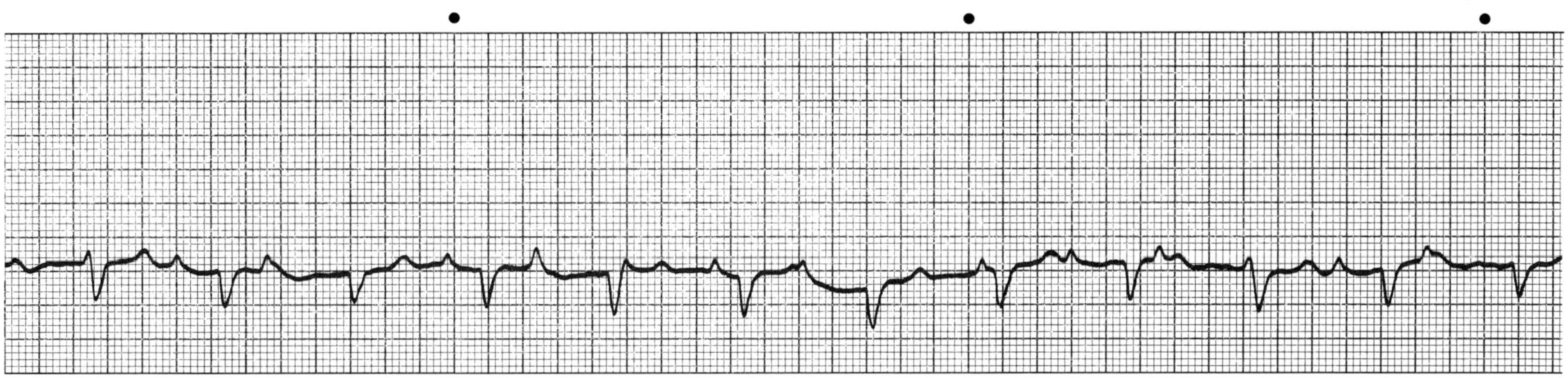

Question: This rhythm strip was recorded from a 19-year-old domestic shorthair cat that had no clinical signs.

1. What is the rhythm diagnosis?
2. What is the best therapeutic approach?

Case 79

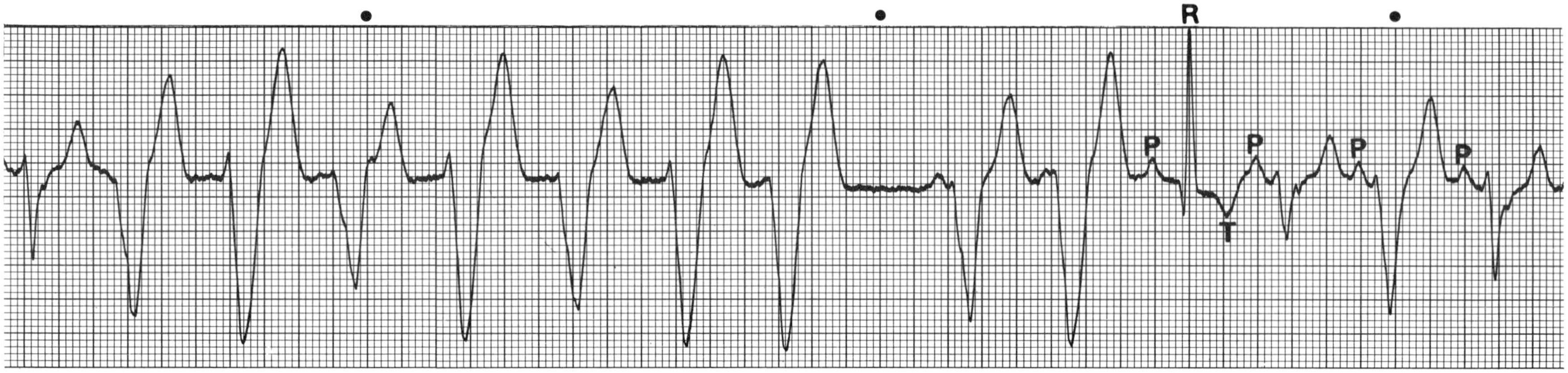

Answer: Multiform ventricular tachycardia. Heart rate is approximately 180 beats/min. The ventricular tachycardia is classified as multiform because of the varying configuration of ventricular ectopic complexes. The fourth complex from the end of the strip is a capture complex. A normal sinus impulse has reached the AV junction in a recovered state, thereby capturing the ventricles for one complex. The last three complexes represent different degrees of fusion: simultaneous activation of the ventricles by a sinus impulse (the P wave just preceding) and a ventricular ectopic focus. Ventricular tachycardia is generally considered one of the most serious of all tachyarrhythmias. With gastric dilatation volvulus or traumatic myocarditis, ventricular ectopic activity often occurs 12 to 36 hours after the event. Treatment in this dog should begin as soon as possible. Acid-base and electrolyte abnormalities should be corrected. The treatment of choice is lidocaine administered intravenously, first as a bolus and then as a constant intravenous infusion. Other therapeutic drugs include procainamide, quinidine, tocainide, mexiletine, and propafenone. Electrical cardioversion is indicated when the animal is in a hemodynamic crisis and when lidocaine or procainamide fails.

Case 80

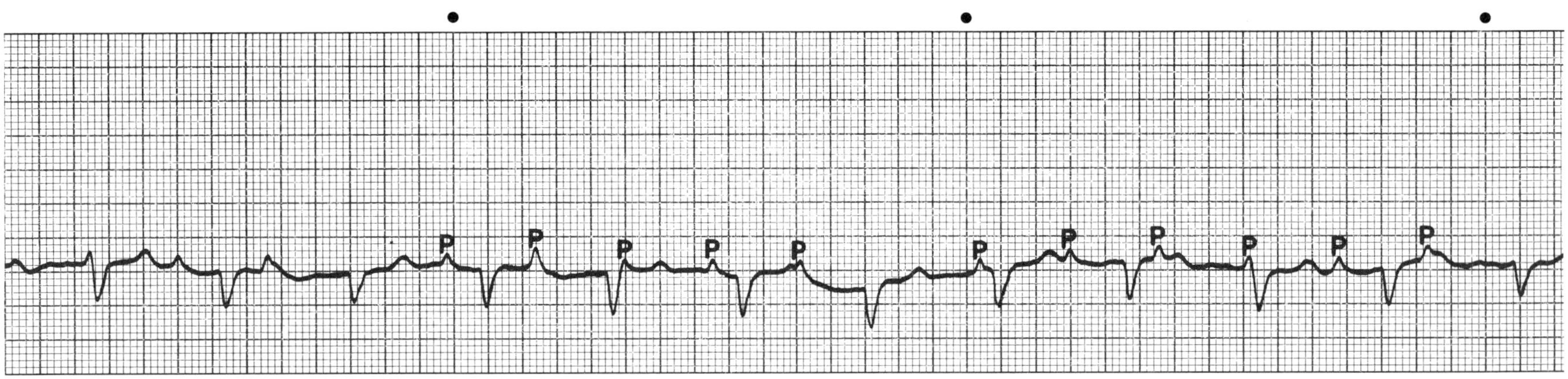

Answer: Complete AV block. Atrial heart rate is 220 beats/min; ventricular heart rate is 160 beats/min. No association exists between P waves and QRS complexes. The ECG can be evaluated by identifying two consecutive P waves and then plotting out the remaining P waves. The two most common causes of AV dissociation are complete AV block and ventricular tachycardia. The ventricular rate is 160 beats/min. This rate is relatively rapid for a ventricular escape rate and slow for ventricular tachycardia. No capture complexes are present. Complete AV block is the most likely diagnosis. Degeneration and fibrosis of the AV conduction system is the most common cause of complete AV block in geriatric cats. The enhanced ventricular escape rate may be associated with increased levels of sympathetic tone. Because the ventricular rate is normal and the cat has no clinical signs, no treatment is needed.

Case 81

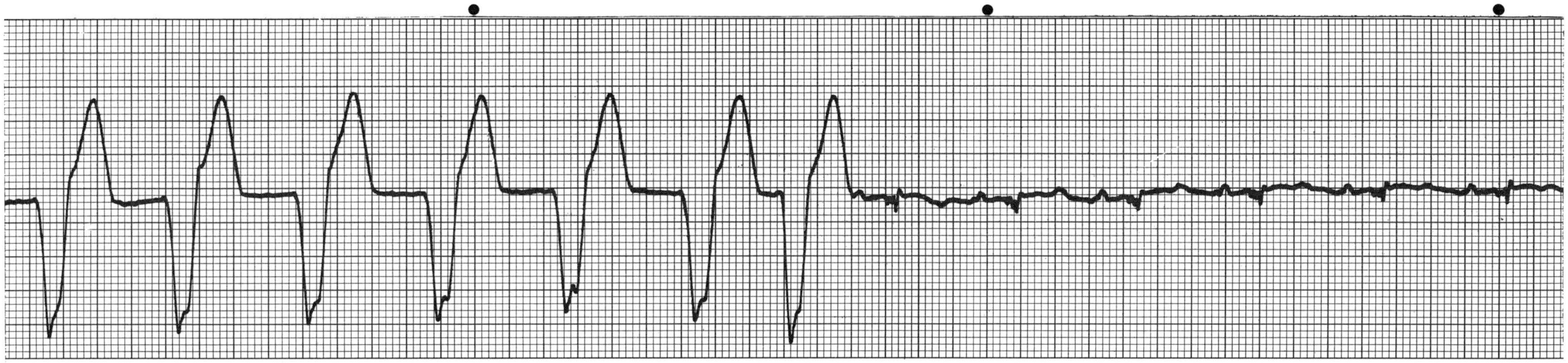

Question: This ECG was recorded from a dog with pericardial effusion. Severe ascites was present.

1. What is the rhythm diagnosis?
2. What is the best therapeutic approach?

Case 82

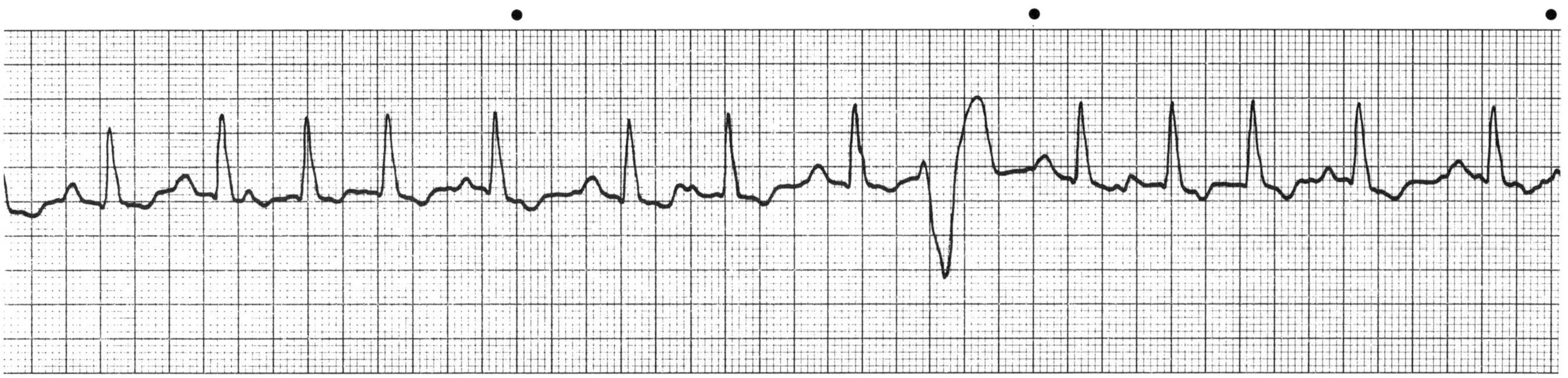

Question: This rhythm strip was recorded from an 11-year-old Chihuahua with mitral valvular insufficiency and congestive heart failure.

1. What is the rhythm diagnosis?
2. What is the best therapeutic approach?

Case 81

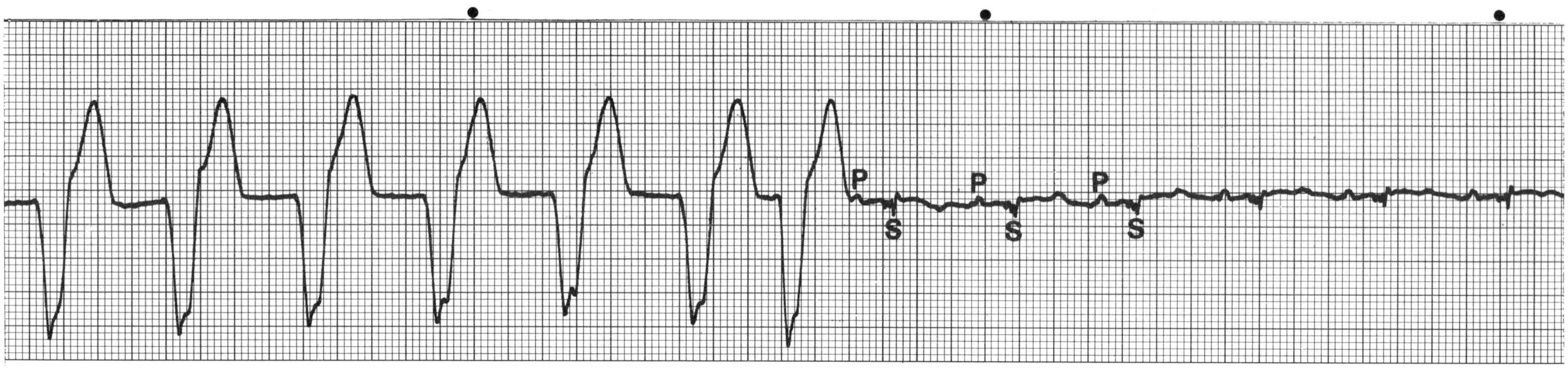

Answer: Paroxysmal ventricular tachycardia. Heart rate is approximately 155 beats/min. The first seven complexes on this rhythm strip represent ventricular tachycardia. Note the small P-QRS-T sinus complexes that eventually dominate the rhythm. The small complexes are compatible with the pericardial effusion that was diagnosed on an echocardiographic study. The severe ventricular arrhythmia in this case could indicate underlying myocardial injury secondary to a neoplasm, a common cause of pericardial disease. Ventricular arrhythmias can be classified as benign, complex, and malignant. Antiarrhythmic agents are administered for ventricular tachycardia, especially with serious structural heart disease. Treatment of choice is lidocaine administered intravenously, first as a bolus and then as a constant intravenous infusion. If this dog had not had major heart disease, the ventricular tachycardia probably would not have been life threatening. Thus, one should adhere to the following common advice: "Look at the patient, not just the ECG."

Case 82

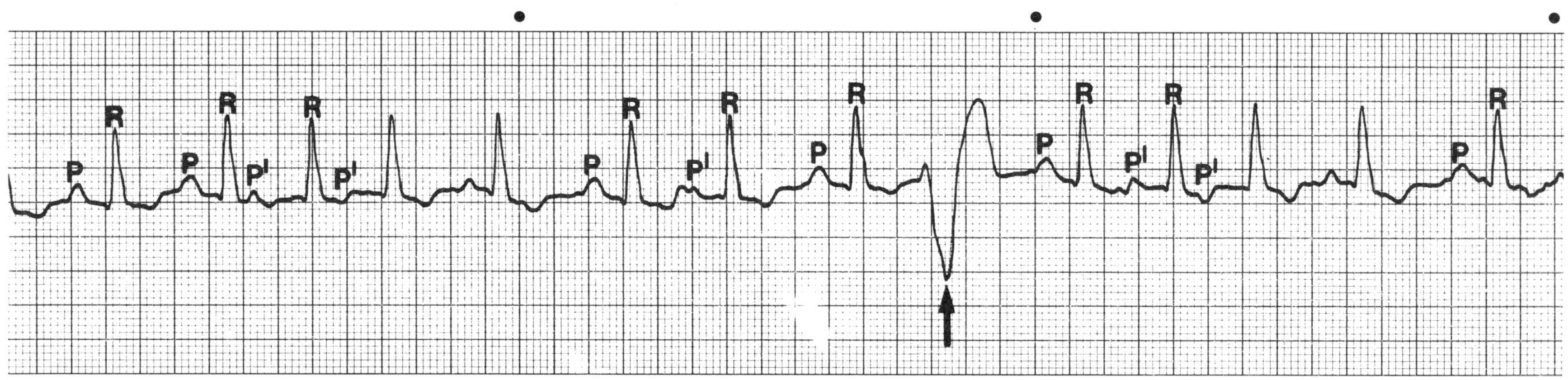

Answer: Sinus rhythm with frequent atrial premature complexes and one ventricular premature complex (arrow). Heart rate is approximately 180 beats/min. The atrial premature complexes (P′/R) are probably secondary to atrial distention caused by mitral valvular insufficiency. The appearance of the P′ waves of the premature complexes differs from that of the sinus P waves. The ventricular premature complex indicates possible ventricular wall injury associated with distention and inadequate perfusion. The predominant arrhythmia is supraventricular. In dogs with congestive heart failure associated with degenerative valve disease, supraventricular arrhythmias should be treated with digoxin. Ventricular premature complexes do not occur with sufficient frequency to warrant antiarrhythmic therapy at this time. Treatment of the heart failure often eliminates or reduces the frequency of ventricular premature complexes. A follow-up ECG should be performed in 1 week to reassess the arrhythmias.

Case 83

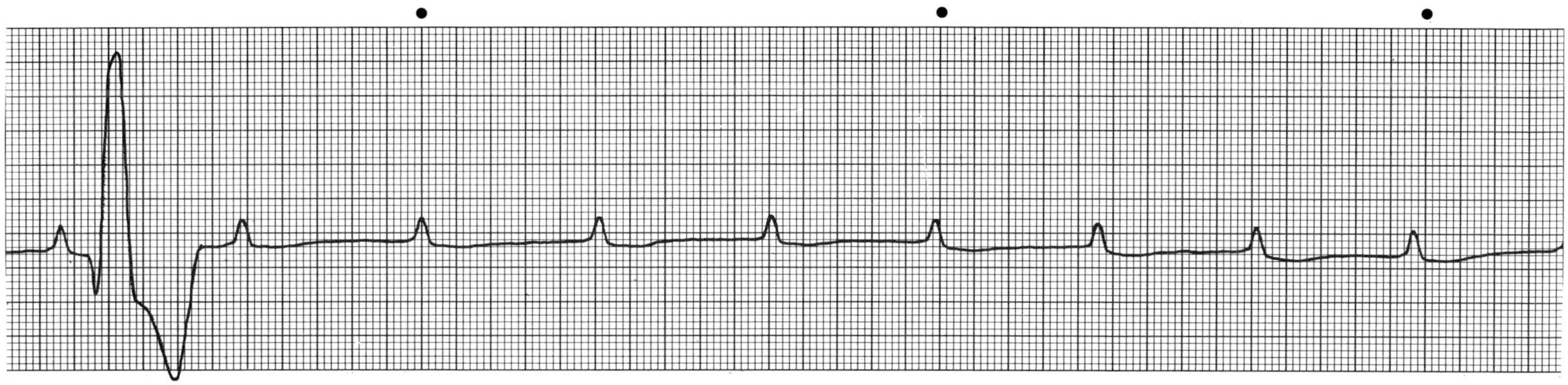

Question: A 10-year-old German Shepherd with a history of frequent collapsing episodes over the past 24 hours was examined. The dog also had a recent history of lameness in the left forelimb.

1. What is the rhythm diagnosis?
2. What is the best therapeutic approach?
3. What infectious disease has been reported to be associated with this rhythm, especially in humans?

Case 84

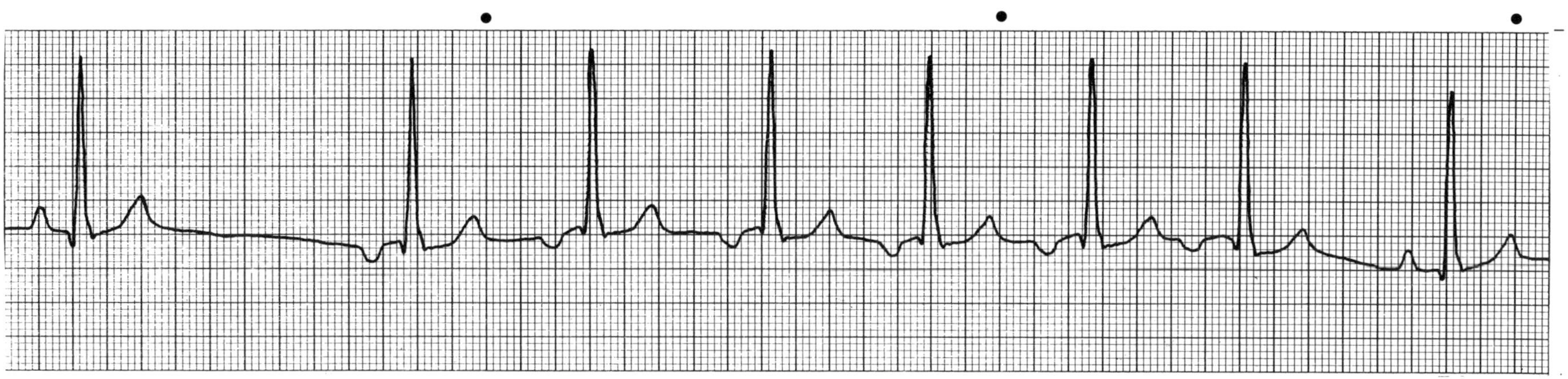

Question: This lead II ECG was obtained from a 10-year-old German Shepherd being treated for chronic heart failure with digoxin, furosemide, and enalapril. The dog was doing well.

1. What is the rhythm diagnosis?
2. What is the most likely underlying disorder?
3. What is the best therapeutic approach?

Case 83

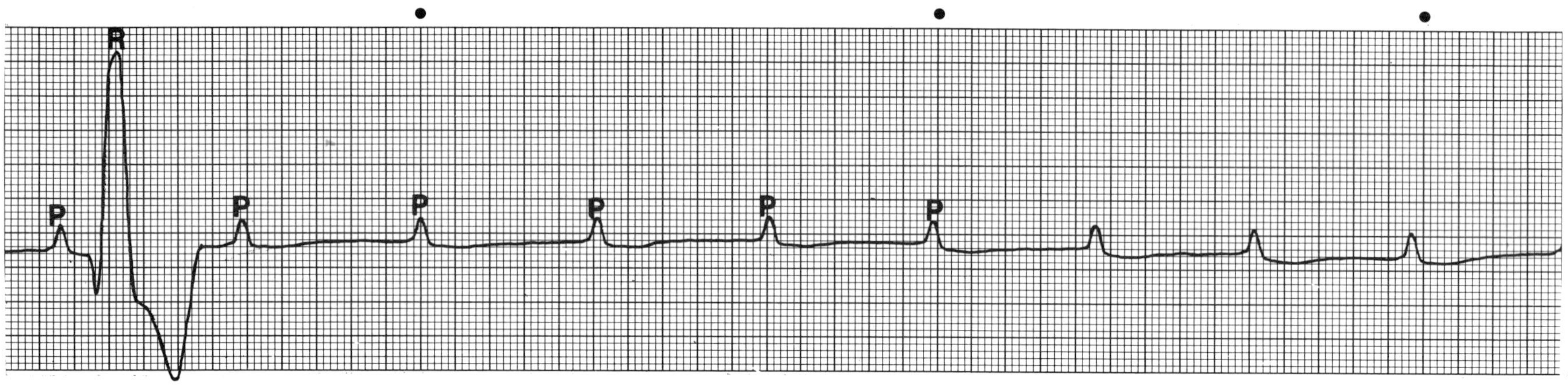

Answer: Complete (third-degree) AV block. Atrial heart rate is 125 beats/min. An artificial cardiac pacemaker is required in animals with symptomatic complete AV block. Lyme disease can cause myocarditis leading to complete AV block. Other conditions associated with complete AV block include idiopathic fibrosis of the AV conduction system in geriatric dogs, hypertrophic cardiomyopathy, bacterial endocarditis, myocardial infarction, and congenital defects. Drugs, including atropine, isoproterenol, and dobutamine, may not be effective in re-establishing AV conduction. Isoproterenol and dobutamine may elevate the heart rate by increasing the rate of the ventricular escape pacemaker. Complete AV block is characterized by regularly occurring P waves that are totally independent of the slow ventricular escape rhythm. Because no other QRS complexes are present, the actual relationship of the P waves to the QRS complexes cannot be determined. Advanced second-degree AV block with left bundle-branch block should be considered.

Case 84

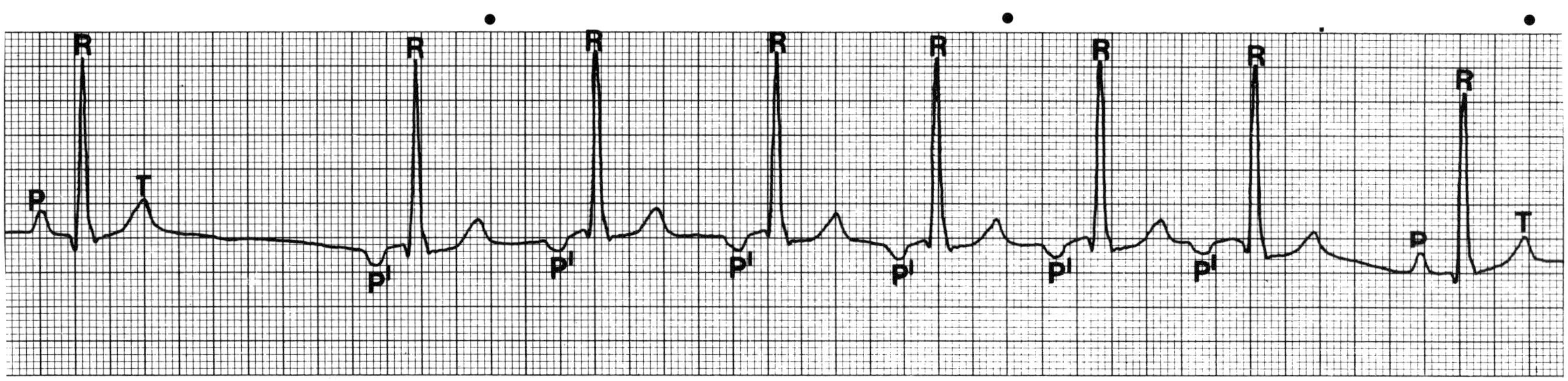

Answer: Sinus rhythm with an AV junctional escape rhythm. The first and last complexes are normally conducted sinus P-QRS complexes. Heart rate is 120 beats/min. Digoxin toxicity is the most likely cause of this arrhythmia. The digoxin should be stopped for 48 to 72 hours, followed by a repeat ECG and reassessment of treatment. Arrhythmias originating in the AV junction commonly occur with digoxin toxicity, possibly by the mechanism of delayed after-depolarizations. AV junctional rhythms have negative P′ waves with retrograde conduction from the AV junction to the basal portion of the atria. The negative P′ waves may occur before, during, or after the QRS complex, depending on the conduction speed retrograde from the AV junction through the atria and antegrade to the ventricles. Arrhythmias originating in the AV junction may also occur in animals with all types of progressive heart disease.

Case 85

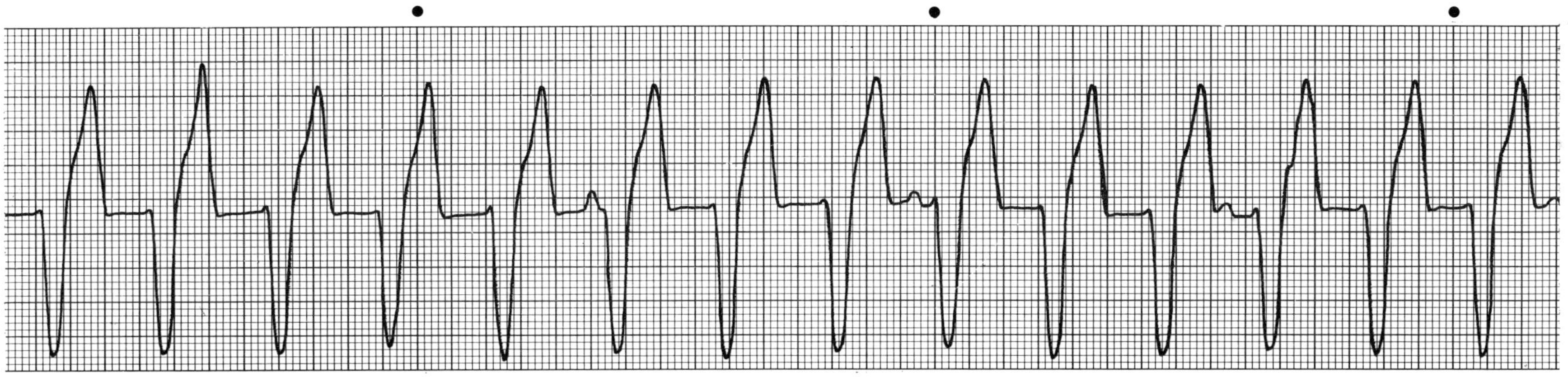

Question: This lead II preoperative ECG was obtained from a 4-year-old Airedale that was being prepared for orthopedic surgery 24 hours after being hit by a car. The dog appeared clinically stable, and a regular cardiac rhythm was heard on auscultation. Jugular venous pulsations were evident.

1. What is the rhythm diagnosis?
2. What is the best therapeutic approach?

Case 86

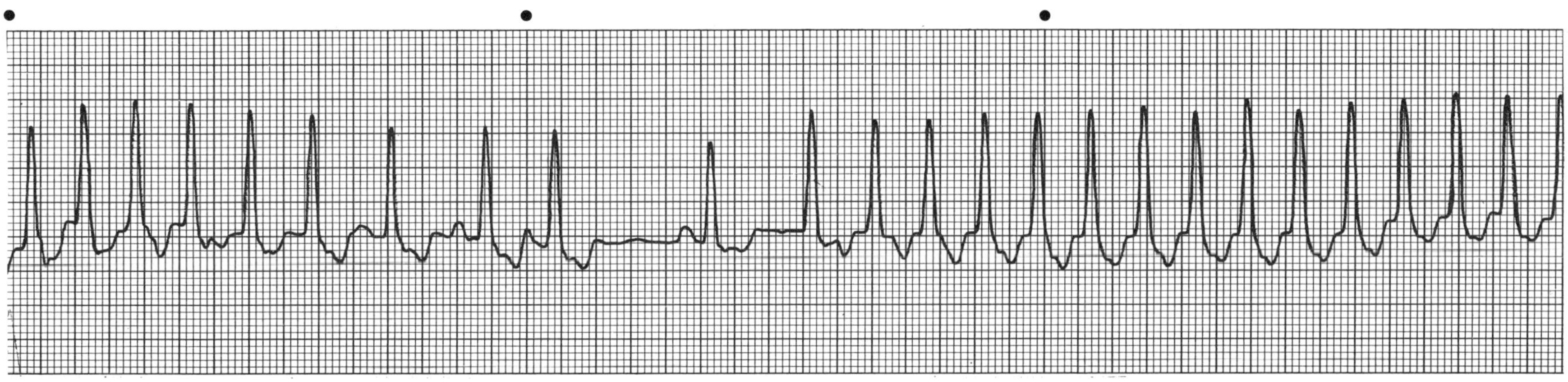

Question: This ECG was obtained from a 5-year-old King Charles Cavalier Spaniel that was being examined because of a fast heart beat that the owner noticed while holding the dog.

1. What is the rhythm diagnosis?
2. What is the most likely underlying disorder?
3. What is the best therapeutic approach?

Case 85

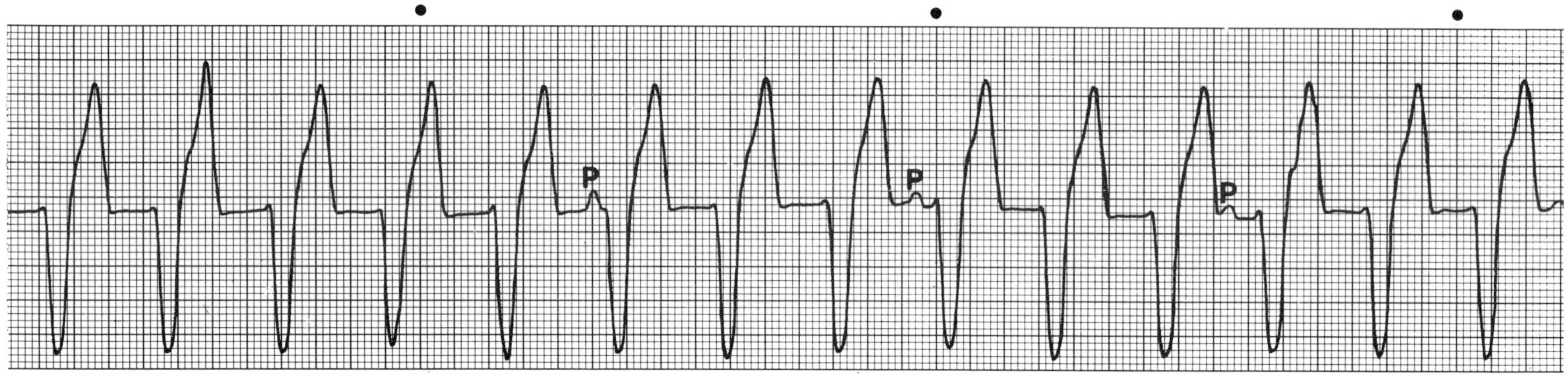

Answer: Sustained ventricular tachycardia. Heart rate is 190 beats/min. Ventricular tachycardia can be an electrically unstable rhythm and proceed to ventricular fibrillation. Also, ventricular tachycardia may promote hypotension and poor cardiac output. A bolus of lidocaine is needed to attempt conversion of the ventricular tachycardia to sinus rhythm before surgery. If successful, a lidocaine infusion can be administered during surgery to maintain sinus rhythm. Wide and bizarre QRS complexes that have no fixed relationship to visible P waves (AV dissociation) are the hallmark of ventricular tachycardia. The other P waves are hidden in the QRS complexes or T waves. Other diagnostic clues used to diagnose ventricular tachycardia (not on this ECG) include normal sinus (capture) beats, which are compared to bizarre QRS complexes, and fusion beats, which are QRS complexes intermediate in size and morphology between ventricular premature complexes and sinus beats. A rapid conversion of the wide complex tachycardia by a lidocaine bolus is also a quick diagnostic maneuver that can confirm or refute the diagnosis of ventricular tachycardia.

Case 86

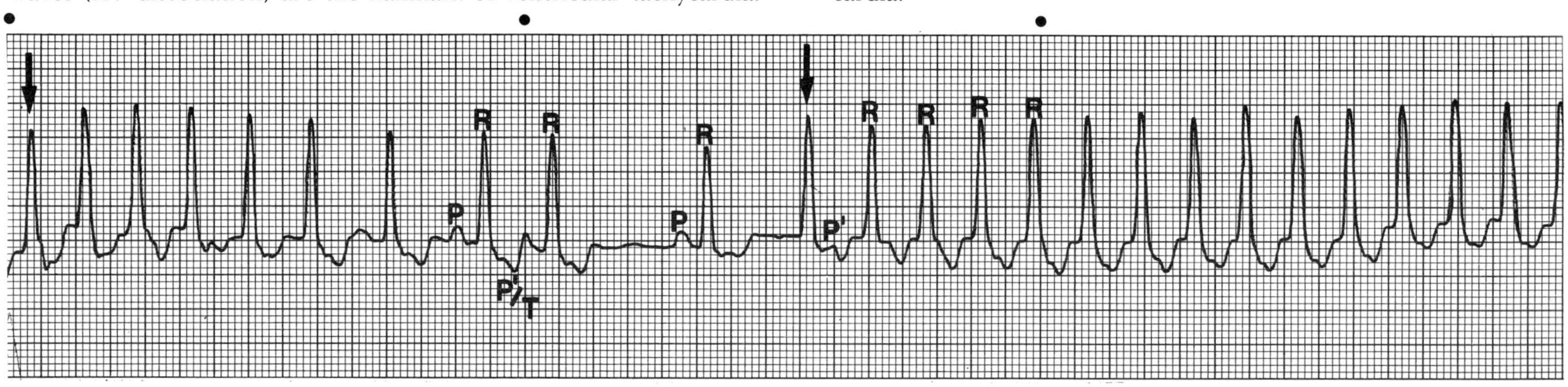

Answer: Sinus rhythm with an atrial premature complex (P′/T) and paroxysmal supraventricular tachycardia (after arrows). Heart rate is variable with rates approaching 400 beats/min during periods of tachycardia. Mitral valvular insufficiency with progressive dilation of the left atrium is common in this breed. The fact that the QRS complexes during the tachycardia resemble the QRS complexes of the sinus beats is a hallmark of supraventricular tachycardia. Abnormal atrial myocardial cell automaticity and AV nodal re-entry may cause this arrhythmia. The potential re-entrant circuit is formed by a functional separation of the AV node into two pathways. One pathway (beta) has slower conduction and a shorter refractory period than does the other (alpha). Typically, an atrial premature complex approaches the AV node and is blocked in the fast pathway but conducts anterograde even more slowly than normal in the slow pathway. Then the impulse reaches the distal part of the fast pathway after it has repolarized and is conducted retrograde back to the proximal portion of the AV node, where the impulse can again excite the slow pathway. This re-entrant circuit can simultaneously activate the atria and ventricles. A vagal maneuver or drugs (e.g., digoxin, diltiazem, propranolol, and adenosine) can slow or block conduction of the re-entrant circuit by their effect on the slow pathway, thereby terminating the arrhythmia. Drugs that block retrograde conduction by the fast pathway (e.g., procainamide and quinidine) may occasionally be required to terminate this type of AV nodal re-entrant supraventricular tachycardia.

Case 87

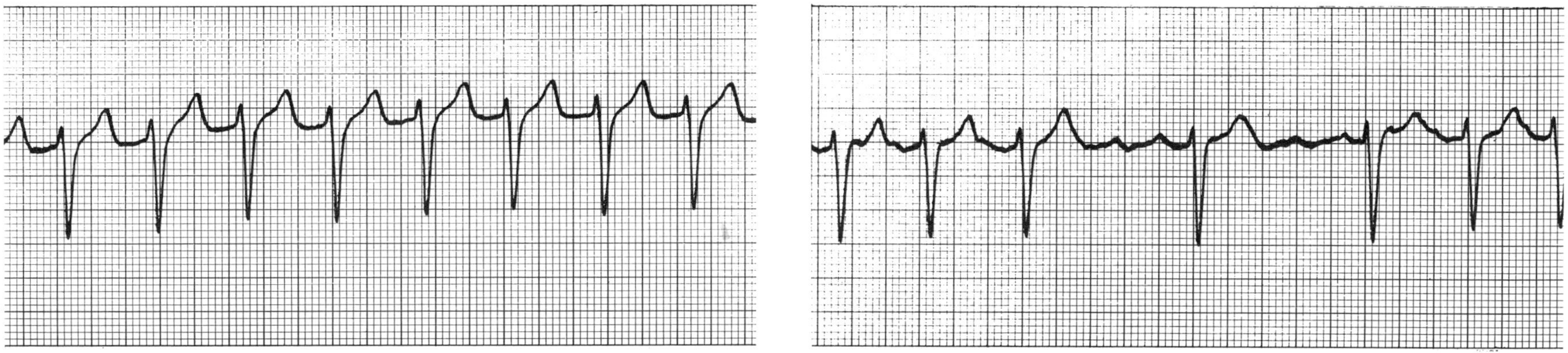
A B

Question: This series of two separate rhythm strips was recorded from a cat with hypertrophic cardiomyopathy. Dyspnea and 2 episodes of fainting were reported over the last 48 hours

1. What is the rhythm diagnosis in strip A?
2. What procedure was performed in strip B?
3. What is the subsequent rhythm diagnosis?
4. What is the best therapeutic approach?

Case 88

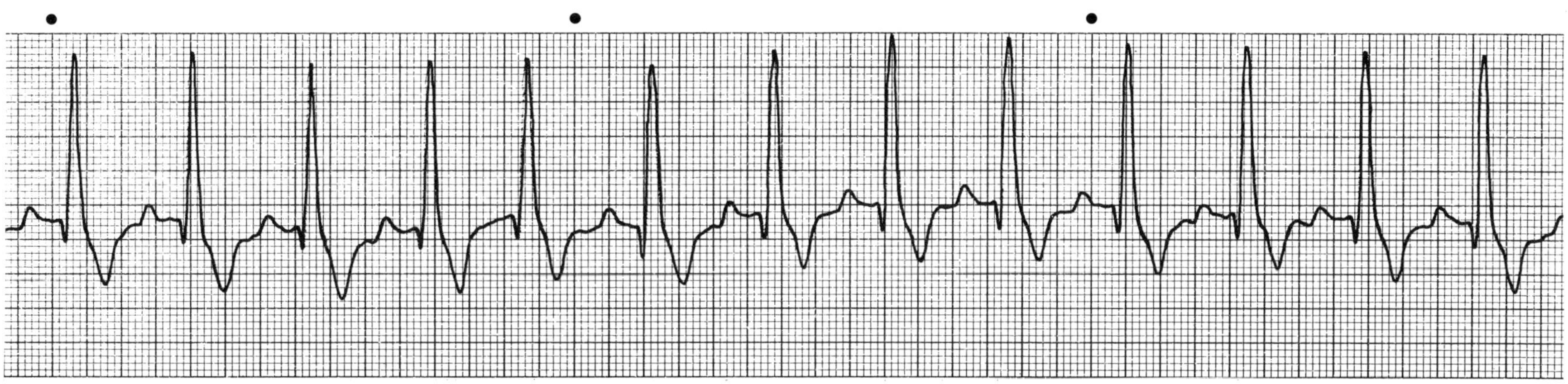

Question: This lead II ECG was recorded from a 9-year-old Great Dane with a history of coughing and exercise intolerance.

1. What is the rhythm diagnosis?
2. What is the most likely underlying disorder?
3. What is the best therapeutic approach?

Case 87

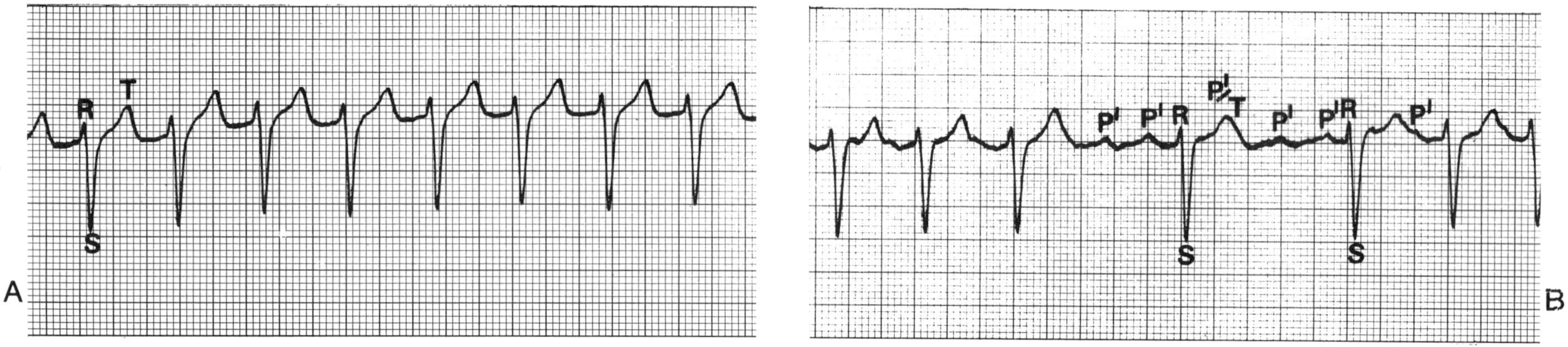

Answer: Atrial flutter. Atrial heart rate is 460 beats/min in strip B. In strip A, a regular ventricular rhythm at a ventricular rate of 230 beats/min is present. P waves cannot be seen. This strip does not reveal whether the underlying rhythm is ventricular or supraventricular. Strip B was the result of ocular pressure. The increase in vagal tone effects AV conduction, with the P′-like waves (F waves) now clearly seen with different conduction ratios. Strip A then represents 2:1 AV conduction with P waves hidden in the QRS-T complexes. The large negative QRS complexes represent enlargement of the heart chamber and/or an intraventricular conduction defect, based on the evaluation of other limb lead recordings. Atrial tachycardia and atrial flutter basically do not differ, except for the atrial rate and the presence of flutter waves in atrial flutter. Atrial flutter usually occurs at atrial rates greater than 300 to 350 beats/min. The term supraventricular tachycardia is used when atrial flutter cannot be differentiated from atrial tachycardia. Propranolol and diltiazem are useful in treating and preventing atrial arrhythmias in hypertrophic cardiomyopathy.

Case 88

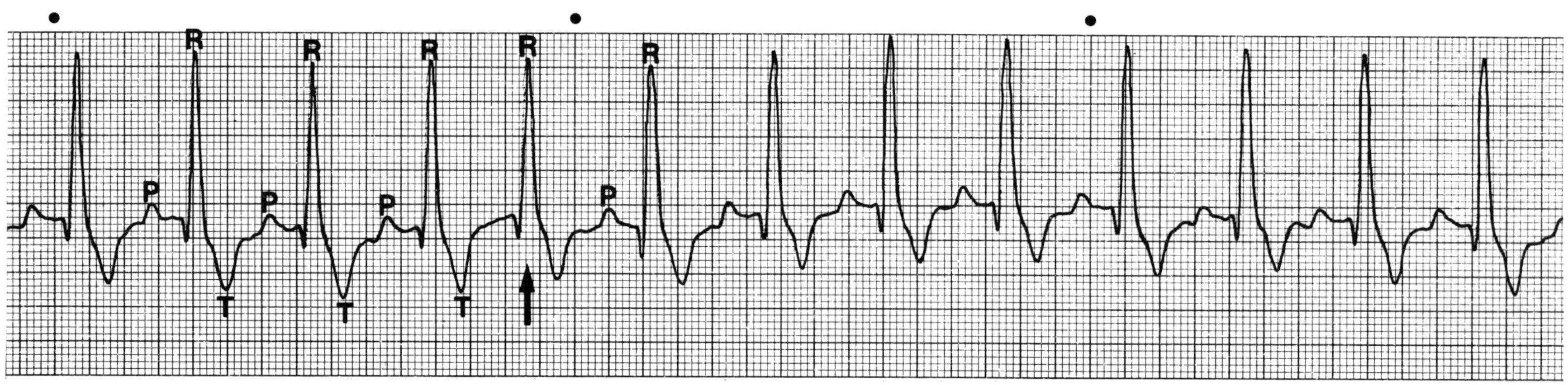

Answer: Sinus tachycardia with one atrial premature complex. Heart rate is 175 beats/min. Sinus tachycardia is the predominant rhythm. The fifth complex (arrow) is an atrial premature complex. The premature complex appears similar to the sinus complexes and is followed by a noncompensatory pause. These characteristics are consistent with atrial premature complex. The associated P wave is probably lost in the T wave of the preceding complex. The atrial premature complex and sinus tachycardia, coupled with the history of coughing and exercise intolerance, suggest congestive heart failure. Heart failure in this breed is often associated with dilated cardiomyopathy. Thoracic radiographs confirmed heart failure, and the arrhythmia was treated with digoxin.

Case 89

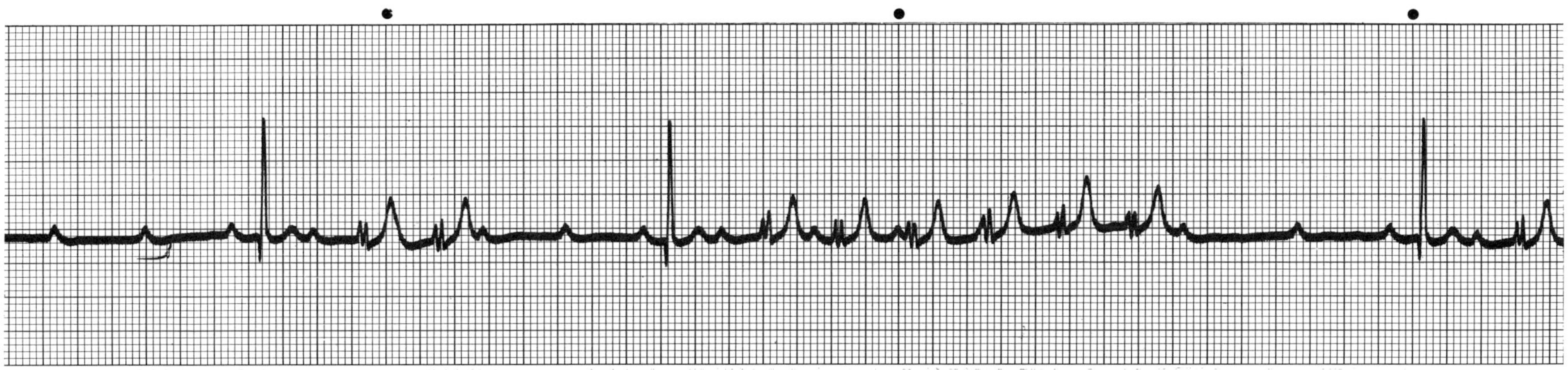

Question: This lead II ECG was obtained from a 4-year-old Irish Setter diagnosed with Lyme disease. Paper speed: 25 mm/sec.

1. What is the rhythm diagnosis?
2. What is the most likely underlying disorder?
3. What is the best therapeutic approach?

Case 90

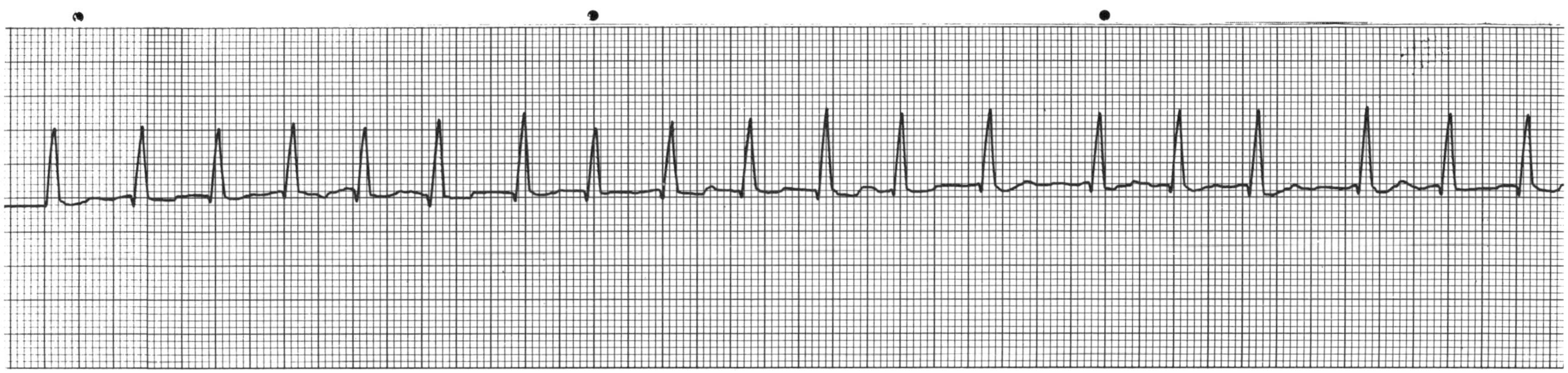

Question: This lead II rhythm strip was recorded from a cat. Severe dyspnea was present.

1. What is the rhythm diagnosis?
2. What is the most likely underlying disorder?
3. What are the hemodynamic effects of this cardiac arrhythmia?

Case 89

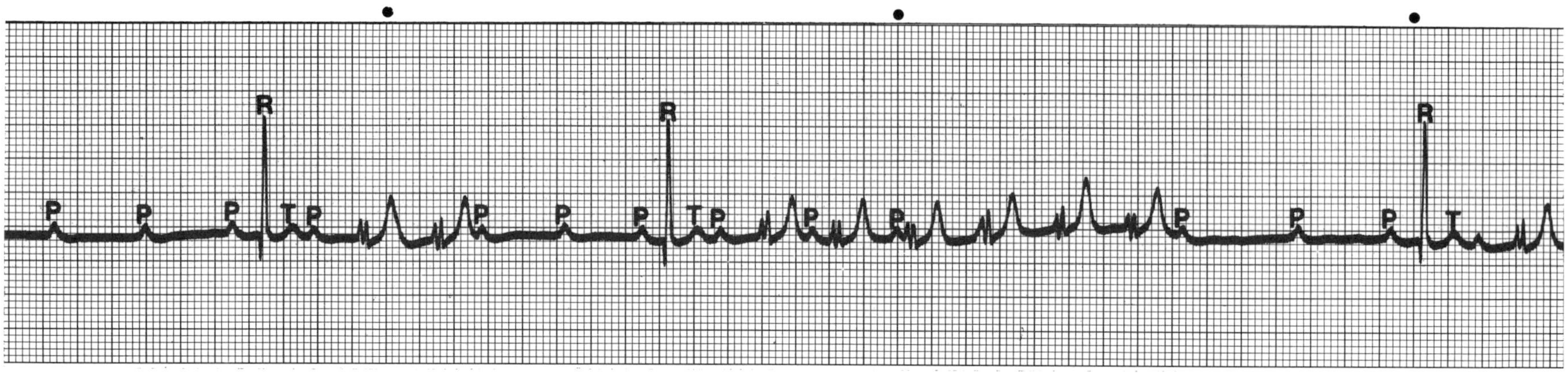

Answer: Sinus rhythm with advanced second-degree AV block and paroxysmal ventricular tachycardia. Heart rate is variable. Lyme carditis is the most likely underlying disorder. Treatment for Lyme disease is the best therapeutic approach. If signs of marked weakness or syncope occur, oral or parenteral anticholinergics can be employed. Persistent syncope requires a temporary or permanent cardiac pacemaker and possibly antiarrhythmic medication if the ventricular tachycardia persists. Without a pacemaker, procainamide or quinidine may abolish the ventricular arrhythmia, but the underlying advanced AV block would remain, with a resultant decrease in cardiac output. Sinus beats are labeled P-R-T. The P waves not followed by QRS complexes are typical of second-degree AV block. The QRS complexes that differ from the sinus QRS complexes but are not associated with P waves are ventricular premature complexes. Three or more ventricular premature complexes in succession are termed paroxysmal ventricular tachycardia. Advanced AV block usually resolves with antibiotics in humans with Lyme carditis.

Case 90

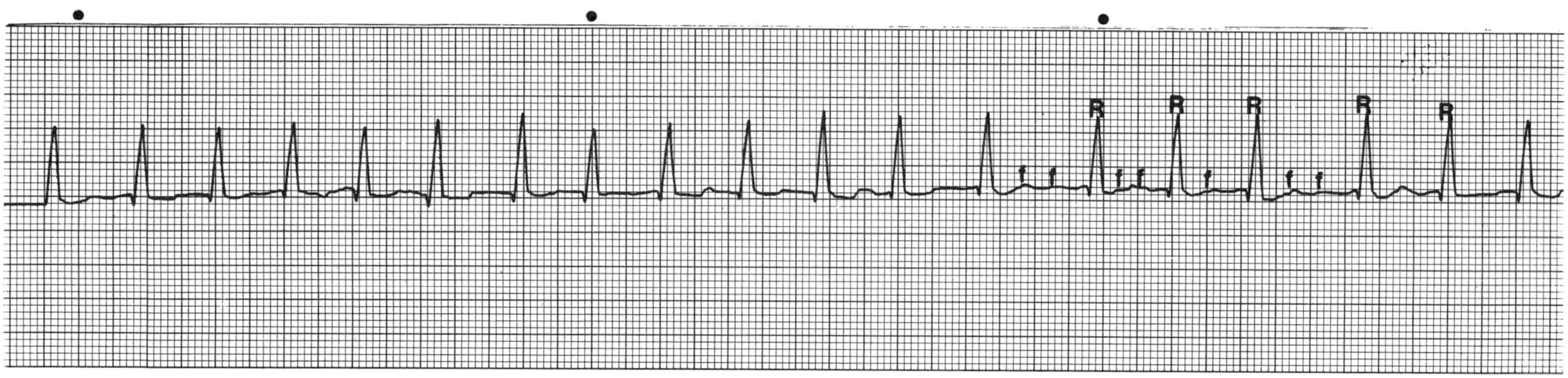

Answer: Atrial fibrillation. Heart rate is 240 to 260 beats/min. Atrial fibrillation is rare in cats and is primarily associated with hypertrophic cardiomyopathy. Hypertrophic cardiomyopathy causes a chronic increasing resistance to left ventricular filling, eventually resulting in severe left atrial enlargement and atrial fibrillation. The electrocardiographic features of atrial fibrillation include a rapid and totally irregular ventricular rhythm and sinus P waves that are replaced by fibrillating f waves. The QRS complexes vary in amplitude in this case, because numerous supraventricular impulses arrive so early that parts of the ventricle are not yet completely recovered. The loss of the "atrial kick" contribution to ventricular filling, combined with the rapid heart rate, may substantially reduce cardiac output and cause congestive heart failure. A rapid ventricular response and atrial fibrillation may cause a 20% reduction in renal blood flow and a pronounced reduction in blood flow to the coronary arteries (as much as 40%). Drugs of choice for atrial fibrillation include digoxin, propranolol, and diltiazem. Furosemide and a low-salt diet are also indicated for the severe state of cardiac failure usually present.

Case 91

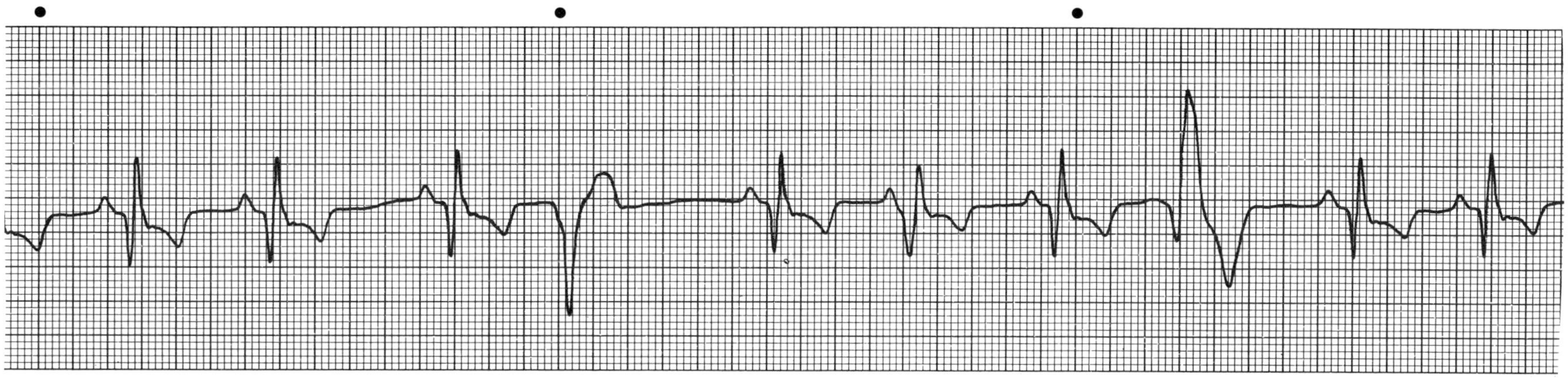

Question: This lead II ECG was obtained from a 4-year-old Doberman Pinscher that was examined because of dyspnea and lethargy.

1. What is the rhythm diagnosis?
2. What is the most likely underlying disorder?
3. What is the best therapeutic approach?

Case 92

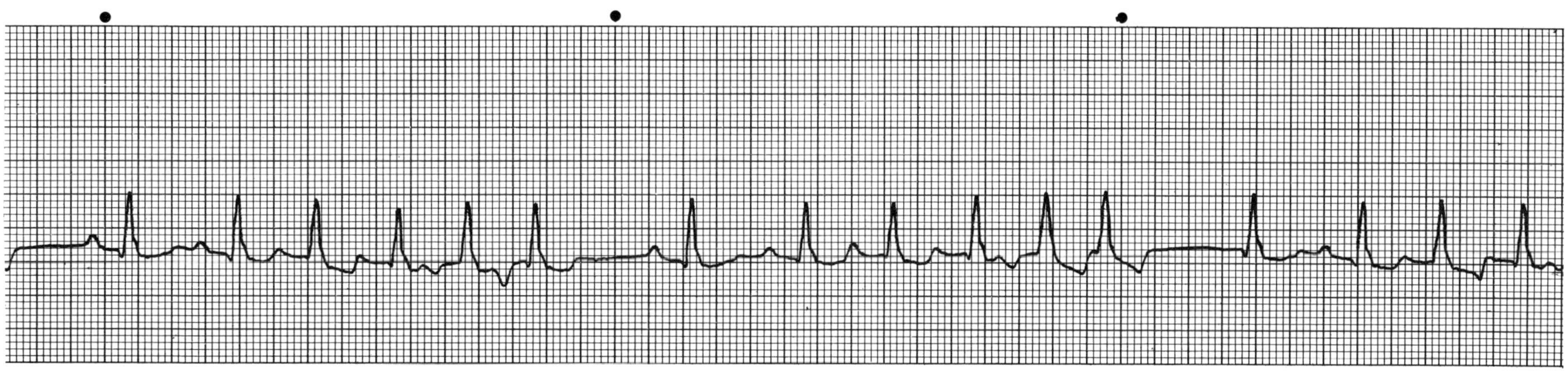

Question: This lead II ECG was obtained from a 9-year-old mixed-breed Terrier with a 2-year history of chronic obstructive pulmonary disease.

1. What is the rhythm diagnosis?
2. What is the most likely underlying disorder?
3. What is the best therapeutic approach?

Case 91

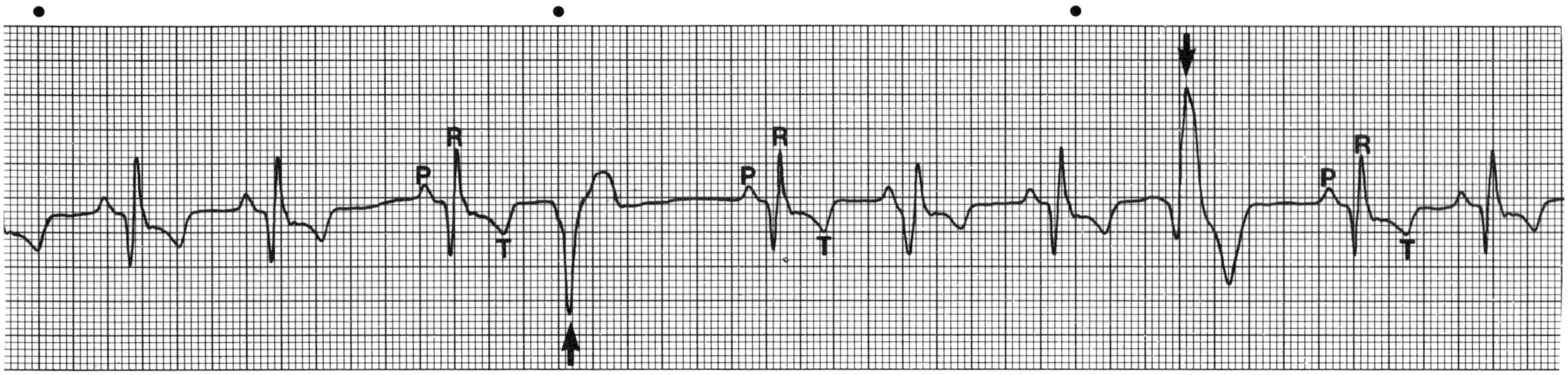

Answer: Sinus rhythm with multiform ventricular premature complexes (arrows). Heart rate is approximately 140 beats/min. Premature complexes of variable shape are termed multiform. Dilated cardiomyopathy is commonly associated with ventricular arrhythmias. Treatment depends on the presence or absence of congestive heart failure. If the dog has clinical signs (e.g., dyspnea, weakness, syncope) without congestive heart failure, ventricular antiarrhythmic agents (e.g., procainamide, quinidine, or tocainide) can be administered. Serial ECGs are important to document improvement or worsening (proarrhythmia) of the arrhythmia. In animals with congestive heart failure, the initial approach includes administration of digoxin, furosemide, and vasodilators. Ventricular arrhythmias require stabilization before digoxin can be initiated. Digoxin shortens the ventricular myocardial cell transmembrane action potential refractory period and may worsen ventricular arrhythmias.

Case 92

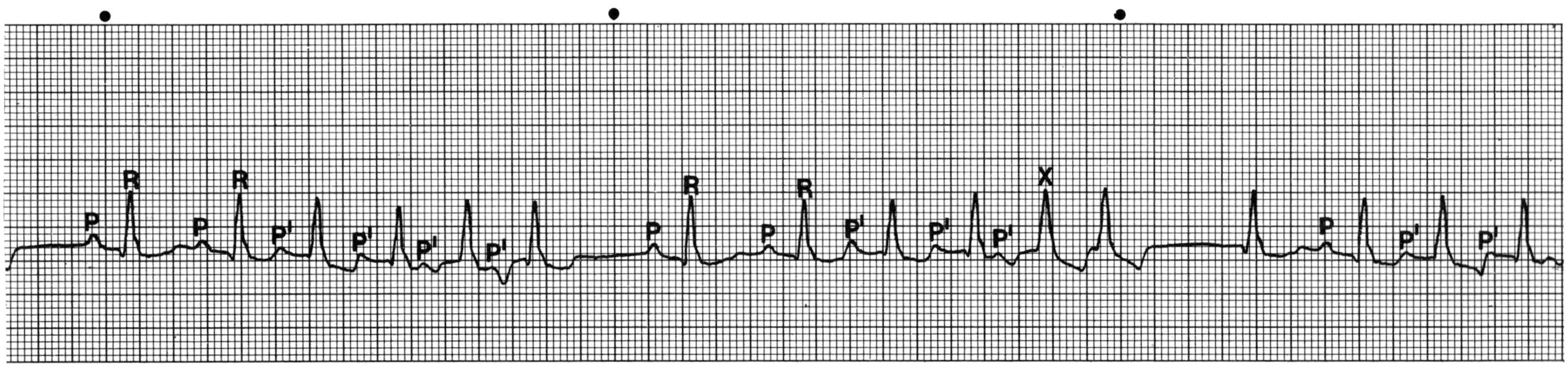

Answer: Sinus rhythm with multifocal atrial premature complexes and paroxysmal supraventricular tachycardia. Heart rate is 200 to 220 beats/min. Right atrial dilation caused by chronic obstructive pulmonary disease is the most likely underlying disorder. Digoxin or diltiazem is an effective drug for treating this arrhythmia. Frequent atrial premature complexes are likely to have adverse hemodynamic consequences. The premature P′ waves, with different P′-to-P′ intervals support the multifocal origin of the atrial premature complexes. Notice that the QRS complexes following the P′ waves resemble the QRS complexes following the sinus P waves, a characteristic typical of an atrial arrhythmia. The QRS complex labeled X is slightly wider than the other QRS complexes, probably because of aberrant ventricular conduction in the left bundle-branch network. The finding of aberrant ventricular conduction following an atrial premature complex may also indicate ventricular myocardial disease in this dog.

Case 93

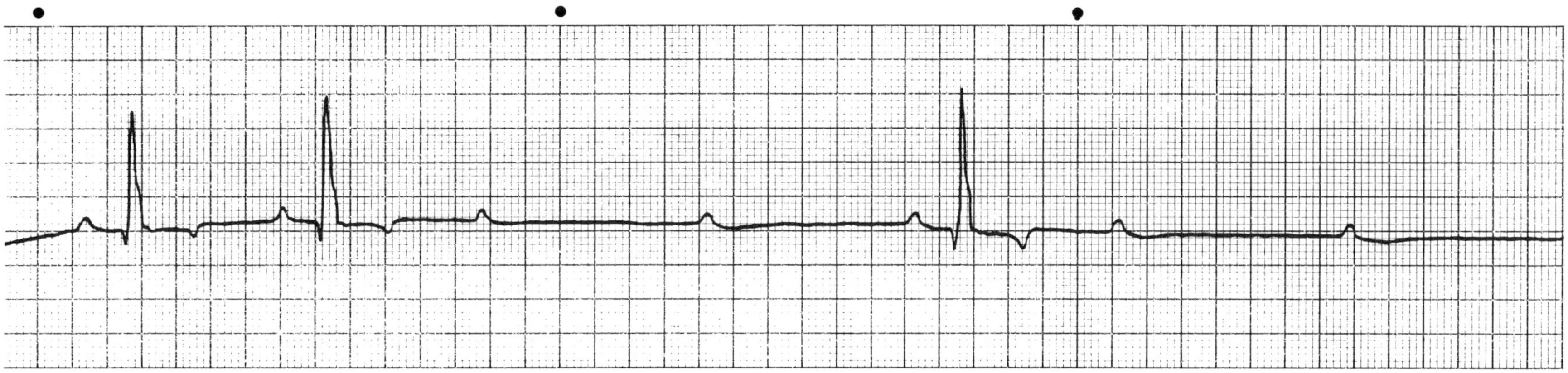

Question: This lead II ECG was obtained from a 14-year-old Wheaten Terrier with a 24-hour history of weakness and collapse.

1. What is the rhythm diagnosis?
2. What is the best therapeutic approach?

Case 94

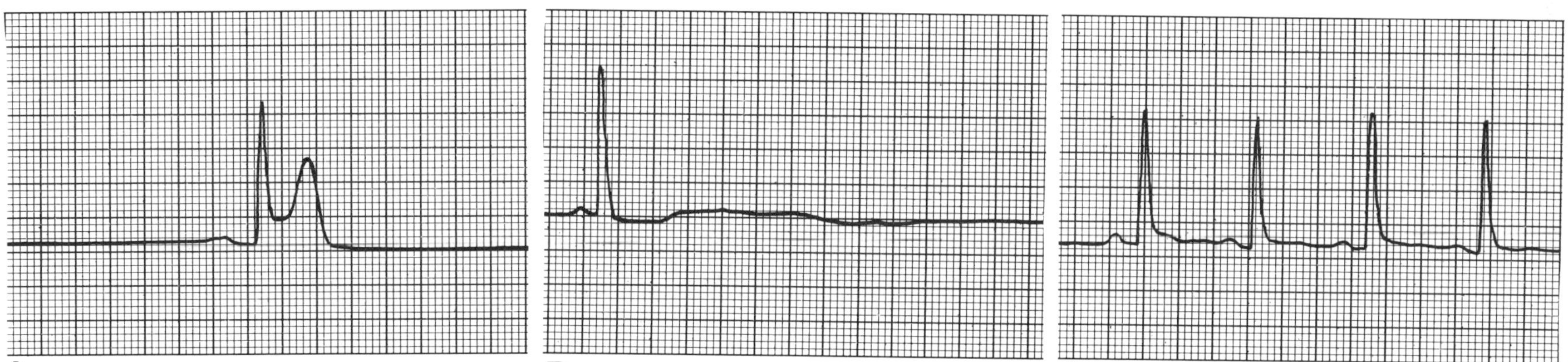

A B C

Question: These rhythm strips were recorded from a 6-year-old cat that had been anesthetized with halothane for a cystotomy. Strip A was taken intraoperatively after respiratory arrest and at the onset of marked bradycardia, strip B was taken minutes after treatment, and strip C was taken 1 hour later.

1. What is the rhythm diagnosis?
2. What is the most likely underlying disorder?
3. What is the best therapeutic approach?

Case 93

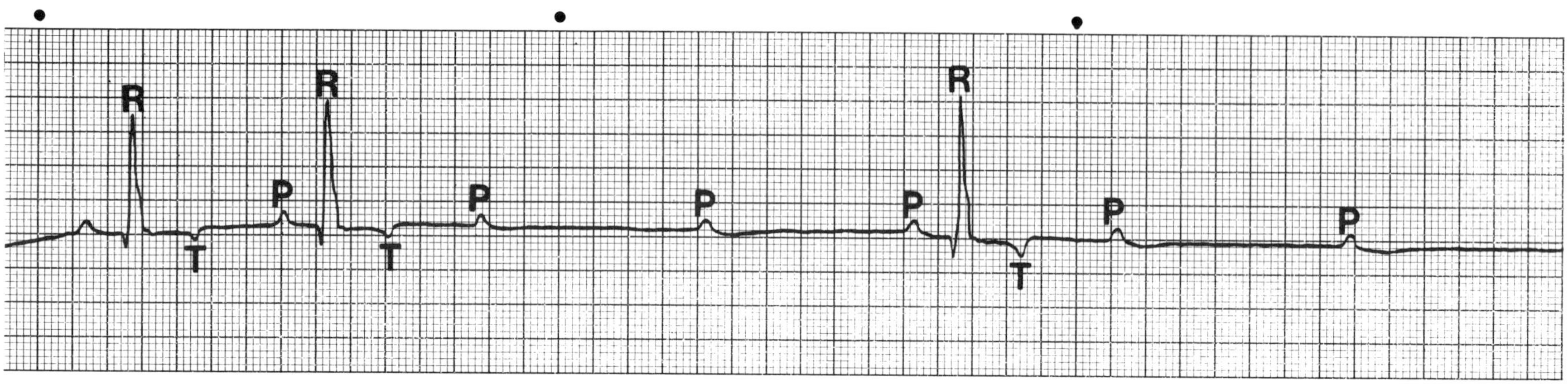

Answer: Sinus rhythm with frequent second-degree AV block. Heart rate is approximately 40 to 50 beats/min. An atropine response test should be performed (atropine administered intramuscularly followed by a repeat ECG in 30 minutes) to determine if the AV block is related to high vagal tone or to AV conduction system disease. If the response to atropine is favorable with an elevation in heart rate, anticholinergics can be administered orally. A poor response to atropine supports the need for a permanent cardiac pacemaker. Idiopathic fibrosis of the AV conduction system is the most common cause of advanced AV block in geriatric dogs and cats. Intermittent P waves not followed by QRS complexes are the hallmark of second-degree AV block.

Case 94

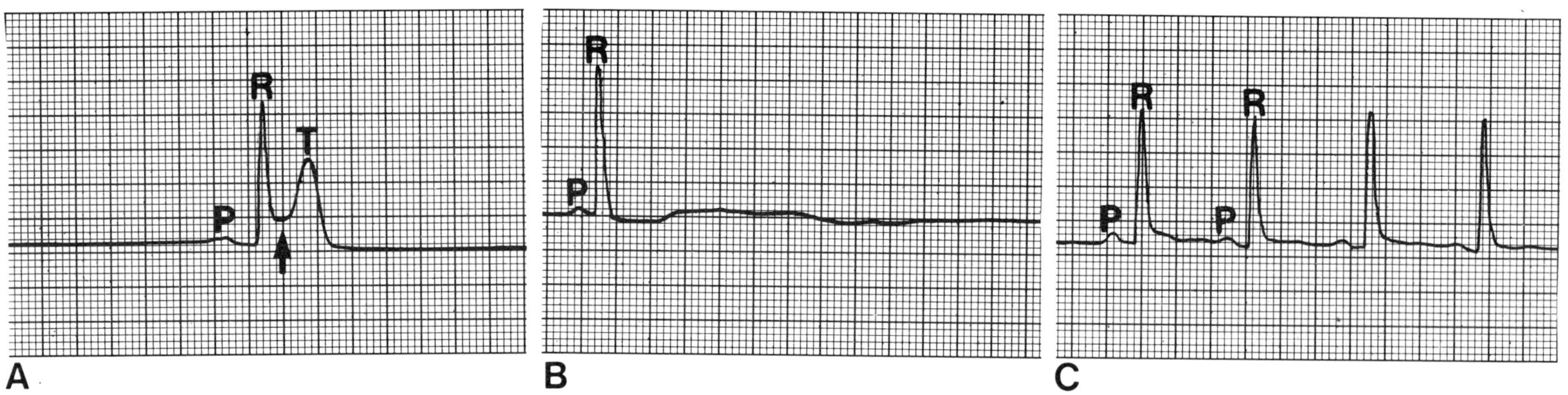

Answer: Strips A and B. Sinus bradycardia. Strip C. Sinus rhythm. Heart rate is 180 beats/min. Strip A shows sinus bradycardia with severe S-T segment elevation (arrow) and a prominent T wave. These changes suggest myocardial hypoxia-ischemia. The anesthetic was discontinued, and positive pressure ventilation with 100% oxygen was instituted. Atropine was administered for the bradycardia. Epinephrine was not used initially because the cat had been anesthetized with halothane. Halothane sensitizes the myocardium to sympathetic stimulation, and thus, epinephrine could have induced ventricular tachycardia. Fortunately, the condition of the cat improved without epinephrine. The complex in strip B shows resolution of the hypoxic changes. Strip C shows normal rate and rhythm. The wide P waves and the tall and wide QRS complexes may indicate left heart enlargement. The problems encountered during surgery may have been associated with cardiomyopathy in this cat.

Case 95

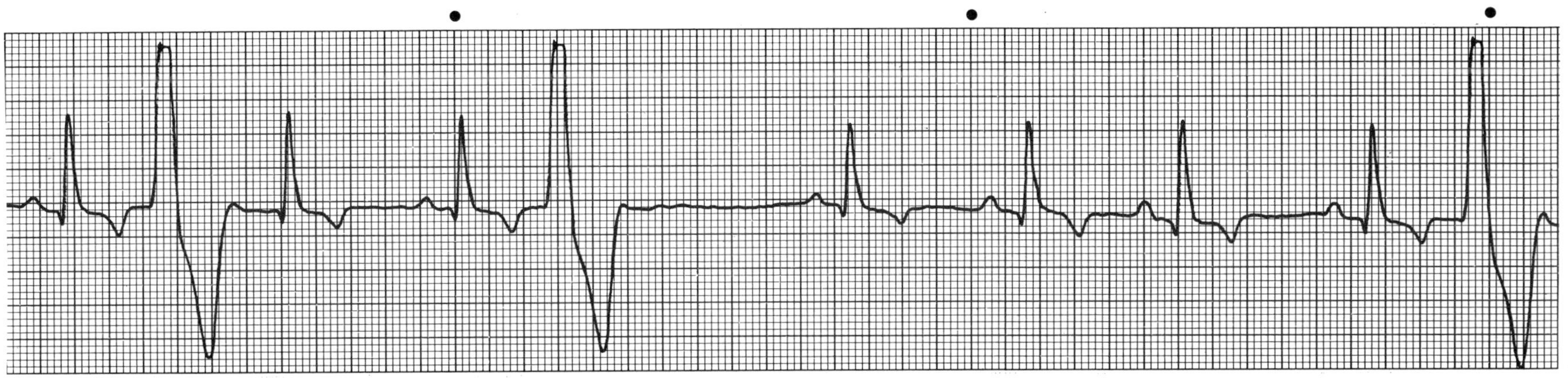

Question: This rhythm strip was recorded from a 5-year-old Beagle that had been hit by a car.

1. What is the rhythm diagnosis?
2. What is the best therapeutic approach?

Case 96

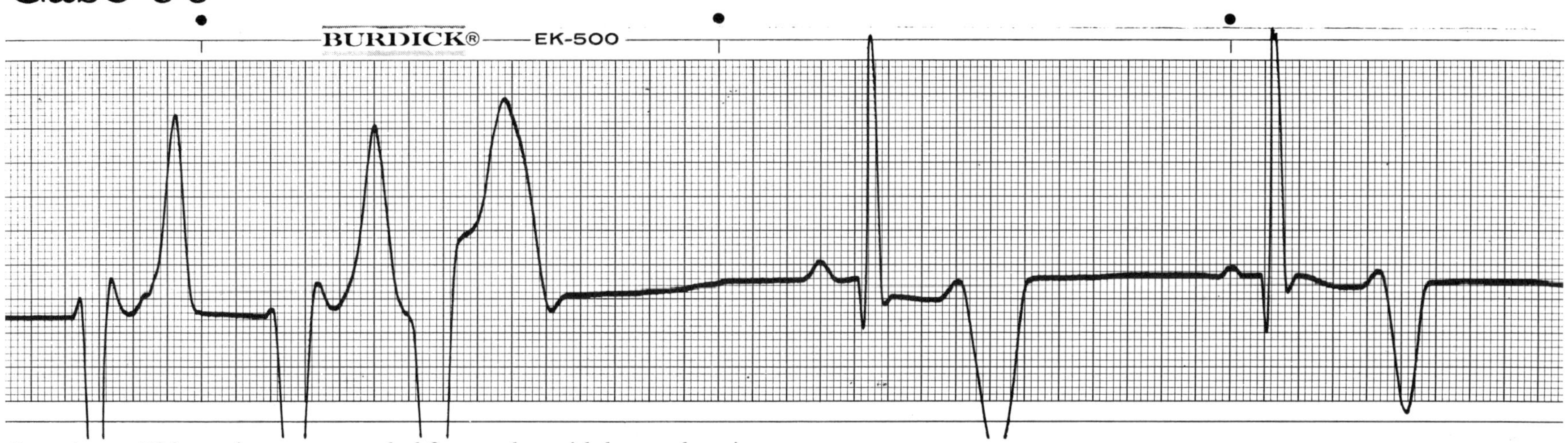

Question: This tracing was recorded from a dog with hypocalcemia. An arrhythmia was auscultated on physical examination.

1. What is the rhythm diagnosis?
2. What is the most likely underlying disorder?
3. What is the best therapeutic approach?
4. What abnormality is compatible with the hypocalcemia?

Case 95

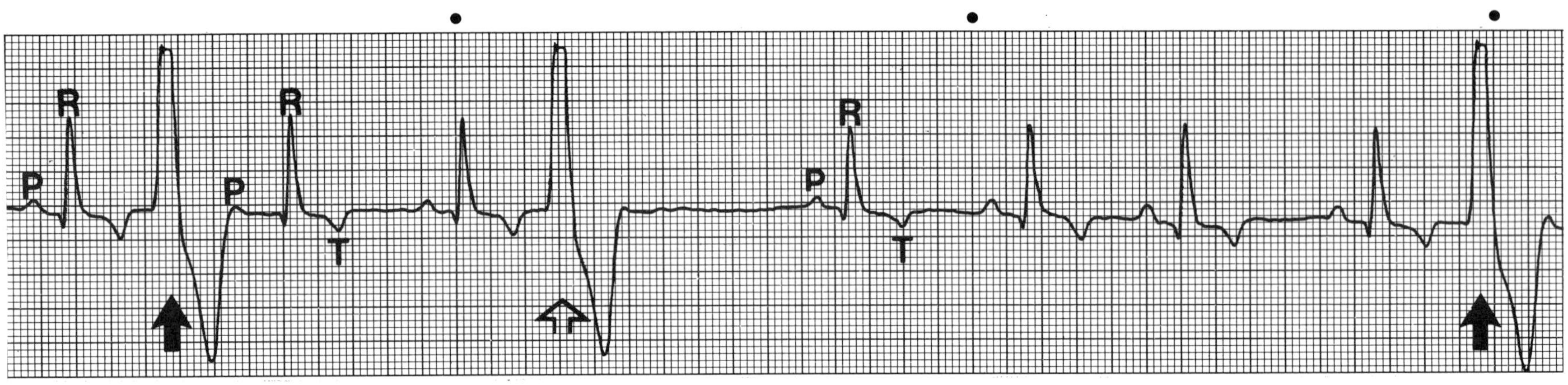

Answer: Sinus arrhythmia with frequent ventricular premature complexes. Heart rate is approximately 130 beats/min. Three ventricular premature complexes are identified by the arrows. The ventricular premature complexes are wide and bizarre and are not associated with P waves. The P-R interval of the third complex from the left is longer than that of the other sinus complexes, thus demonstrating the concept of concealed conduction. An impulse from the preceding ventricular premature complex travels retrograde through the conduction system and penetrates the AV node, thereby delaying conduction through the AV node of the subsequent sinus complex. A pause follows the second ventricular premature complex (open arrows). The pause is probably caused by a sinus impulse that was blocked at the AV node because it originated during the repolarization of the ventricular premature complex. The AV node is refractory because of concealed conduction from the preceding ventricular premature complex.

Case 96

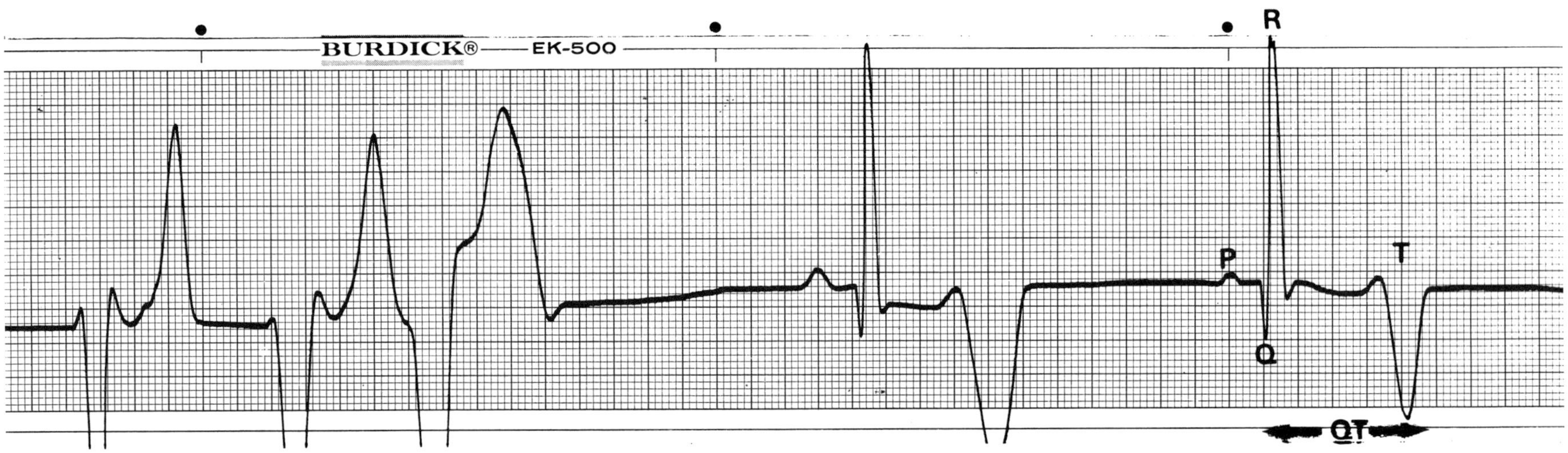

Answer: Ventricular premature complexes and prolongation of the Q-T interval. The heart rate is variable. The first three complexes are ventricular premature complexes (VPCs). A shortened Q-T interval can occur with hypercalcemia. The Q-T intervals are prolonged in the two sinus complexes. The possible causes for the hypocalcemia should include hypoparathyroidism, renal failure with phosphorus retention, eclampsia in the lactating bitch, ethylene glycol toxicity, and pancreatitis. Therapy is directed at the underlying disorder. A prolonged Q-T interval has greater significance than a shortened Q-T interval because of the effect of prolonging the relative refractory period. The relative refractory period includes the T wave, which is the vulnerable period of the ventricles. If a ventricular premature complex falls within that period, ventricular fibrillation can result. This dog obviously is at risk for a serious ventricular arrhythmia.

Case 97

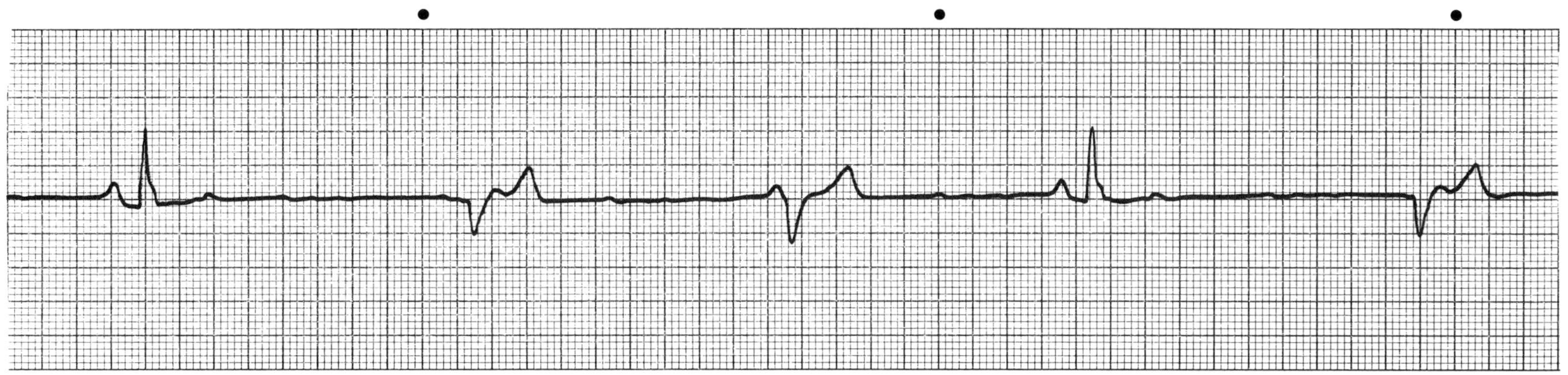

Question: This lead II ECG was obtained from an 11-year-old female Miniature Schnauzer examined because of frequent collapsing episodes.

1. What is the rhythm diagnosis?
2. What is the most likely underlying disorder?
3. What is the best therapeutic approach?

Case 98

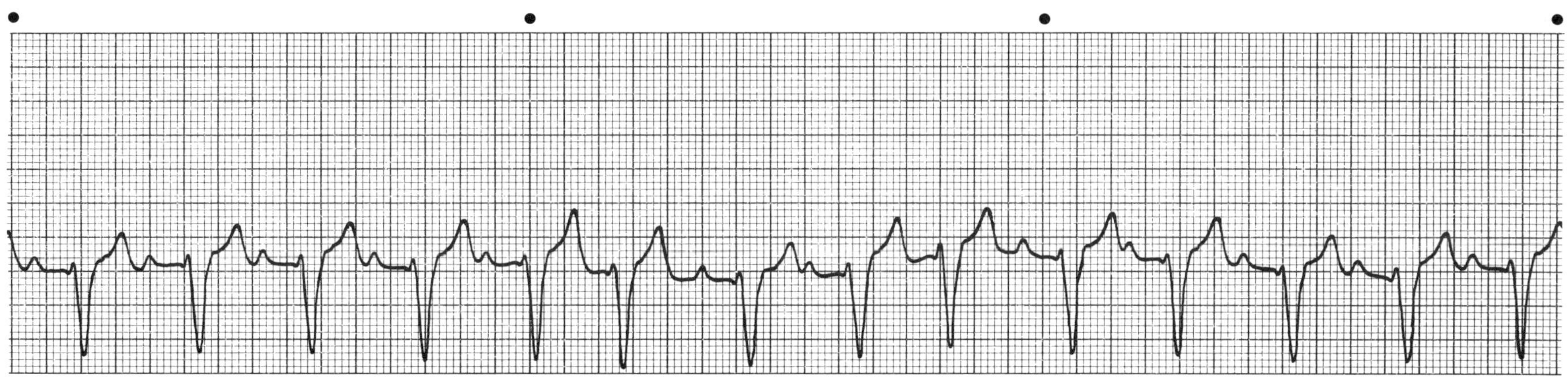

Question: This rhythm strip was recorded from a 6-month-old Beagle with a crescendo-decrescendo murmur heard loudest at the left heart base. The dog had no clinical signs. Leads I and III were also negative.

1. What is the rhythm diagnosis?
2. What are common causes of this arrhythmia?
3. What is the most likely underlying disorder?
4. What is the best therapeutic approach?

Case 97

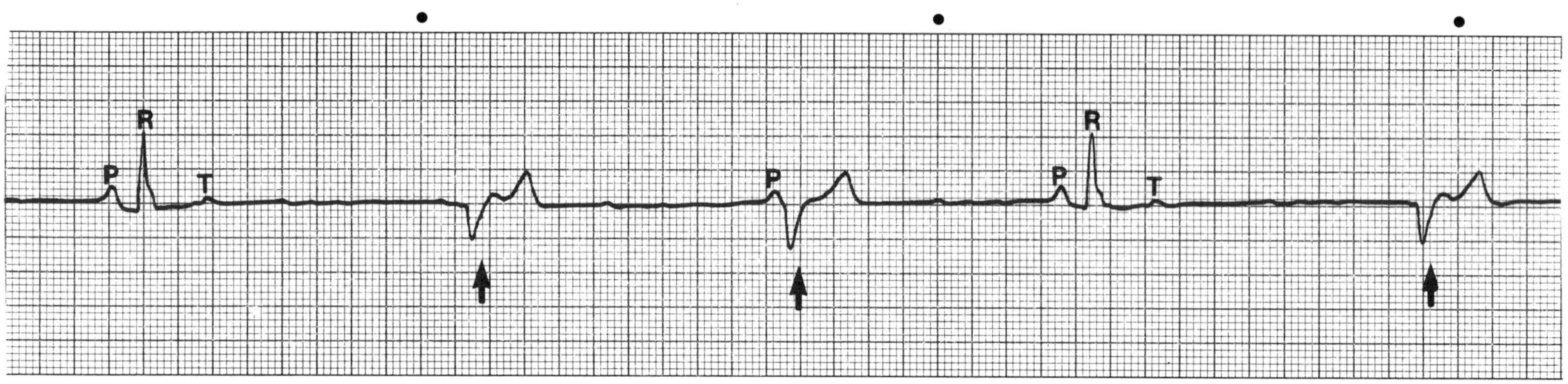

Answer: Sinus bradycardia and sinus arrhythmia with ventricular escape beats. Heart rate is 60 beats/min. Sick sinus syndrome is the most likely underlying disorder. Anticholinergics (e.g., propantheline) and bronchodilators may be effective in controlling the collapsing episodes. A permanent cardiac pacemaker is required when syncope persists. The ventricular escape beats (arrows) have bizarre QRS complexes that are not associated with the P waves. They should not be confused with or treated as ventricular premature complexes. Ventricular escape beats occur after a pause, whereas ventricular premature complexes are premature and are often closely coupled with the previous sinus beats.

Case 98

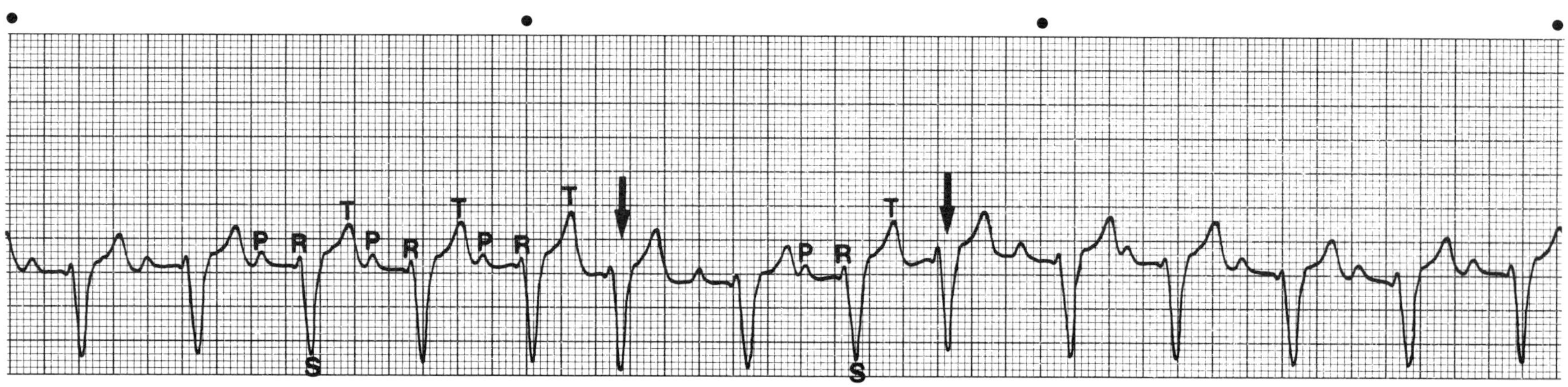

Answer: Sinus rhythm with two atrial premature complexes. Heart rate is 180 beats/min. Two atrial premature complexes (arrows) are present in the middle of the strip. Atrial premature complexes usually accompany atrial distention. The QRS complexes of the premature complexes are similar in morphology to the sinus QRS complexes. The history in this dog suggests a congenital cardiac defect. The breed and murmur suggest pulmonic stenosis, which is consistent with the right-axis deviation on the ECG. Other congenital defects that cause right ventricular enlargement include tetralogy of Fallot, right-to-left ventricular septal defect, and right-to-left shunt patent ductus arteriosus. The wide QRS complexes and the right axis may be compatible with right bundle-branch block. Thoracic radiographs are needed. Echocardiography may be necessary for a definitive diagnosis. A dog with occasional atrial premature complexes and no clinical signs requires no treatment. Prognosis is guarded because of the major ECG abnormalities in a young animal.

Case 99

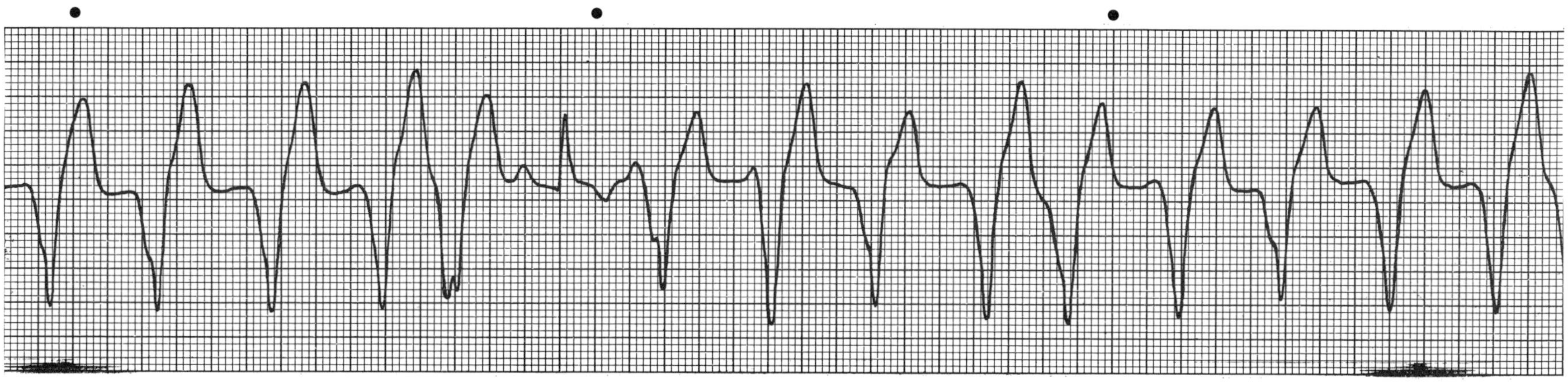

Question: This rhythm strip was recorded from a 4-year-old Samoyed that was examined because of vomiting.

1. What is the rhythm diagnosis?
2. What is the best therapeutic approach?

Case 100

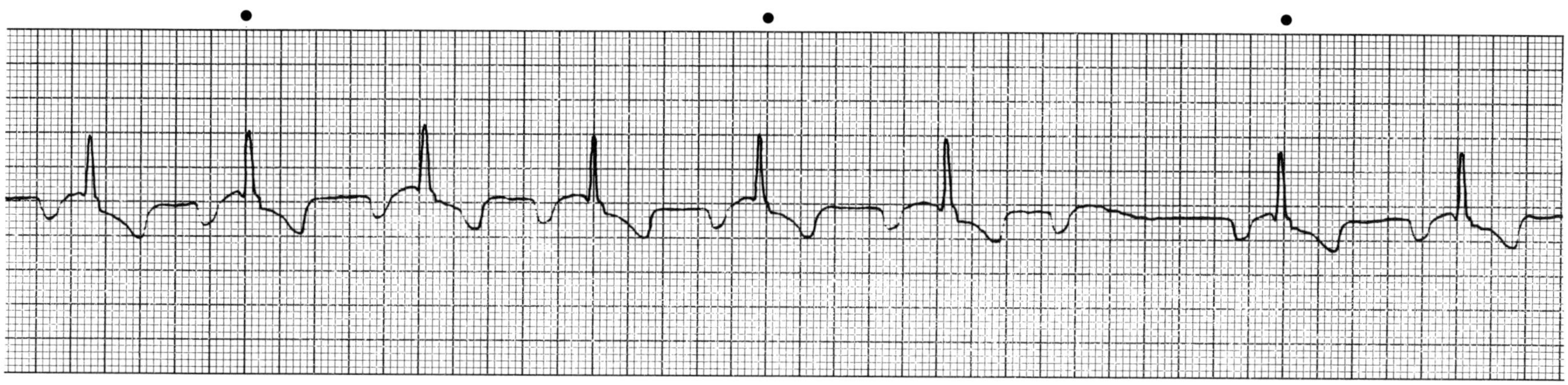

Question: This lead II ECG was obtained from an anorectic, lethargic, 13-year-old male Dachshund that had been successfully treated for congestive heart failure for 3 years. He was receiving digoxin, furosemide, and captopril.

1. What is the rhythm diagnosis?
2. What is the best therapeutic approach?

Case 99

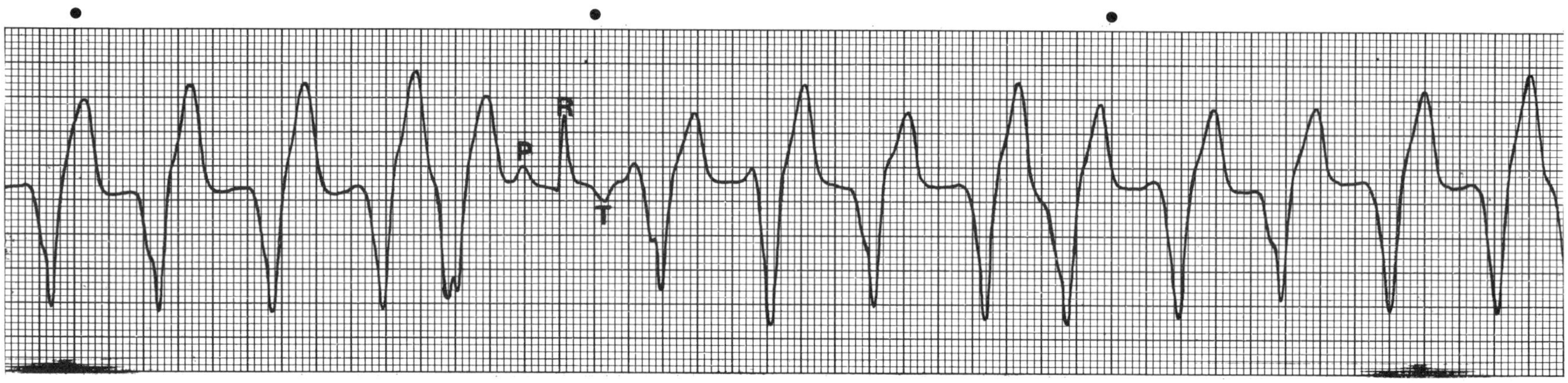

Answer: Paroxysmal ventricular tachycardia. Heart rate is approximately 180 beats/min. The ventricular premature complexes are negative, wide, and bizarre and are not associated with P waves. The appearance of three or more ventricular premature complexes in a row is termed ventricular tachycardia. Ventricular tachycardia is generally a regular rhythm. Irregular ventricular tachycardia, as in this case, can be explained by intermittent exit block out of the Purkinje system. When irregular, aberrant-appearing complexes are present without P waves, the other major differential diagnosis is atrial fibrillation with bundle branch block. The presence of a sinus or fusion beat confirms ventricular tachycardia as the abnormal rhythm. In the absence of a sinus or fusion beat, the more irregular the rhythm, the more likely the diagnosis is atrial fibrillation. The wider the complexes, the more likely the diagnosis is ventricular tachycardia. The rhythm in this instance was stabilized with lidocaine. The dog was kept on a lidocaine infusion while treatment with injectable procainamide was initiated. When the vomiting resolved, the procainamide was given orally and continued for 10 days. The arrhythmia in this dog was associated with pancreatitis.

Case 100

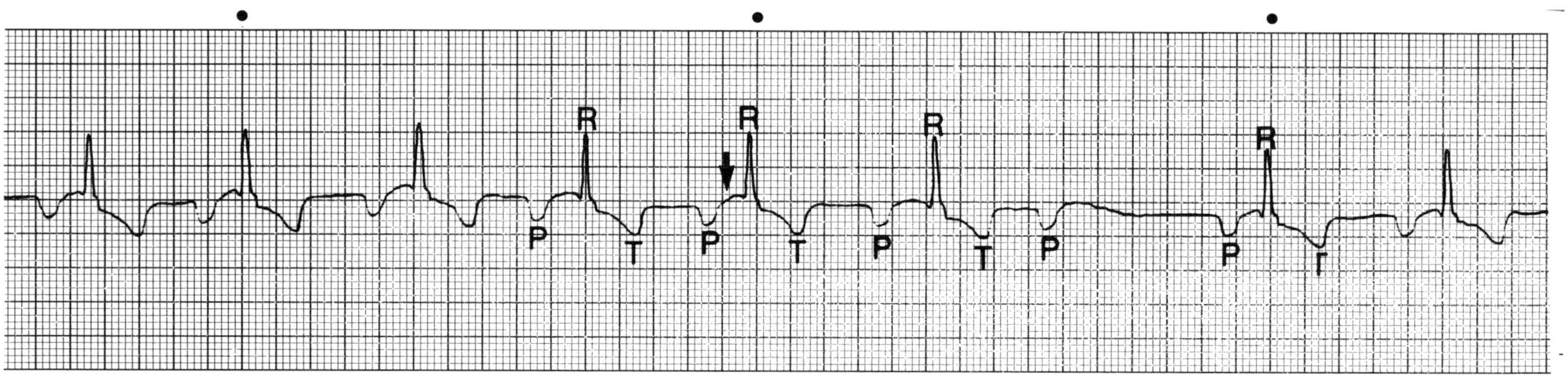

Answer: AV junctional rhythm with occasional Mobitz type I (Wenckebach) second-degree AV block. Heart rate is variable. Arrhythmias originating in the AV junction commonly occur in dogs with digoxin toxicity. The digoxin should be stopped for 48 to 72 hours, followed by a repeat ECG and reassessment of treatment. Renal function should be monitored. Negative P waves are the hallmark of AV junctional arrhythmias. Notice the progressive lengthening of the two P-R intervals before the blocked P wave (not followed by a QRS complex). Following this blocked P wave, the P-R interval shortens to its original value. In dogs with Mobitz type I (Wenckebach) second-degree AV block with a normal QRS complex, the block is usually at the level of the AV node, above the His bundle. The typical form of AV Wenckebach periodicity is characterized by progressive prolongation of the P-R interval, with the greatest incremental increase following the second conducted P wave. The prolongation of the P-R interval is typically in progressively decreasing increments, resulting in a progressively shorter R-R interval. This typical form is not reflected in this ECG, which shows atypical Mobitz type I AV block. Other atypical manifestations of type I AV block include several P-R intervals of the same duration and an unexpected decrease of a P-R interval (arrow). Type I Wenckebach periodicity and block may complicate conduction from any ectopic pacemaker, including the AV node and Purkinje system.

Case 101

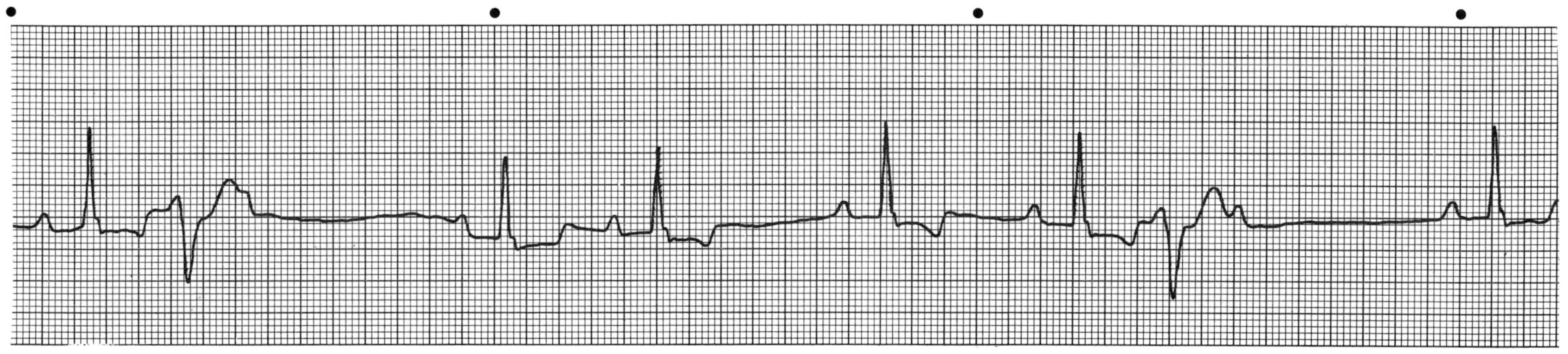

Question: This ECG was obtained from an asymptomatic 11-year-old Cocker Spaniel. An irregular heart rhythm was heard on auscultation, and an ECG was advised.

1. What is the rhythm diagnosis?
2. What is the most likely underlying disorder?
3. What is the best therapeutic approach?

Case 102

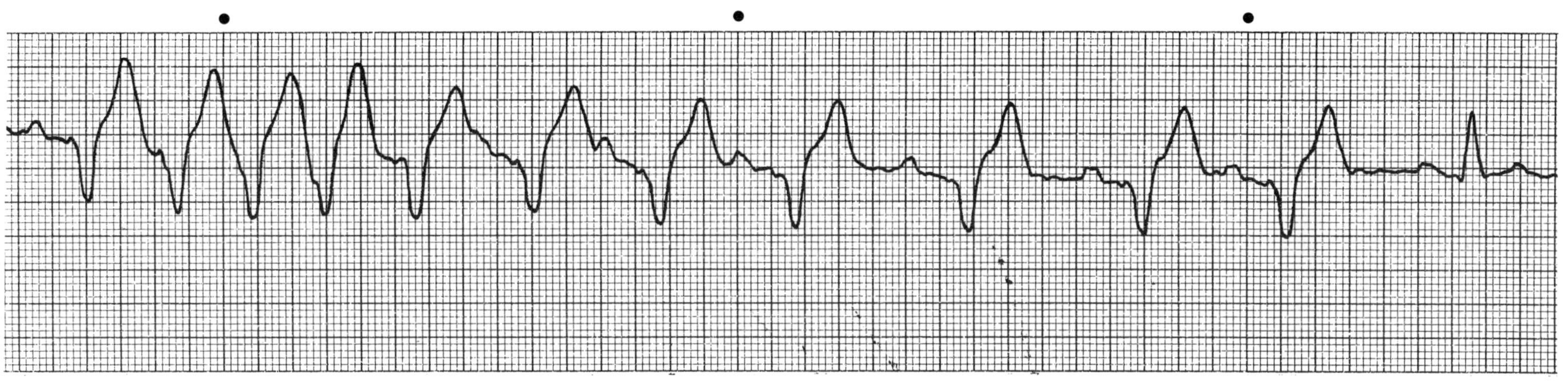

Question: This lead II ECG was obtained from a 5-year-old mixed-breed dog that was examined because of syncope.

1. What is the rhythm diagnosis?
2. What is the best therapeutic approach?

Case 101

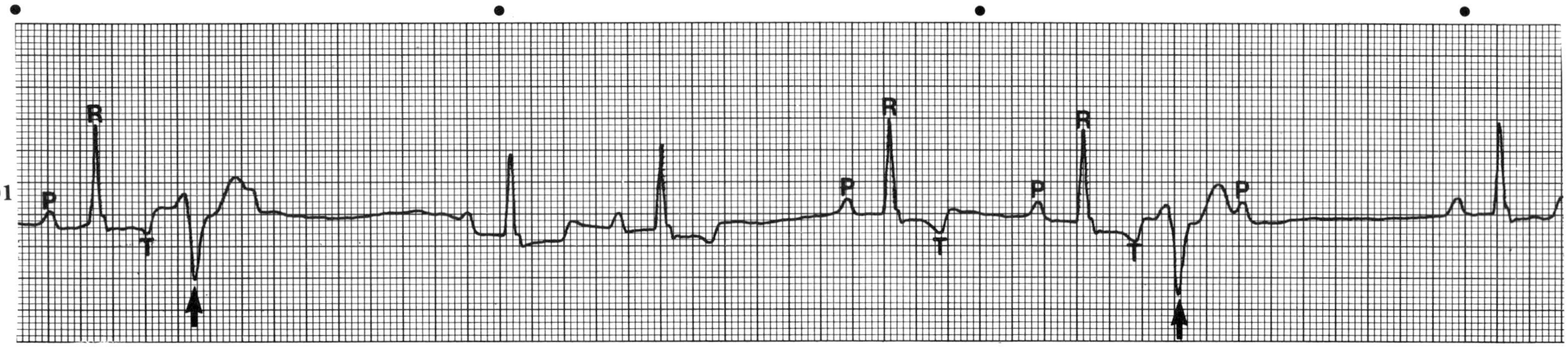

Answer: Sinus arrhythmia with ventricular premature complexes (arrows). The P-R interval is slightly prolonged (normal value, 0.13 sec). Heart rate is approximately 100 beats/min. Idiopathic myocarditis most likely accounts for the ventricular premature complexes. Antiarrhythmic drugs are not required in a dog with no clinical signs. Negative, wide, and bizarre QRS complexes not associated with P waves are the hallmark of ventricular premature complexes. The ventricular premature impulses (second arrow) can travel retrograde and depolarize the AV node (concealed conduction). The following P waves enter the AV node in its refractory period and are blocked. Concealed conduction is not detected on the ECG, but is deduced by its effect on the subsequent sinus beat.

Case 102

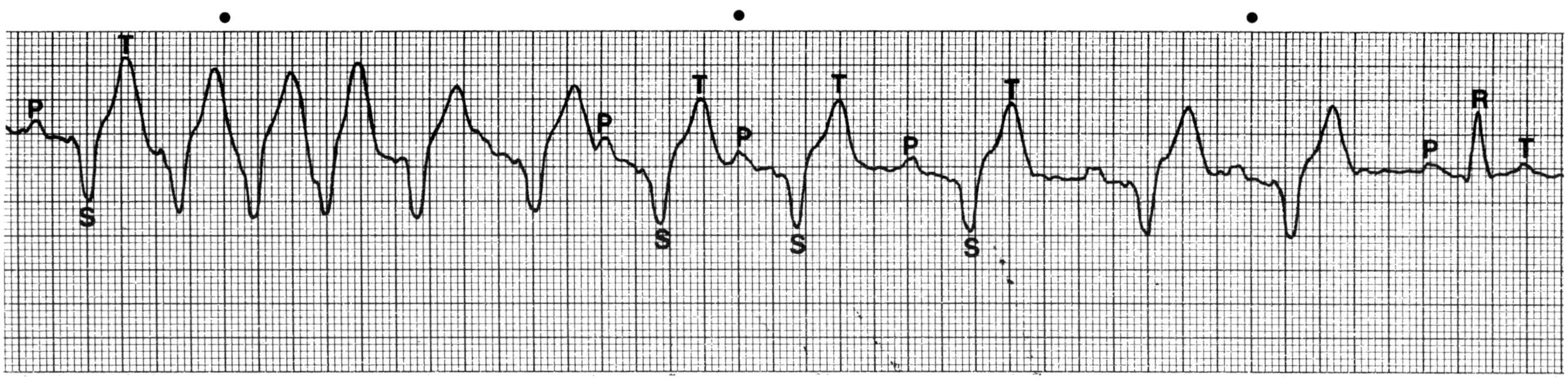

Answer: Sinus rhythm with intermittent, rate-related right bundle-branch block and paroxysmal supraventricular tachycardia. Heart rate is 120 to 180 beats/mins. If progressive mitral valvular insufficiency or dilated cardiomyopathy and/or congestive heart failure is evident, digoxin is the preferred drug for treating the arrhythmia. If the size of the heart is normal and no congestive heart failure exists, diltiazem or propranolol is an appropriate alternative. The first sinus beat (labeled) has a right bundle-branch block pattern. Right bundle-branch block is recognized by prolongation of the QRS complex, consistent P-R interval, and deep and wide S wave in leads I, II, III, aVF, and the left precordial chest leads. The second through sixth QRS complexes resemble the first QRS complex but occur at different cycles of prematurity, thus supporting the possibility of multifocal atrial premature complexes. The P waves of the atrial premature complexes are fused with the preceding T waves. Sinus rhythm with right bundle-branch block resumes after the sixth QRS complex. The last QRS complex, with a shorter P-R interval, looks different from the preceding QRS complexes and probably represents a return to normally conducted sinus beats. The shorter P-R interval and normally shaped QRS complex can be explained, because the last P wave-to-P wave interval is the longest in the strip, thereby allowing extra time for refractory period recovery of the AV node and right bundle-branch Purkinje fibers.

Case 103

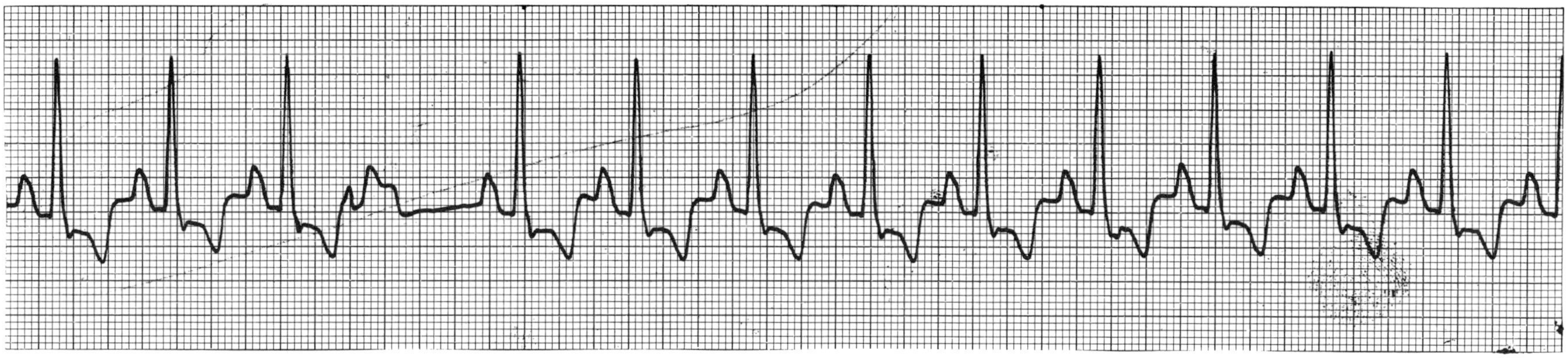

Question: This tracing was recorded from a dog with mitral valvular insufficiency and no major clinical signs.

1. What is the rhythm diagnosis?
2. Can you explain all the deflections that occur in the pause of this rhythm strip?

Case 104

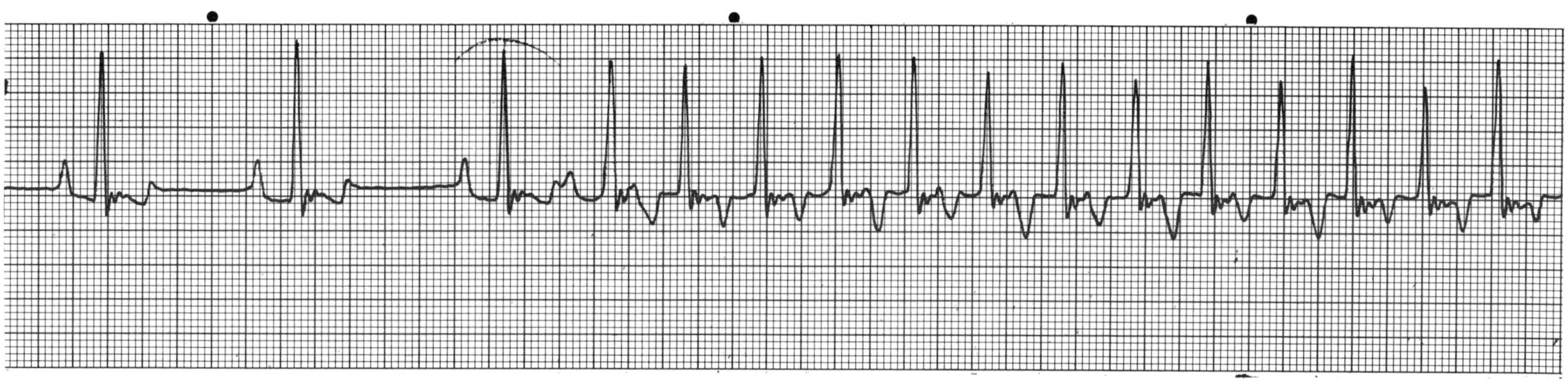

Question: This ECG was obtained from a 4-year-old male Poodle with a history of tracheal collapse. He was being examined because of recent fainting episodes.

1. What is the rhythm diagnosis?
2. What is the best therapeutic approach?

Case 103

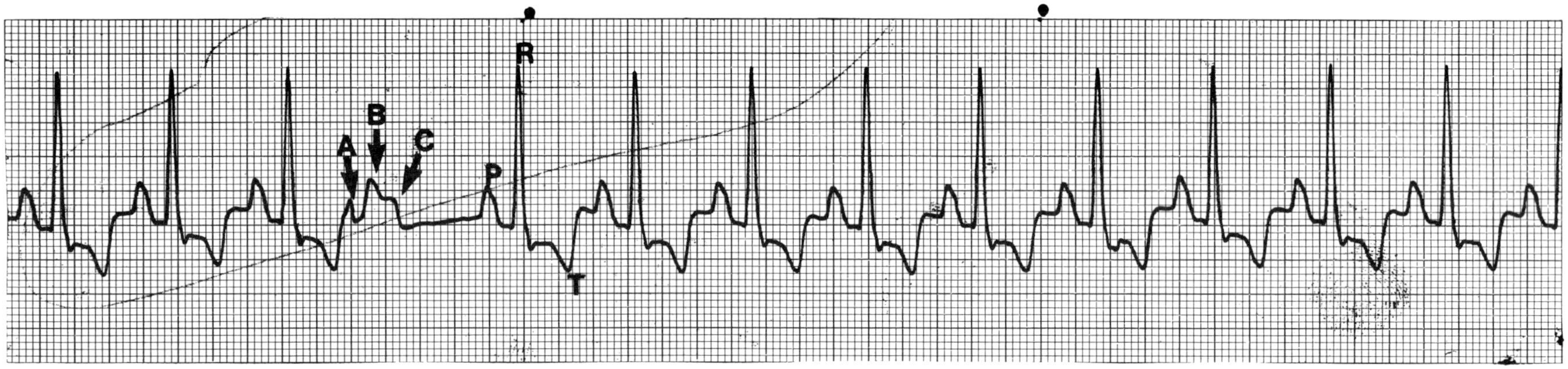

Answer: Ventricular premature complex. Heart rate is 175 beats/min. The fourth complex in this rhythm strip represents an abnormality that is difficult to analyze. The diagnosis of some arrhythmias can be difficult because the routine surface ECG provides only a limited understanding of the electrophysiologic events. The pause in this lead II rhythm strip is caused by a premature complex. B represents the normal atrial P wave (from the SA node) that does not conduct to the ventricle because either the AV node or the ventricle is refractory to the event labelled A. Although A does not activate the atria, it nevertheless is visible and, thus, must represent ventricular activation. Because it does not look the same as conducted sinus beats, it must be a ventricular premature complex. Thus, A is the QRS and C is the T wave of the ventricular premature complex.

Case 104

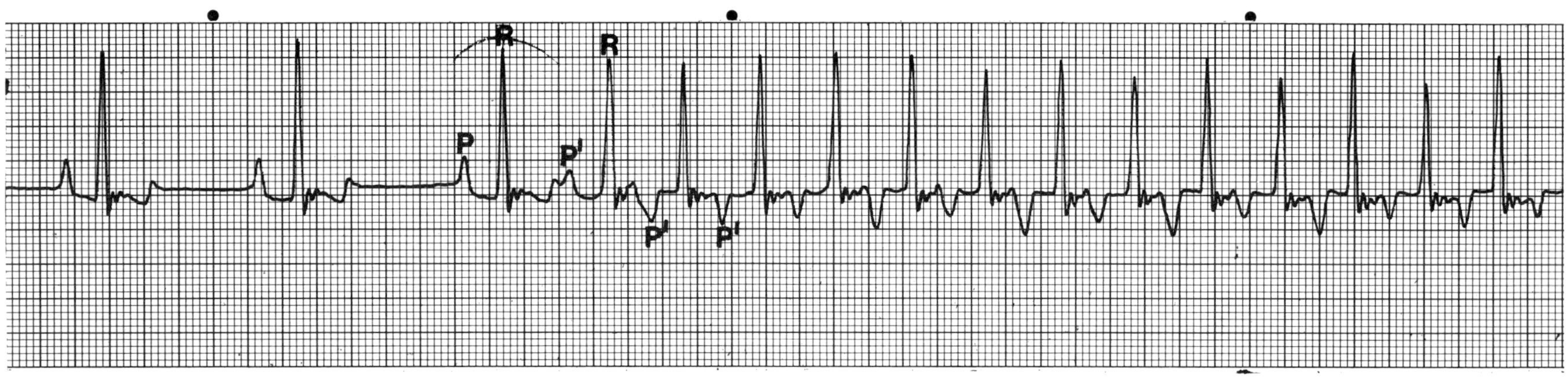

Answer: Sinus rhythm with paroxysmal re-entrant supraventricular tachycardia. Heart rate is variable, approaching 370 beats/min during tachycardic episodes. The narrow QRS complex during the tachycardia, which appears similar to the QRS complexes of the sinus beats, is the key diagnostic feature of supraventricular tachycardia. Digoxin, diltiazem, or propranolol, either alone or in combination, may be effective in controlling this arrhythmia. The mechanism responsible for the production of this paroxysmal tachycardia is complex. The mechanism for most cases of supraventricular tachycardia is probably AV nodal re-entry, but ectopic automatic atrial tachycardias may also occur. In re-entrant tachycardia, the P′ wave morphology is retrograde (inverted) except for the initiating atrial premature complex (first P′), which is upright. The initiating beat is also associated with AV nodal conduction delay. Abrupt termination of a supraventricular tachycardia by carotid massage or other vagal maneuvers favors a re-entrant mechanism. Notice the variation in amplitude of the QRS complex (QRS alternans) during the tachycardia. The exact cause of QRS alternans during supraventricular tachycardia remains controversial, although suspected mechanisms include differences in recovery rate of the individual fibers, prolongation of the refractory phase of the heart on an alternating basis, and a retrograde accessory AV pathway in the tachycardia circuit.

Case 105

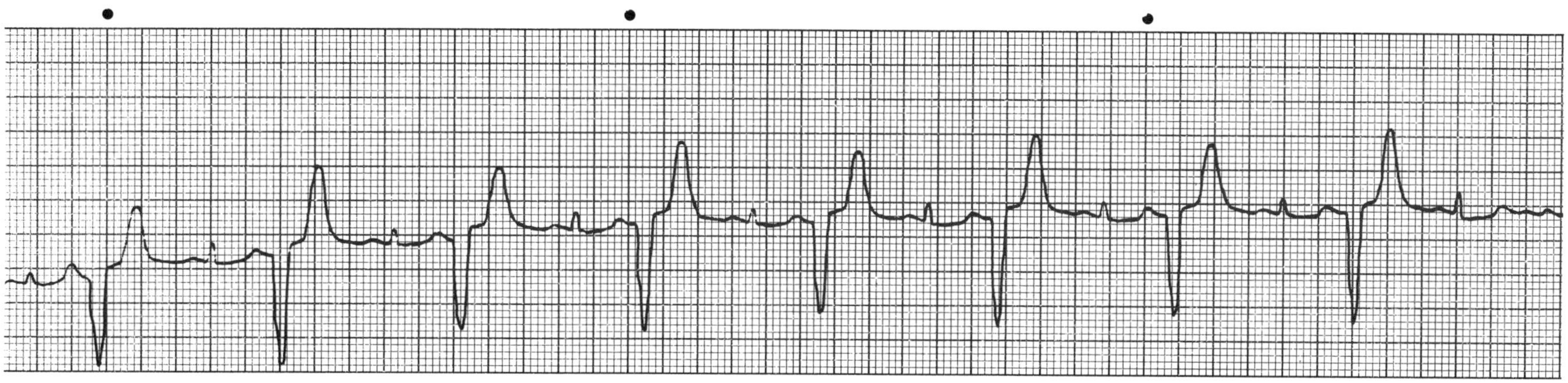

Question: This lead II ECG was obtained from a 14-year-old cat examined because of vomiting. The veterinarian noticed jugular venous pulsations when obtaining a blood sample from the left jugular vein.

1. What is the rhythm diagnosis?
2. What are common causes of this arrhythmia?
3. What is the best therapeutic approach?

Case 106

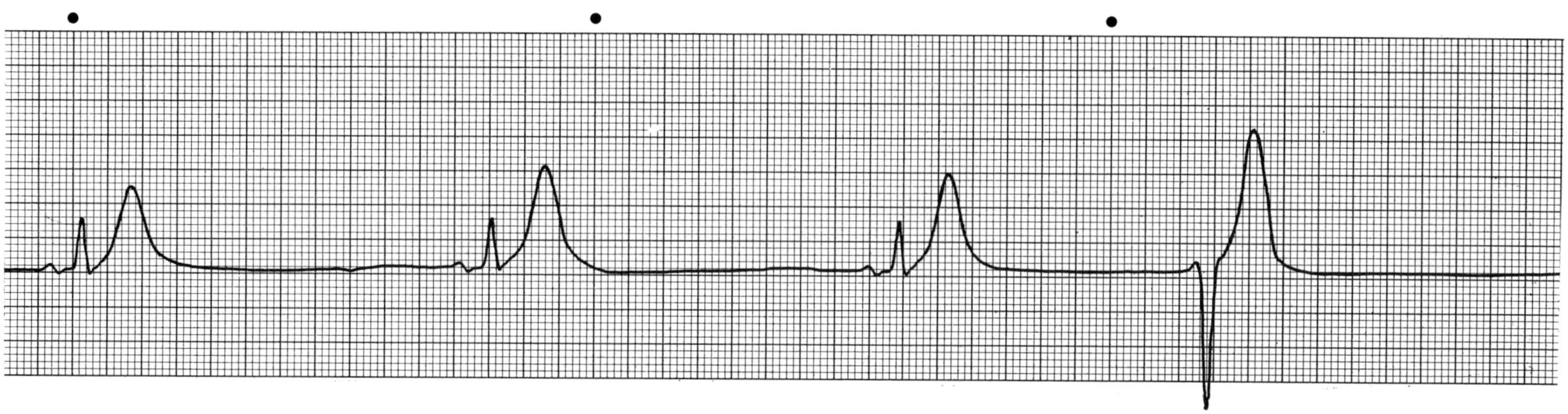

Question: This rhythm strip was recorded from a Standard Poodle after the dog had experienced cardiac arrest and resuscitation.

1. What is the rhythm diagnosis?
2. What is the best therapeutic approach?

Case 105

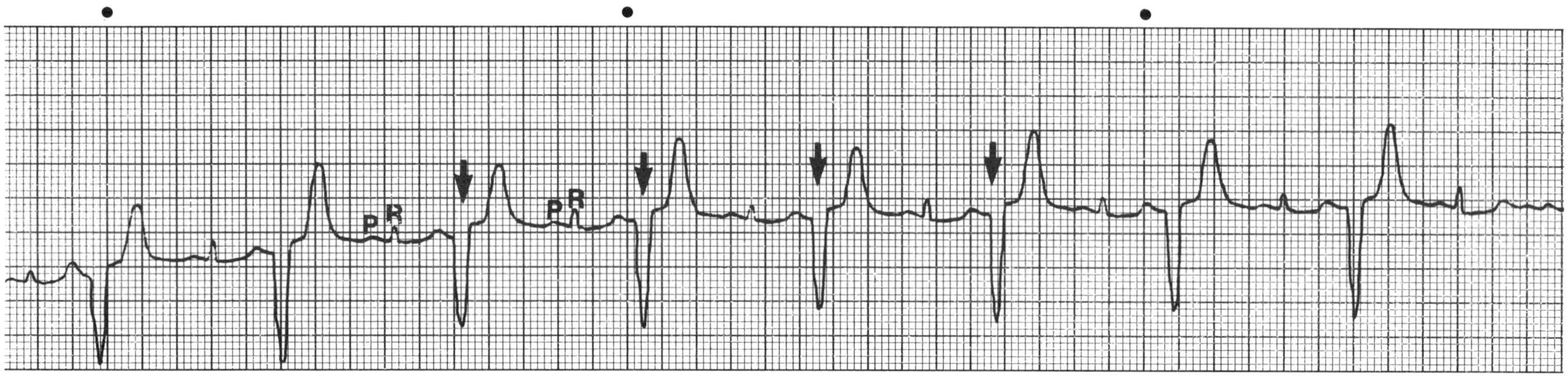

Answer: Sinus rhythm with ventricular premature complexes every other beat (ventricular bigeminy). Heart rate is 230 beats/min. This arrhythmia is not considered dangerous and requires no treatment in a cat with no clinical signs. Ventricular arrhythmias may occur in cats with systemic disease (secondary myocarditis) or cardiomyopathy. A cardiac data base, including thoracic radiographs, complete blood count, and serum chemistry profile, aids in differentiating between primary cardiac and systemic causes of the arrhythmia. Anesthetic induction with thiobarbiturates may also cause transient ventricular bigeminy. Premature wide and bizarre QRS complexes (arrows) that have no association with the atrial rhythm (P waves) are the hallmark of ventricular premature complexes.

Case 106

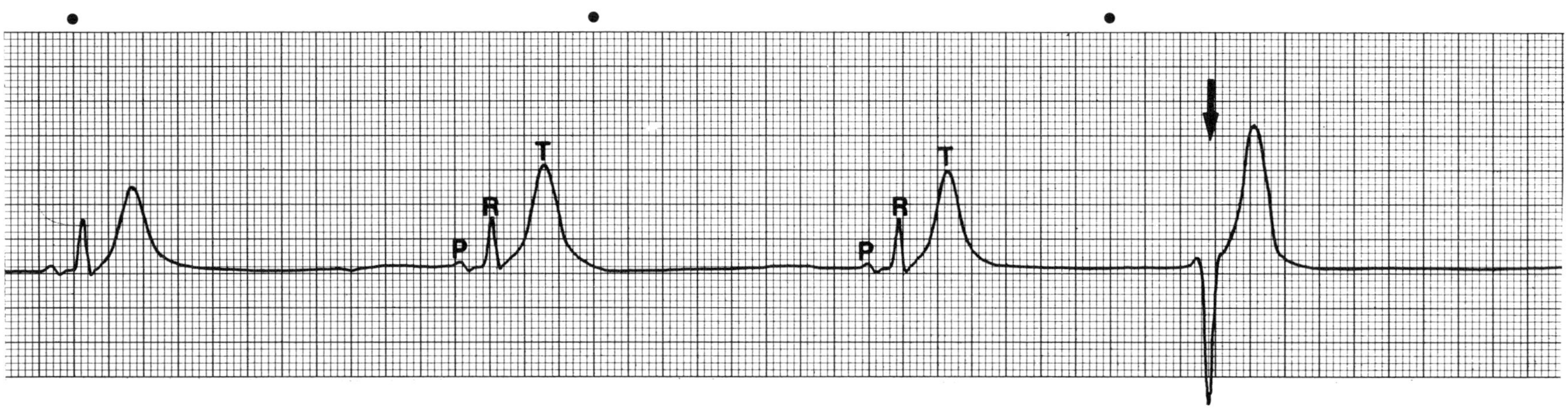

Answer: Sinus bradycardia with one late diastolic ventricular ectopic complex (arrow). Heart rate is approximately 55 beats/min. A slow sinus rhythm is present. The large T waves indicate myocardial hypoxia. The ventricular ectopic complex is consistent with possible underlying myocardial disease. On the basis of the ECG and history, attempts should be made to improve myocardial perfusion and oxygenation. Fluids should be administered intravenously as necessary to improve perfusion without risking overhydration or development of pulmonary edema. The dog should be maintained in an oxygen-enriched environment. Antiarrhythmic medications are not warranted at this time. Attempts to increase the rate may only worsen myocardial hypoxia by increasing myocardial oxygen demand. Frequent monitoring of the ECG in this dog is critical. If the rate drops, atropine or epinephrine may be needed.

Case 107

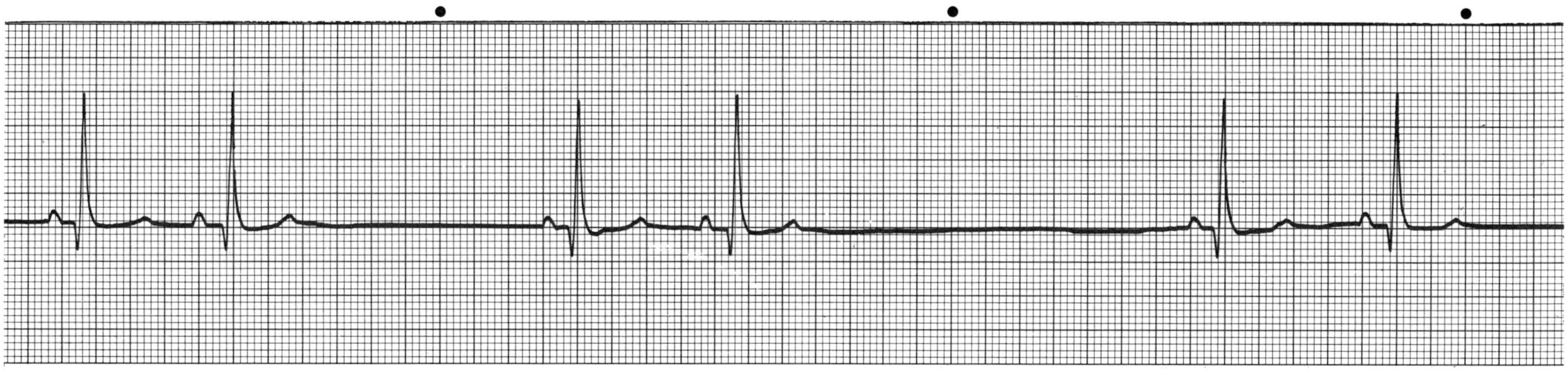

Question: This ECG was recorded from a brachycephalic breed with chronic bronchitis and episodes of fainting.

1. What is the rhythm diagnosis?
2. What is the best therapeutic approach?

Case 108

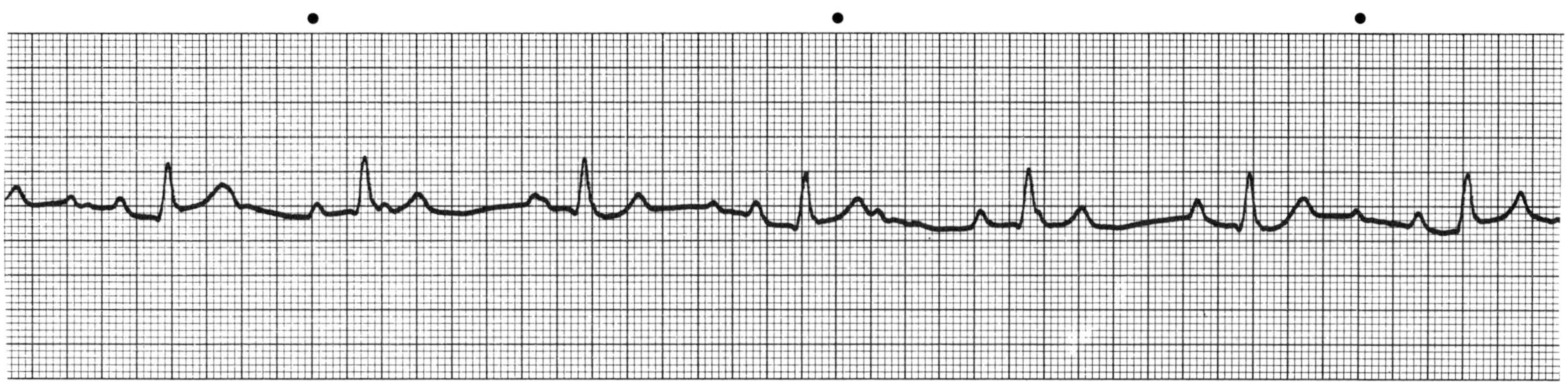

Question: This rhythm strip was received from a dog with severe congestive heart failure.

1. What is the rhythm diagnosis?
2. What is the most likely underlying disorder?

Case 107

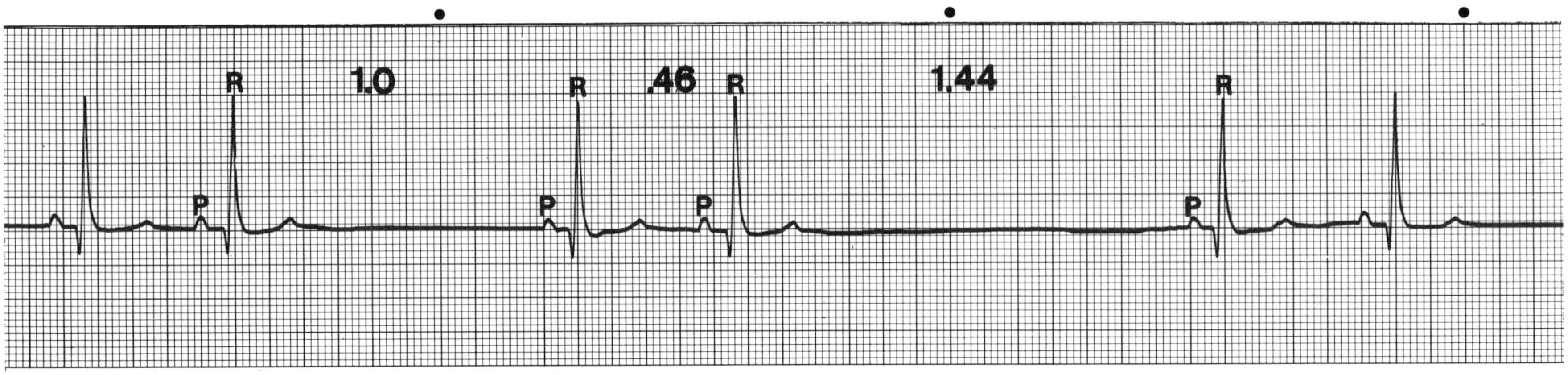

Answer: Intermittent sinus arrest or sinoatrial block. Heart rate is variable. Sinus arrest is the failure of impulses to be formed within the SA node owing to a depression of automaticity in the node. SA block, with the same electrocardiographic pattern, is a disturbance of conduction from a regularly firing SA node. The two conditions are usually difficult to differentiate. The pauses with sinus arrest are twice or greater than twice the normal R-R interval. The pauses (1.0 and 1.44 secs) in this case are greater than twice the normal R-R interval (0.46 secs). Intermittent sinus arrest can be a normal incidental finding in brachycephalic breeds. Inspiration in these breeds causes a reflex decrease in vagal tone, thereby leading to an exaggerated sinus arrhythmia. Ocular or carotid sinus pressure often produces a sinus arrest. Asymptomatic sinus arrest or SA block does not require therapy. If the condition is symptomatic, however, the underlying cause should be treated. The mere administration of bronchodilators to this dog resolved the episodes of fainting. The underlying condition was treated.

Case 108

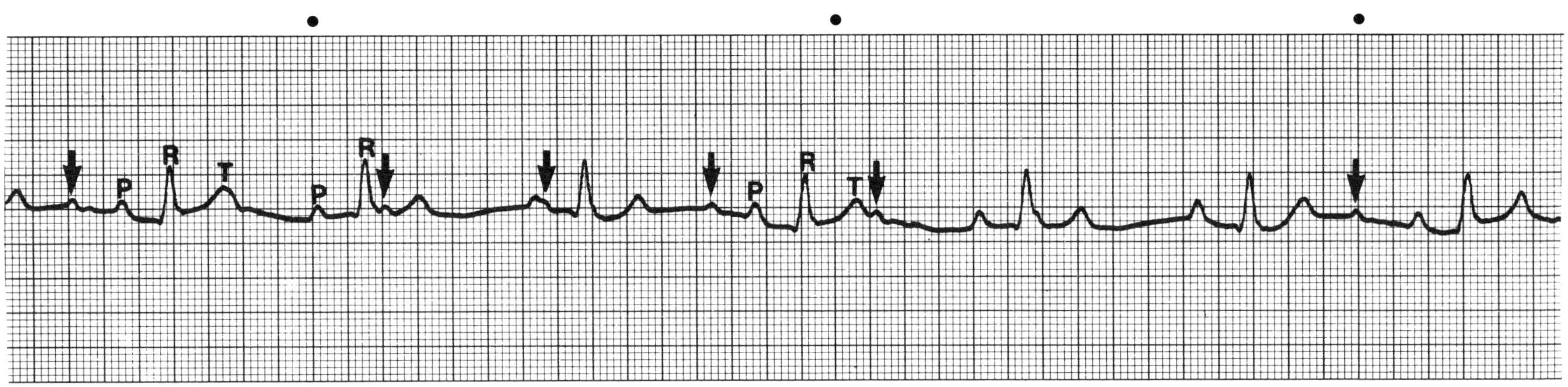

Answer: Atrial dissociation. Heart rate is 100 beats/min. Of the two independent atrial rhythms, one is sinoatrial (P waves) and the other is ectopic atrial (arrows). Both the sinus and the interectopic intervals are constant. The ectopic atrial focus is never conducted to the ventricles; it controls only a part of the atrium because of a probable intra-atrial block in that region. The sinus complexes cannot interfere with the ectopic rhythm, and vice versa. In humans, this arrhythmia is often seen with advanced congestive heart failure. Such an atrial focus could be confused with an artifact, a possible consideration. In this case, however, the arrhythmia was found on repeat ECGs. Most of these independent P waves in humans are actually artifacts produced by the accessory muscles of respiration.

Case 109

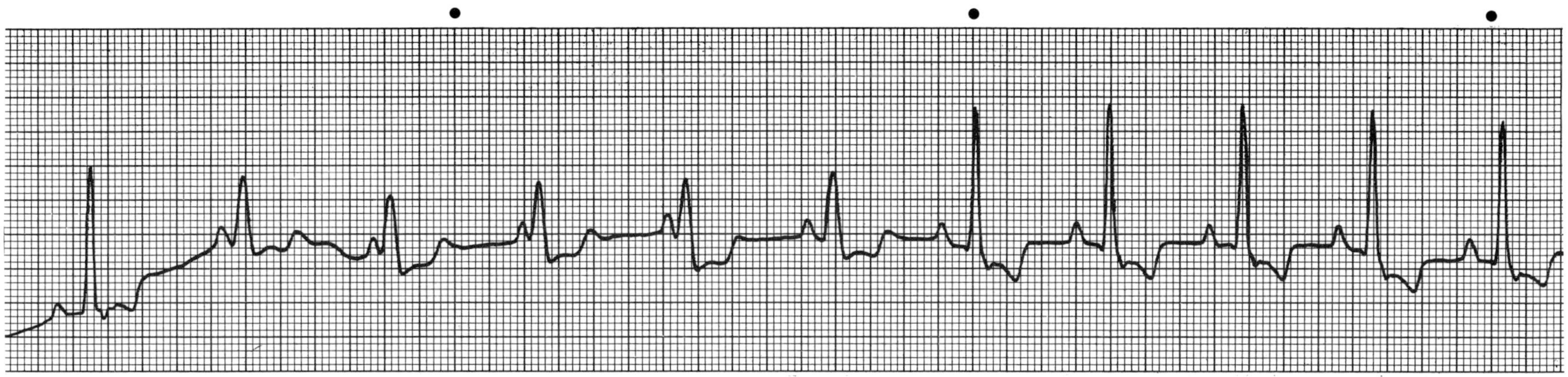

Question: This lead II ECG was obtained from an Irish Setter 24 hours after he had been treated for gastric dilatation.

1. What is the rhythm diagnosis?
2. What is the most likely underlying disorder?
3. What is the best therapeutic approach?

Case 110

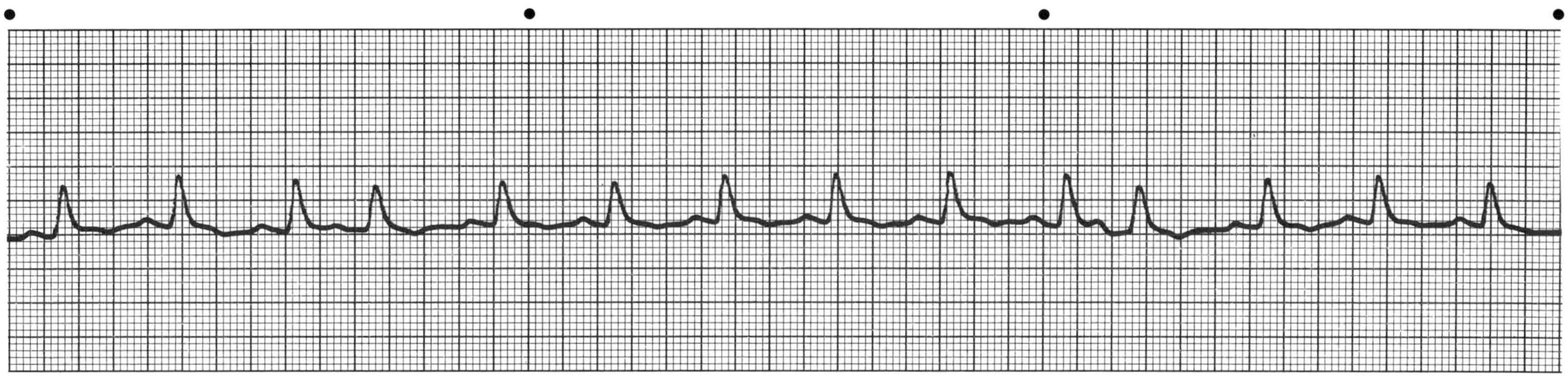

Question: This lead II ECG was obtained from a 3-year-old Boxer with a history of exercise intolerance and an irregular heart rhythm heard on auscultation.

1. What is the rhythm diagnosis?
2. What is the most likely underlying disorder?
3. What is the best therapeutic approach?

Case 109

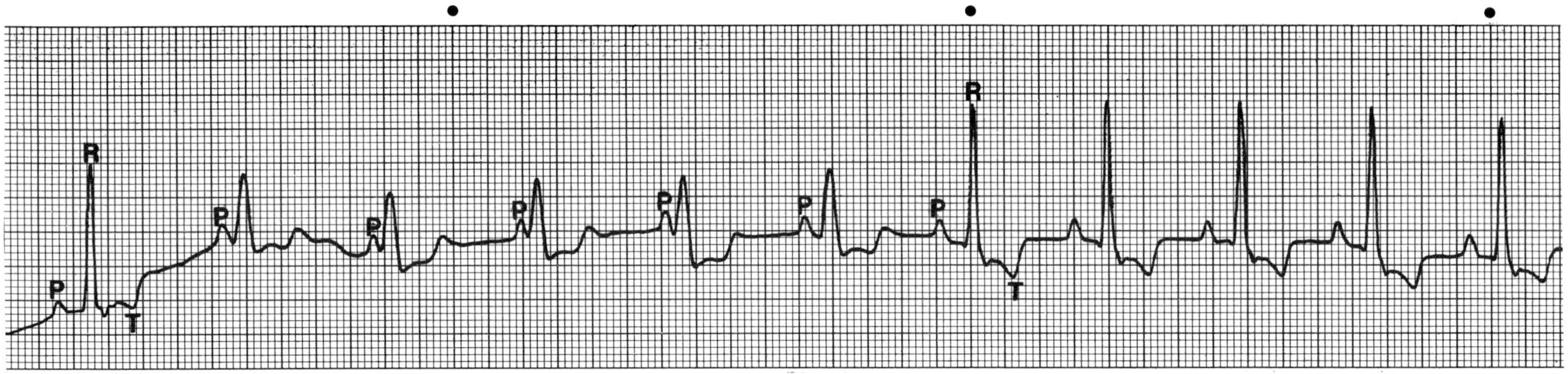

Answer: Sinus rhythm with an accelerated idioventricular rhythm. Heart rate is 150 beats/min. Abnormalities suggested to be responsible for triggering arrhythmias in dogs with gastric dilatation volvulus include acid-base imbalances, electrolyte imbalances, myocardial ischemia, circulating cardiostimulatory substances (e.g., histamine and bradykinins), depressant factors, and autonomic imbalances. Supportive therapy to re-establish normal plasma pH and serum electrolyte concentrations and to maintain adequate blood volume is the initial therapeutic approach. Antiarrhythmic drugs that can be administered alone or in combination to re-establish sinus rhythm include lidocaine (intravenous administration) and procainamide and quinidine (intramuscular administration). If the ventricular rate is < 65 beats/min, the condition is termed a ventricular escape rhythm and may best be treated by speeding up the rate of the sinus beat with atropine rather than by attempting to use antiarrhythmic drugs to suppress the ventricular arrhythmia. The wide and bizarre QRS complexes (when compared with the sinus beat QRS complexes) that have no association with the P waves characterize the ventricular arrhythmia.

Case 110

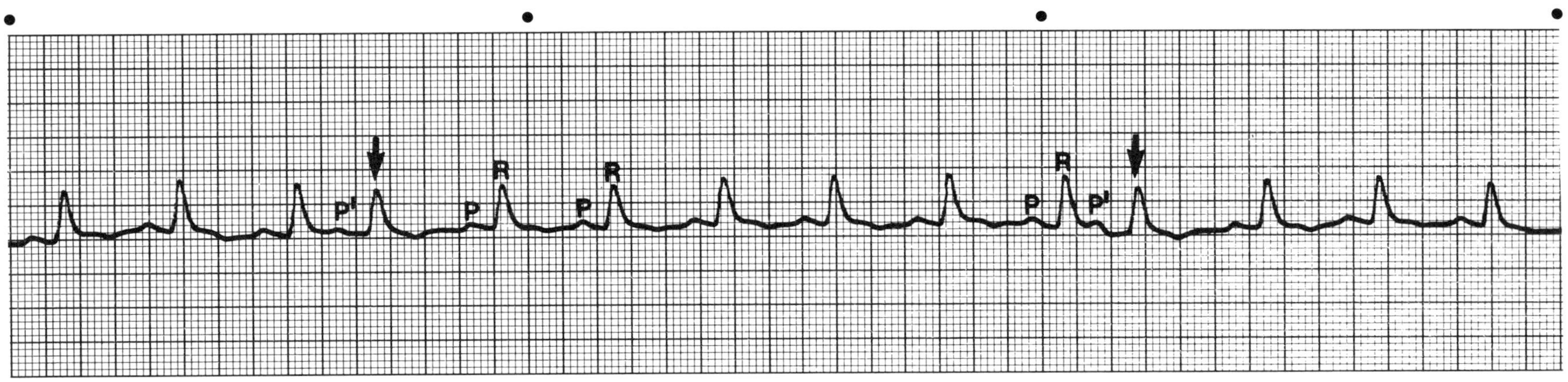

Answer: Sinus tachycardia with atrial premature complexes. Heart rate is 180 beats/min. Cardiomyopathy is the most likely underlying disorder. Digoxin is the drug of choice for treating this atrial arrhythmia. A diuretic and vasodilator may also be required if congestive heart failure is confirmed by thoracic radiographs. The premature QRS complexes (arrows) that resemble the QRS complexes of the sinus beats typify the atrial premature complexes. The premature P′ waves are fused with the preceding T waves and change the shape of the T waves when compared with the other sinus beats. One must first scan the rhythm strip from left to right to avoid missing these atrial premature complexes. Also, the small QRS complexes should be used as a clue to the possible presence of pleural or pericardial effusion.

Case 111

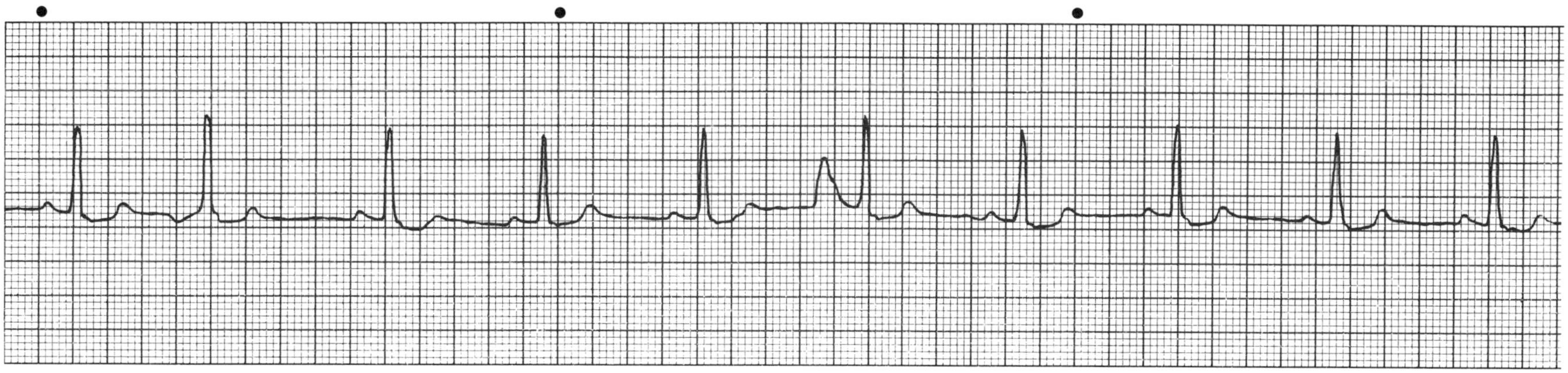

Question: This lead II ECG was obtained from a 7-year-old asymptomatic Miniature Schnauzer with an irregular heart rhythm heard on auscultation.

1. What is the rhythm diagnosis?
2. What is the best therapeutic approach?

Case 112

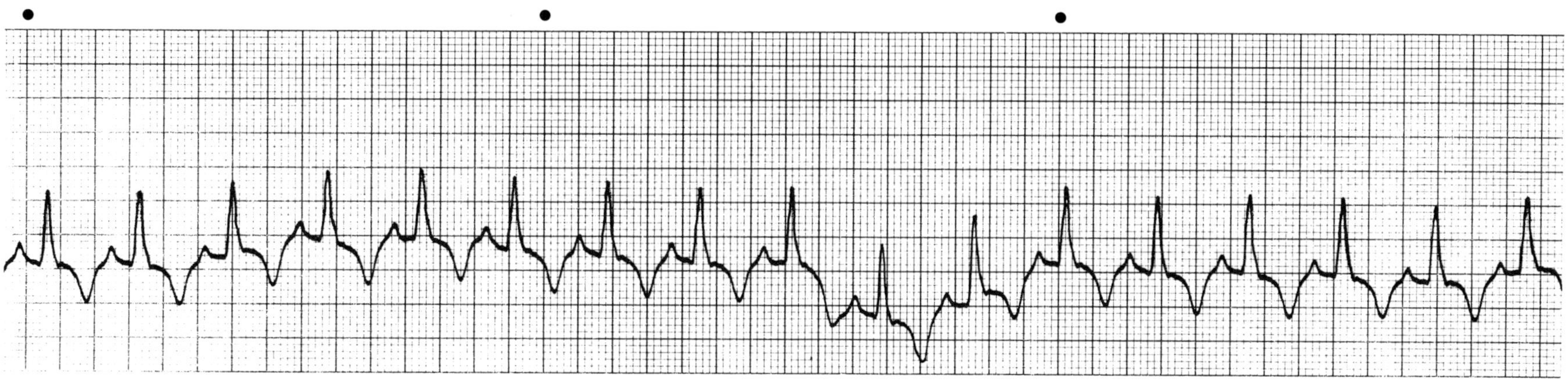

Question: This rhythm strip was recorded from an 11-year-old domestic shorthair cat that was being examined because of aortic thromboembolism and pelvic limb paralysis. Methimazole was being given for hyperthyroidism. Thyroid concentrations had been normal for the past year.

1. What is the rhythm diagnosis?
2. What is the most likely underlying disorder?
3. What is the best therapeutic approach?

Case 111

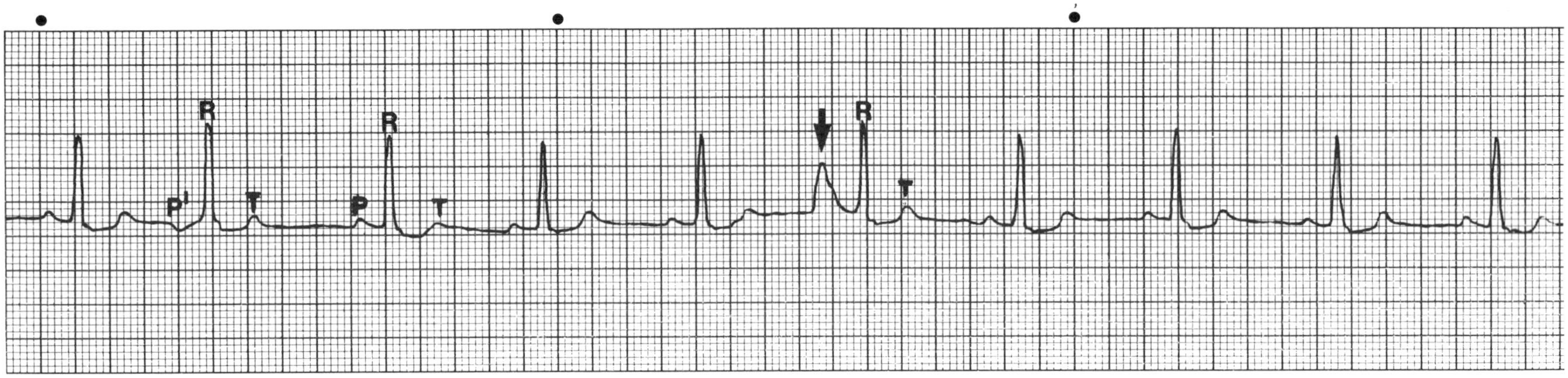

Answer: Sinus rhythm with one atrial premature complex. Heart rate is 140 beats/min. Because the dog is asymptomatic, therapy is not required initially. The QRS complex (second complex) following the premature P′ wave is similar to the QRS complexes of the sinus beats, the hallmark criterion for atrial premature complexes. The complex marked with an arrow is artifact because it neither interrupts the cardiac rhythm nor is followed by a T wave.

Case 112

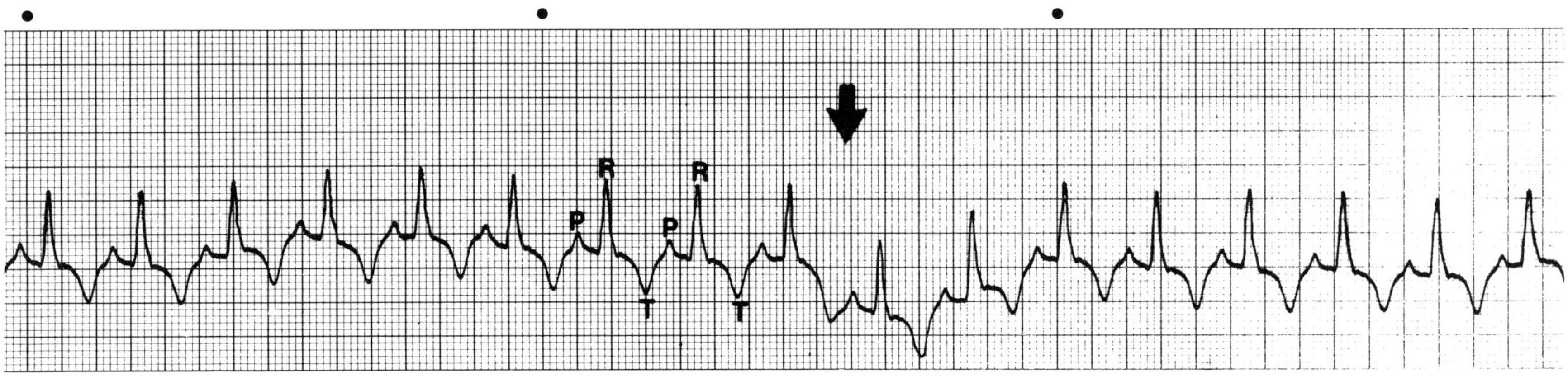

Answer: Sinus rhythm. Heart rate is 215 beats/min. The rhythm is sinus. The tall R waves may indicate left ventricular enlargement. Prominent T waves suggest possible myocardial hypoxia, hyperkalemia, or repolarization changes caused by cardiac enlargement. Motion artifact affects the ECG baseline (arrow). Because the thyroid problem has been well controlled, the ECG enlargement pattern and embolism are probably secondary to cardiomyopathy. Thoracic radiographs and echocardiogram are recommended to determine the underlying cardiac disorder. Antiarrhythmic therapy is not needed. Aspirin and heparin may be useful in treating the embolic problem. Arterial vasodilators may improve collateral circulation.

Case 113

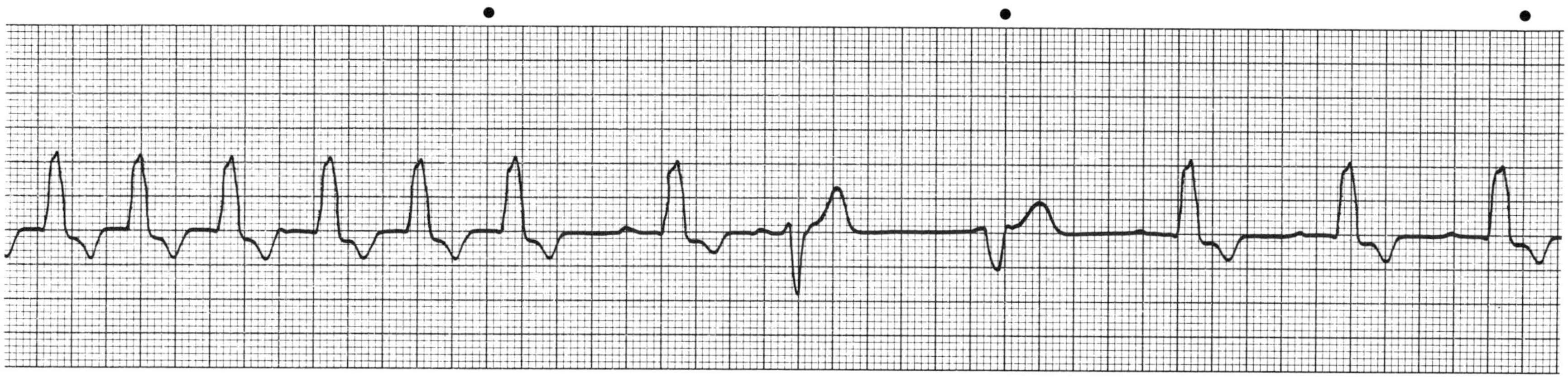

Question: This lead II ECG was obtained from a 5-year-old Boxer examined for collapsing episodes.

1. What is the rhythm diagnosis?
2. What is the best therapeutic approach?

Case 114

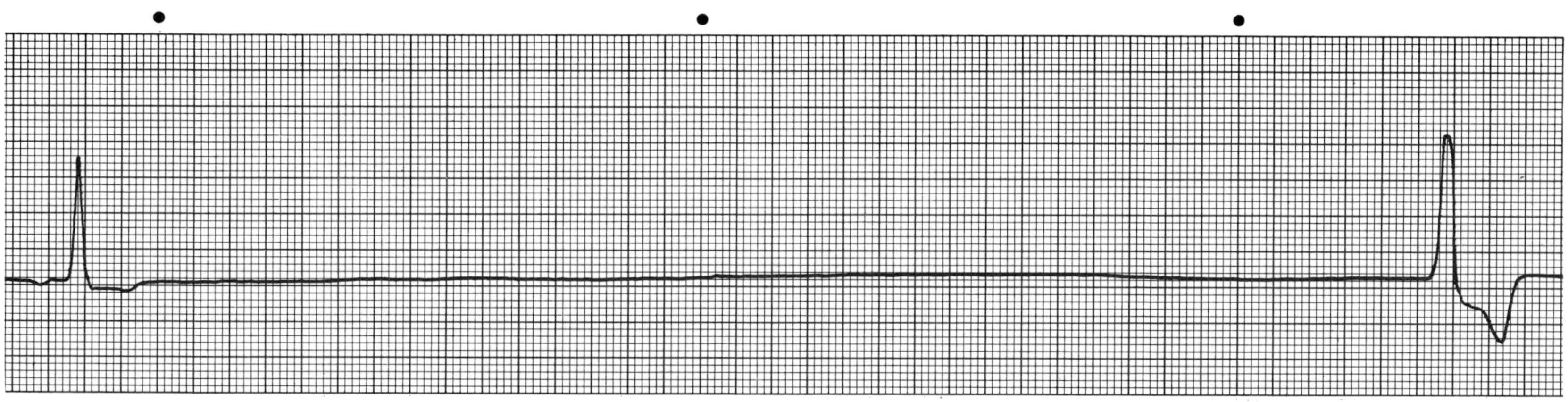

Question: This rhythm strip was recorded from a 14-year-old female Miniature Schnauzer with a history of exercise intolerance and collapse. The dog was being medicated with propantheline bromide.

1. What is the rhythm diagnosis?
2. What is the most likely underlying disorder?
3. What is the best therapeutic approach?

Case 113

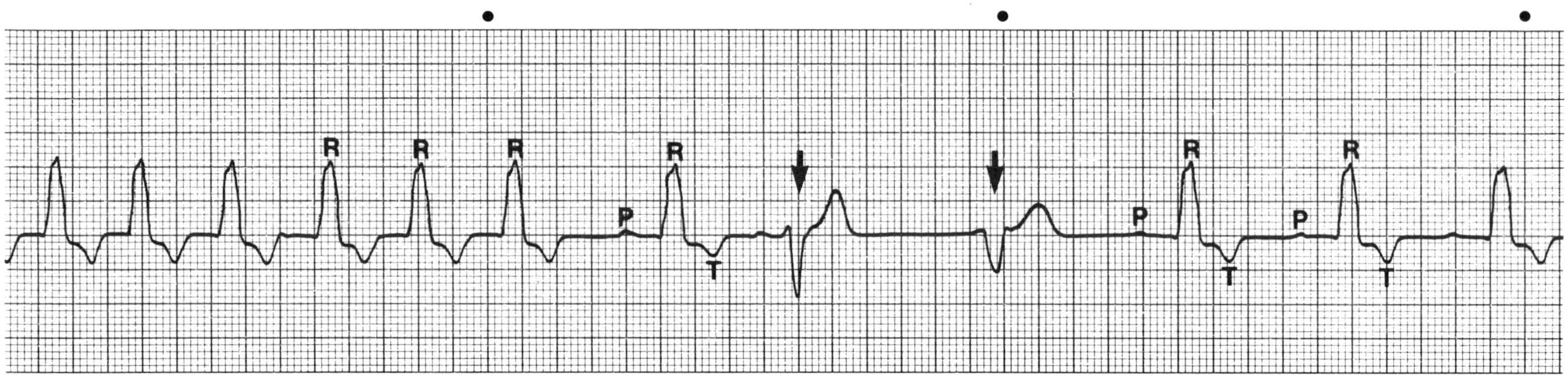

Answer: Sinus rhythm with left bundle-branch block, ventricular premature complexes (VPCs), and paroxysmal supraventricular tachycardia. Digoxin is the drug of choice for this arrhythmia, especially if clinical and radiographic evidence reveals congestive heart failure. Propranolol and diltiazem are alternative antiarrhythmic drugs that can be used to treat the paroxysmal supraventricular tachycardia if congestive heart failure is not evident. The wide complex tachycardia (first six QRS complexes) can be confused with ventricular tachycardia. Ventricular tachycardia is eliminated from the differential diagnosis because when the tachycardia spontaneously terminates, a sinus beat is seen (P-R-T) with a wide QRS complex resembling those during the tachycardia. This wide QRS complex sinus beat supports possible left bundle-branch block by the established criteria of prolonged duration of the QRS complexes, consistent P-R interval, and normal mean electrical axis. The two complexes labelled with arrows appear to be ventricular premature complexes typified by bizarre, premature QRS complexes that are not associated with P waves. The second complex actually occurs after a slightly longer cycle than the sinus beats (last three P waves) and may be a ventricular escape beat rather than a ventricular premature complex.

Case 114

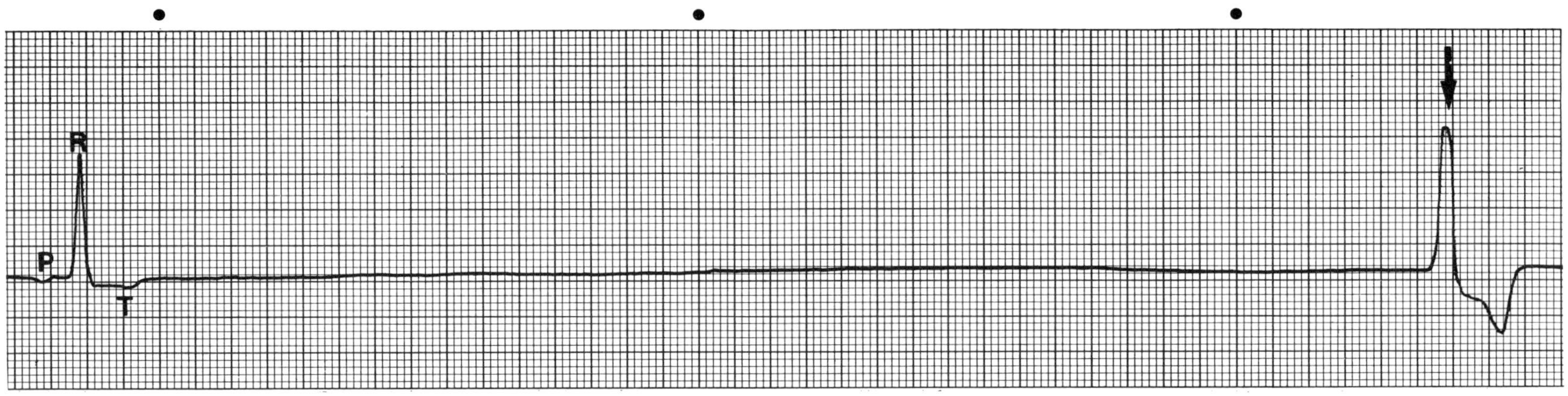

Answer: Long pause of sinoatrial block or sinus arrest followed by a ventricular escape beat (arrow). Sick sinus syndrome is probably present. Sick sinus syndrome is a term given to several electrocardiographic abnormalities of the SA node, including severe sinus bradycardia and severe SA block or sinus arrest. Many animals have recurrent episodes of supraventricular tachycardia. Because the AV junctional pacemaker fails to pace the heart, the term "sick escape pacemaker syndrome" also is used. Abnormalities of the AV junction or bundle branches may also develop. The prolonged sinus pauses may cause hypotension and collapse. Propantheline should be continued and a bronchodilator, such as theophylline, aminophylline, terbutaline, or albuterol, should be administered to raise the heart rate further. Bronchodilators increase sympathetic tone and indirectly stimulate the sinus node and ventricular escape rate. Sinus node disease can be a progressive problem, and implantation of a pacemaker is necessary when the animal no longer responds to medication.

Case 115

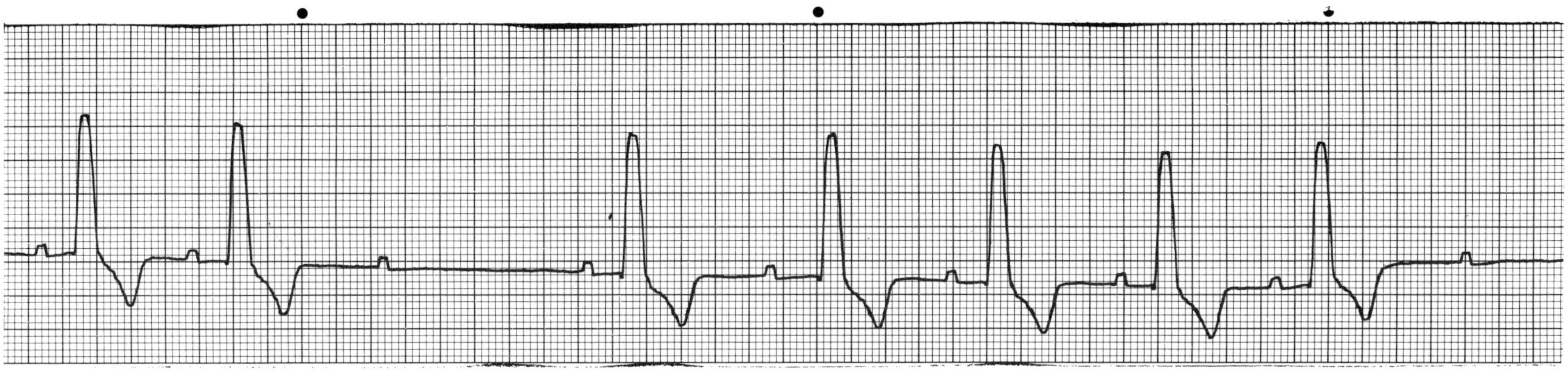

Question: This tracing was recorded from a Miniature Poodle with a history of fainting episodes that had occurred approximately 2 to 3 times a week.

1. What is the rhythm diagnosis?
2. What is the best therapeutic approach?
3. What abnormality other than the arrhythmia helps to determine the cause of the fainting episodes?

Case 116

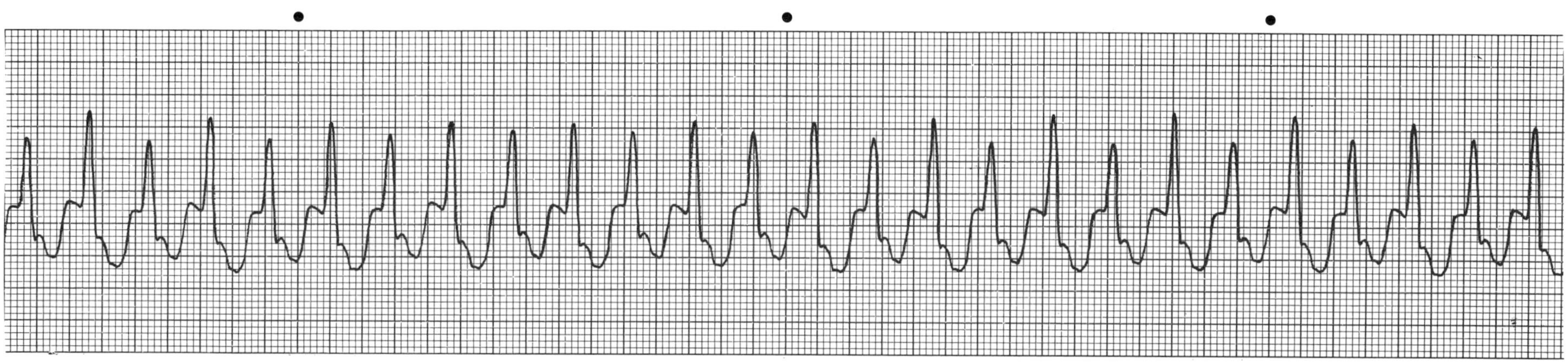

Question: This rhythm strip was recorded from a 2-year-old Poodle with patent ductus arteriosus. The dog was being treated with furosemide and digoxin. A previous ECG had revealed occasional atrial premature complexes. The dog was examined because of weakness.

1. What is the rhythm diagnosis?
2. What are common causes of this arrhythmia?
3. What is the most likely underlying disorder?
4. What is the best therapeutic approach?

Case 115

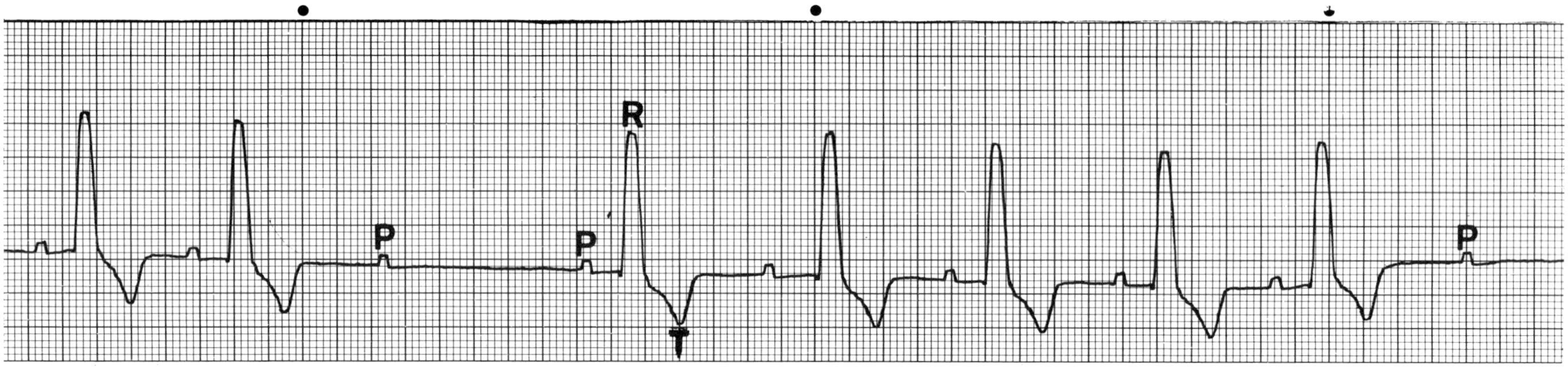

Answer: Second-degree AV block (marked P waves) and left bundle-branch block. The heart rate is variable. Left bundle-branch block is diagnosed by a QRS complex that is wide (0.07 sec or greater) and is positive in leads I, II, III, and aVF and in leads over the left precordium. The presence of first-degree or second-degree AV block in this case may indicate involvement of the right bundle branch. Left bundle-branch block must be differentiated from left ventricular enlargement. The absence of left ventricular enlargement on thoracic radiographs lends support to a diagnosis of left bundle-branch block. The second-degree AV block is Mobitz type II, because no change is evident in the P-R intervals preceding the nonconducted P waves. The fainting episodes in this dog are probably related to periods of more advanced AV block or complete heart block. A 24-hour ambulatory (Holter monitor) ECG may be needed to confirm this hypothesis. If signs do not resolve with anticholinergic drugs, a permanent pacemaker would be indicated.

Case 116

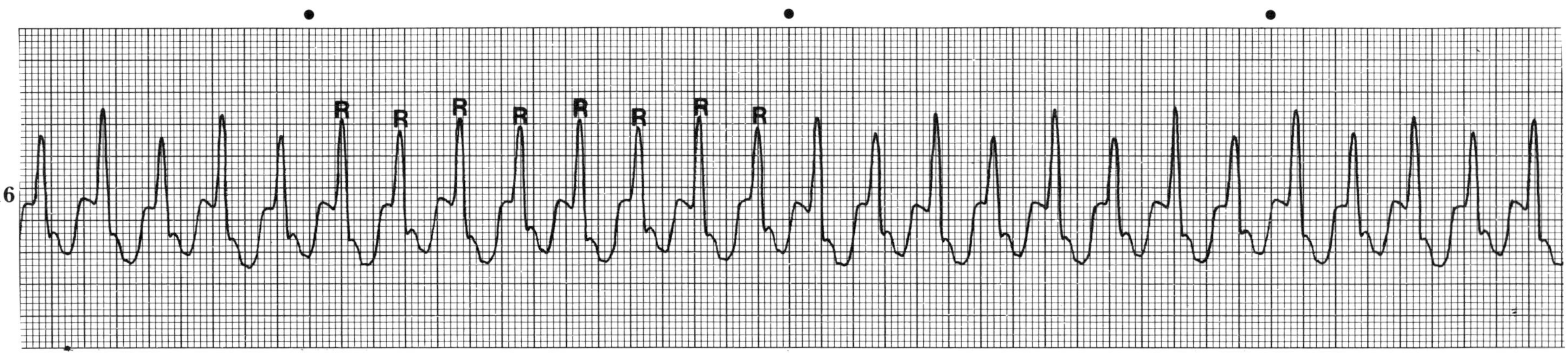

Answer: Supraventricular tachycardia. Heart rate is 320 beats/min. The differential diagnosis for this supraventricular tachycardia should include atrial tachycardia and atrial flutter. Supraventricular tachycardia is generally associated with atrial distention, which would be expected in a dog with patent ductus arteriosus. Supraventricular tachycardia is also seen in animals with digoxin toxicity. This dog, however, had atrial premature complexes before digoxin was prescribed and has had no history of anorexia or vomiting. Electrical alternans is associated with pericardial effusion, supraventricular tachycardia, and alternating bundle-branch block. In a dog with a fast heart rate, electrical alternans results from differences in recovery rate of the individual fibers. A retrograde accessory AV pathway in the tachycardia circuit may be present. Although digoxin is probably not causing the arrhythmia in this dog, the serum digoxin concentration should be determined to rule out toxicity. A vagal maneuver (ocular pressure or carotid sinus massage) should be used to try to break the tachycardia, thereby determining the underlying mechanism. Diltiazem, propranolol, or adenosine should be prescribed to control the arrhythmia.

Case 117

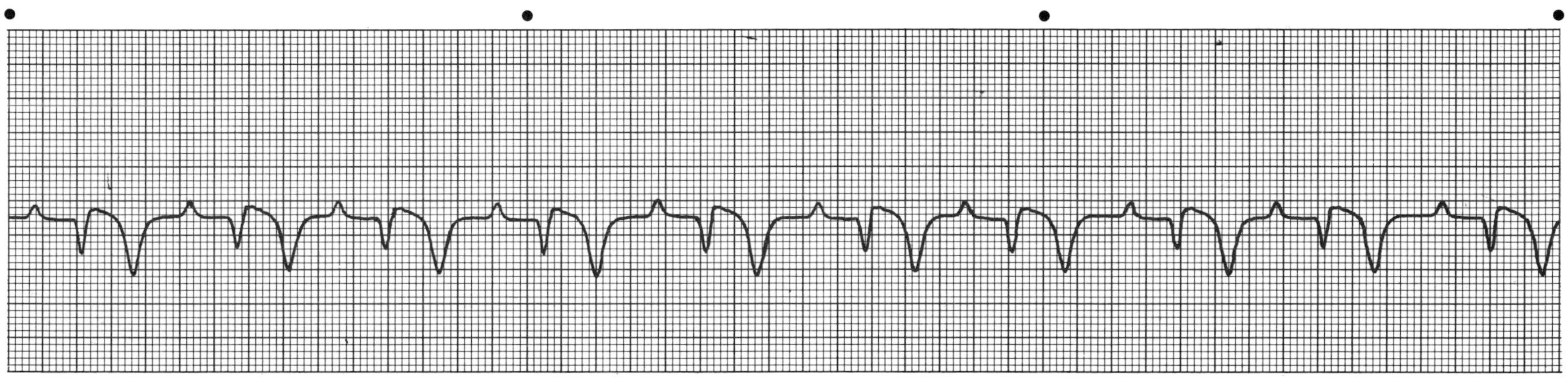

Question: This rhythm strip was recorded from a 4-year-old Coonhound with a history of coughing and ascites. Thoracic radiographs revealed severe right heart enlargement and enlarged pulmonary arteries.

1. What is the rhythm diagnosis?
2. What is the most likely underlying disorder?
3. What is the best therapeutic approach?

Case 118

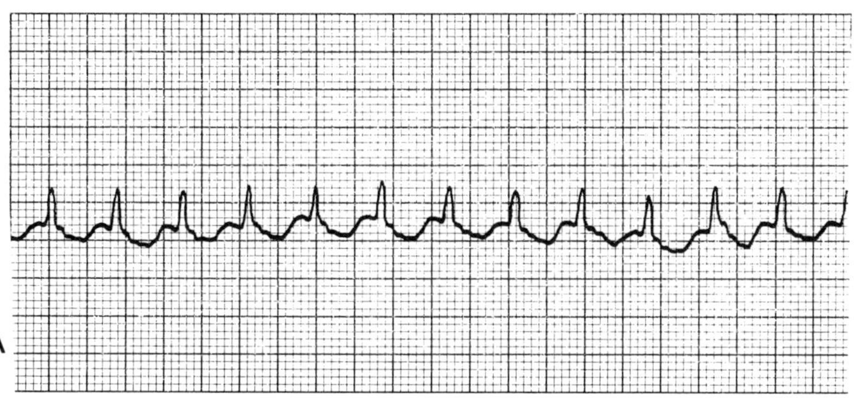

A

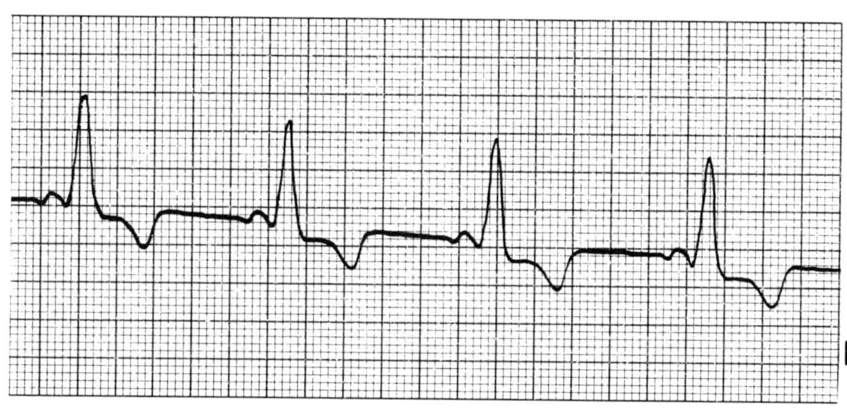

B

Question: This lead II ECG was recorded from a 3-year-old domestic shorthair cat with a history of episodic panting.

1. What is the rhythm diagnosis?
2. What is a common cause of this arrhythmia?
3. What is the most likely underlying disorder?
4. What is the best therapeutic approach?

Case 117

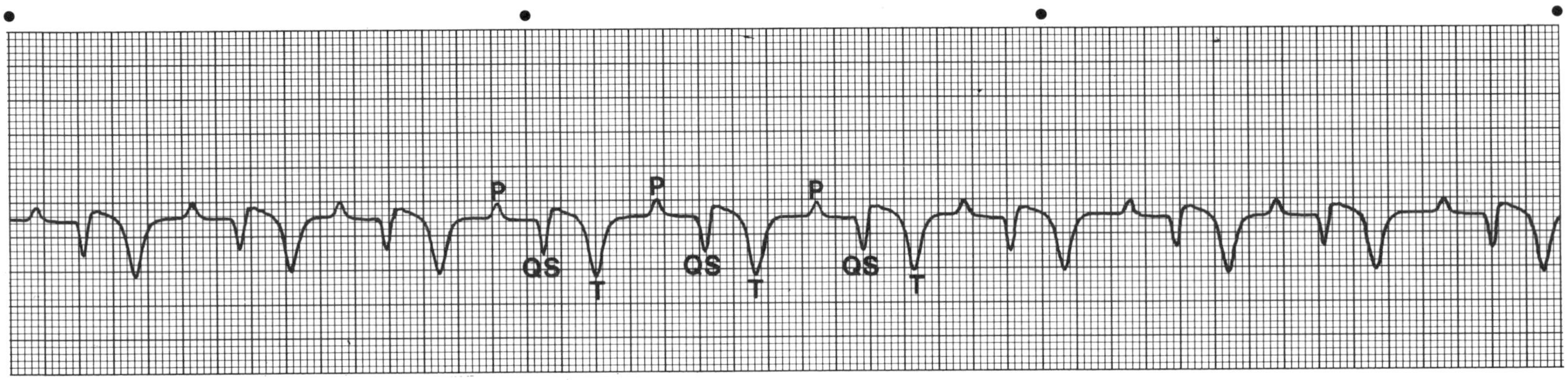

Answer: Sinus rhythm with first-degree AV block. Heart rate is 130 beats/min. First-degree AV block is diagnosed by the slightly prolonged P-R interval (0.14 sec). Leads I and III were negative. The right axis and normal QRS duration may indicate right ventricular enlargement. The large T waves are compatible with myocardial hypoxia or underlying metabolic or electrolyte imbalance. This diagnosis is consistent with the radiographic findings. Right heart enlargement with enlarged pulmonary arteries is probably associated with heartworm disease. A blood sample should be obtained to rule out this disease. First-degree AV block does not cause clinical signs and does not warrant treatment. Administer furosemide for the ascites.

Case 118

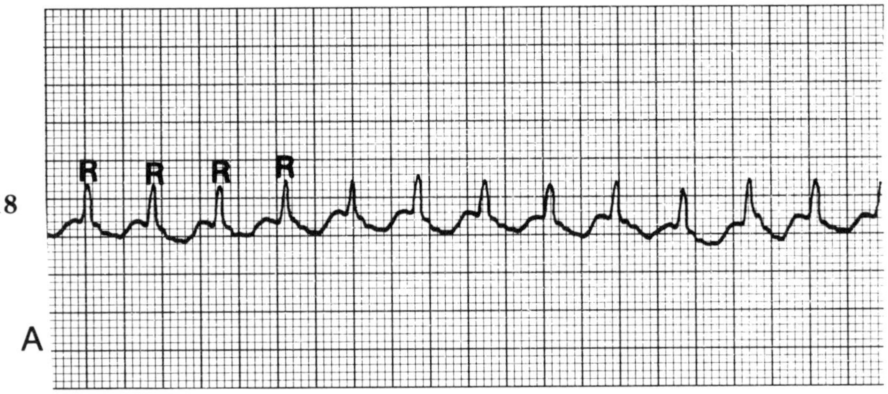

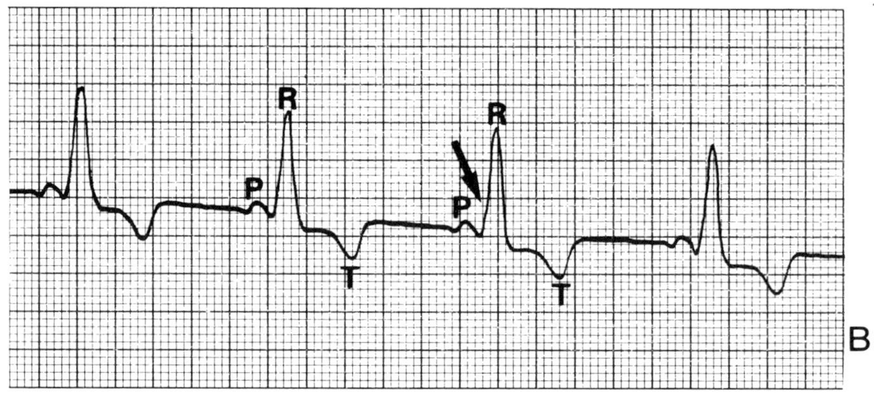

Answer: A. Supraventricular tachycardia. Heart rate is 400 beats/min. B. Sinus rhythm with ventricular pre-excitation. Heart rate is 110 beats/min. The initial ECG reveals a rapid, narrow complex tachycardia that is positive in lead II. These characteristics support the diagnosis of supraventricular tachycardia. Drugs useful for treating supraventricular tachycardia include digoxin, diltiazem, and propranolol. Diltiazem and propranolol have the most rapid onset of action. In this instance, diltiazem was administered orally, and strip B was obtained 1 hour later. The follow-up ECG shows sinus rhythm with a shortened P-R interval. Also apparent is an early slur to the QRS complex (arrow) that is referred to as a delta wave. The short P-R interval is caused by an AV nodal bypass tract that causes early activation of the ventricle. Conduction also occurs normally through the AV node, thereby resulting in a relatively normal QRS complex with a wide base caused by early activation of the ventricle by the bypass tract. Supraventricular tachycardia can be explained by the mechanism of re-entry. A circus movement develops within a re-entrant circuit involving the normal AV nodal pathway and the bypass tract. A narrow complex tachycardia occurs when the circus movement results in impulses passing in the normal direction (antegrade) through the AV node. A wide complex tachycardia occurs when the circus movement results in impulses passing in the reverse direction (retrograde) through the AV node. The combination of short P-R interval, wide QRS complex, delta wave, and supraventricular tachycardia is referred to as Wolff-Parkinson-White syndrome. Once this syndrome is diagnosed, either diltiazem or propranolol should be continued to prevent narrow complex tachycardic episodes.

Case 119

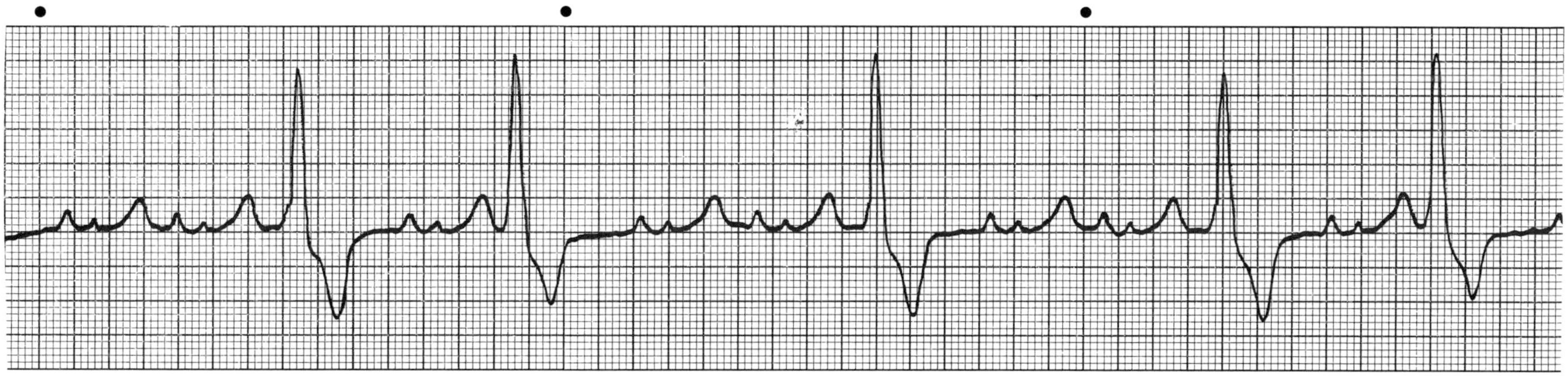

Question: This ECG was obtained from a 9-year-old Pug examined because of cyanosis and severe dyspnea. Thoracic radiographs revealed marked pleural effusion.

1. What is the rhythm diagnosis?
2. What is the best therapeutic approach?

Case 120

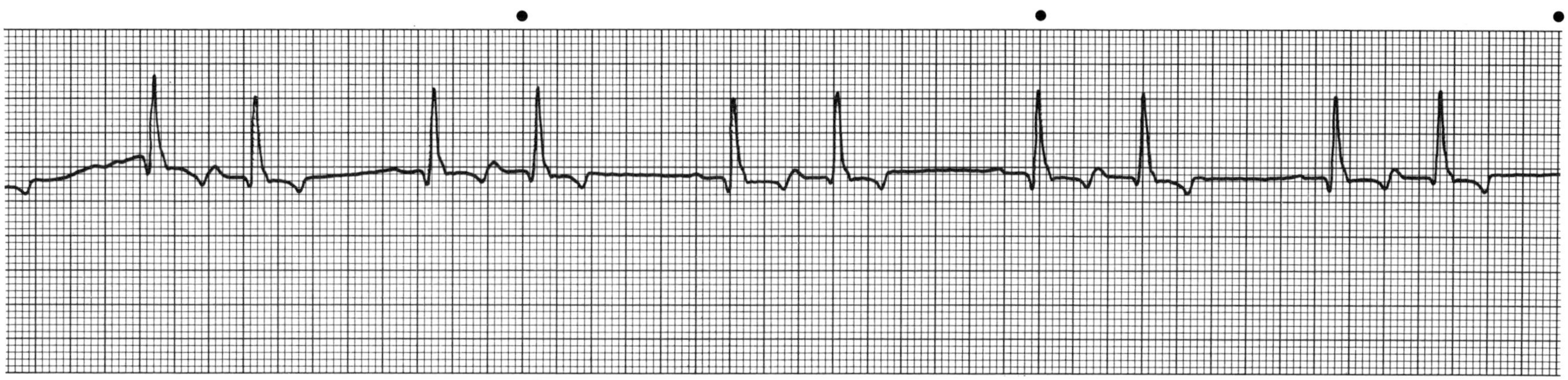

Question: This rhythm strip was recorded from an 8-year-old Boston Terrier with a grade III/VI holosystolic murmur and history of congestive heart failure. The dog was being treated with furosemide.

1. What is the rhythm diagnosis?
2. What is the most likely underlying disorder?
3. What is the best therapeutic approach?

Case 119

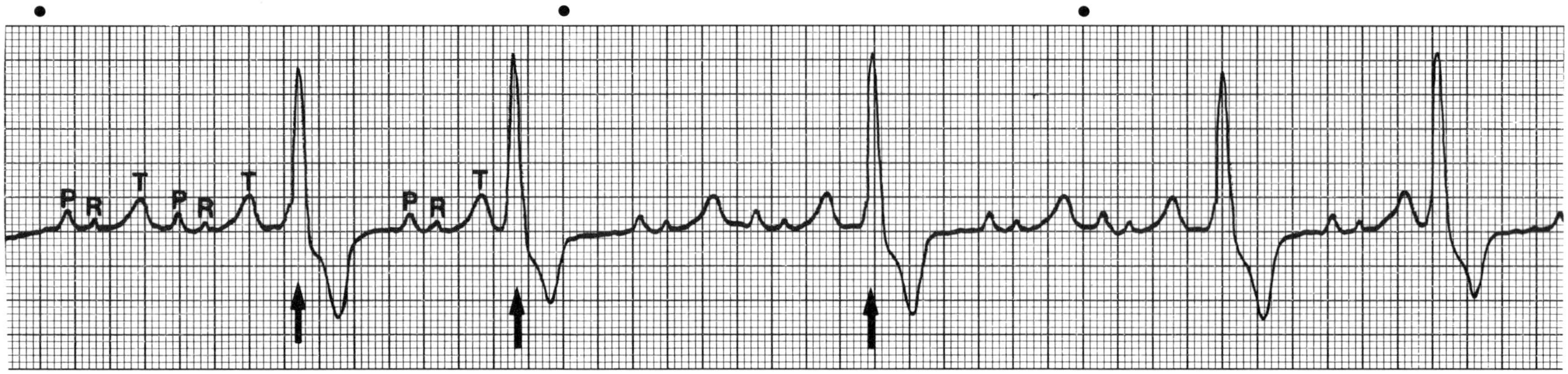

Answer: Sinus rhythm with ventricular premature complexes. Heart rate is approximately 170 beats/min. Before treating with antiarrhythmic drugs, the pleural effusion should be controlled with thoracocentesis and diuretics. An echocardiogram may also aid in diagnosing the underlying disorder. The small QRS complexes are probably caused by the pleural effusion. The ventricular premature complexes (arrows) are characterized by wide and bizarre QRS complexes that are not associated with P waves. The positive polarity of the ventricular premature complexes suggests possible right ventricular origin. If clinical signs persist after the pleural effusion has been controlled, procainamide, quinidine, or tocainide should be administered.

Case 120

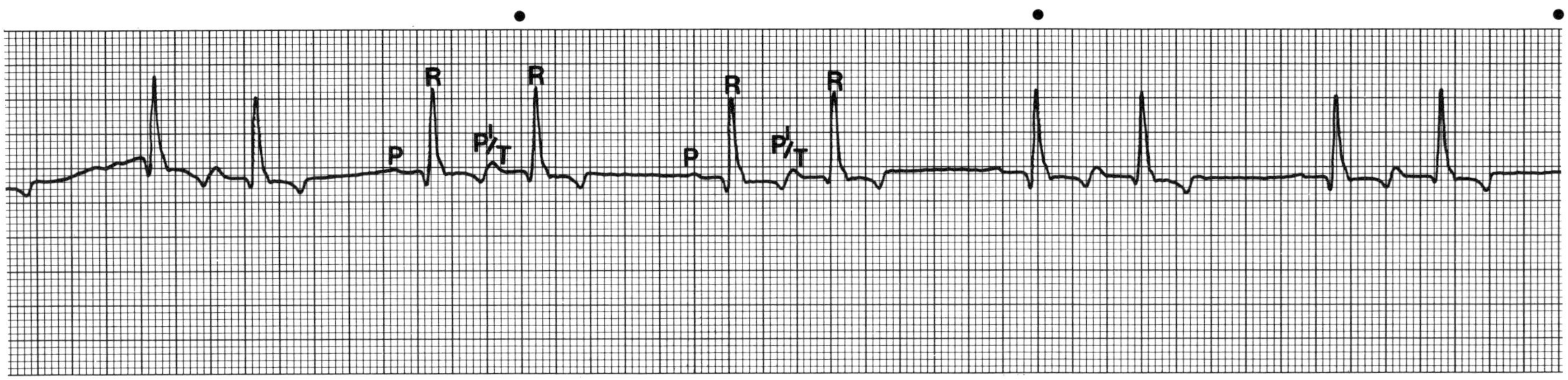

Answer: Sinus rhythm with atrial bigeminy. Heart rate is approximately 140 beats/min. Every other QRS complex occurs prematurely and shares the same configuration as that of the sinus complexes. The premature complexes are atrial premature complexes (atrial bigeminy). The beginning of the P′ wave of the atrial premature complexes is superimposed on the end of the T wave of the sinus complex. The atrial premature complexes are probably secondary to atrial distention caused by degenerative mitral valve disease. Digoxin is indicated because of the high frequency of the atrial premature complexes, coupled with signs of congestive heart failure in this dog. A follow-up ECG should be obtained in 5 to 7 days to monitor the effect of the digoxin.

Case 121

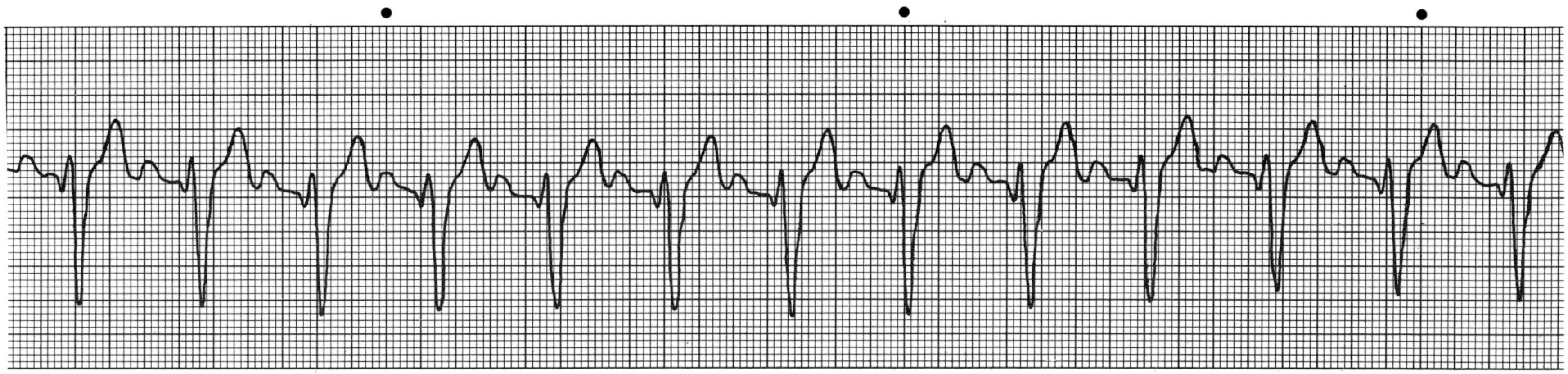

Question: This lead II ECG was obtained from a 12-year-old Standard Poodle that was examined because of a mild cough. A prominent heart murmur was heard on auscultation at the left fifth intercostal space. Leads I, III, and aVF had large, wide S waves.

1. What is the rhythm diagnosis?
2. What is the best therapeutic approach?

Case 122

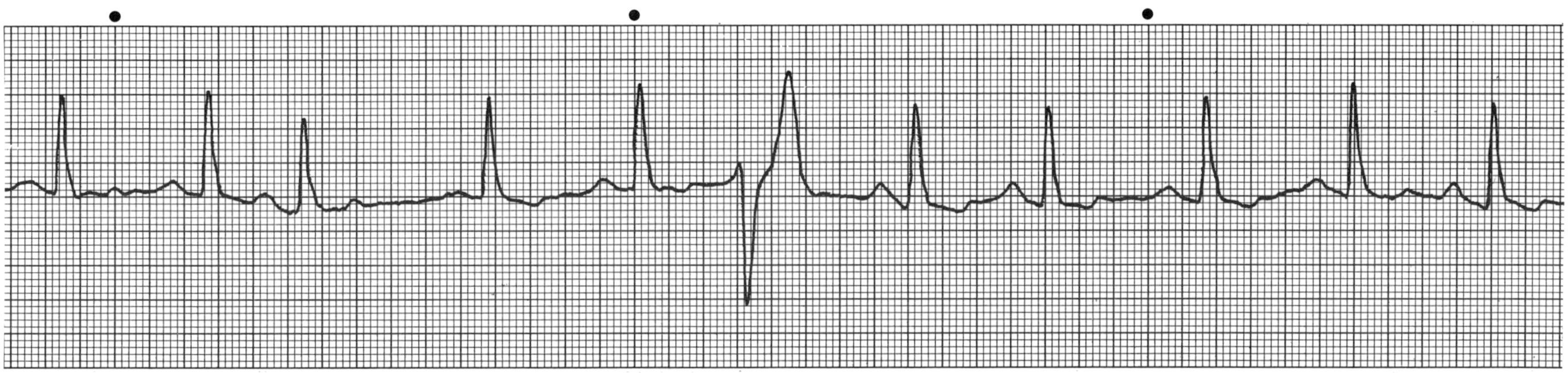

Question: This lead II ECG was obtained from a 10-year-old Wheaten Terrier with a recent history of coughing. A grade V/VI holosystolic murmur over the left fifth intercostal space and lung crackles were heard on auscultation.

1. What is the rhythm diagnosis?
2. What is the most likely underlying disorder?
3. What is the best therapeutic approach?

Case 121

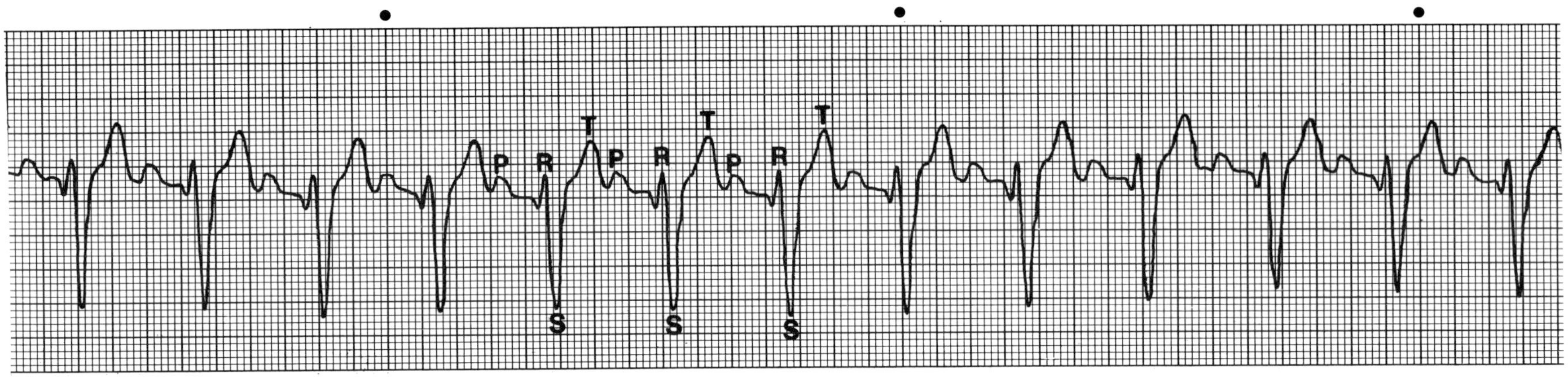

Answer: Sinus rhythm with right bundle-branch block. Heart rate is 180 beats/min. No specific treatment exists for right bundle-branch block. Thoracic radiographs should be taken to rule out congestive heart failure and heartworm disease. Right bundle-branch block is characterized by prolongation of the QRS complex and deep and wide S waves in leads I, II, and aVF, and in left precordial chest leads. The mean electrical axis shows a right axis deviation pattern. Although the wide QRS complexes can be confused with a ventricular arrhythmia, the consistent P-R interval of right bundle-branch block eliminates ventricular tachycardia as a diagnosis.

Case 122

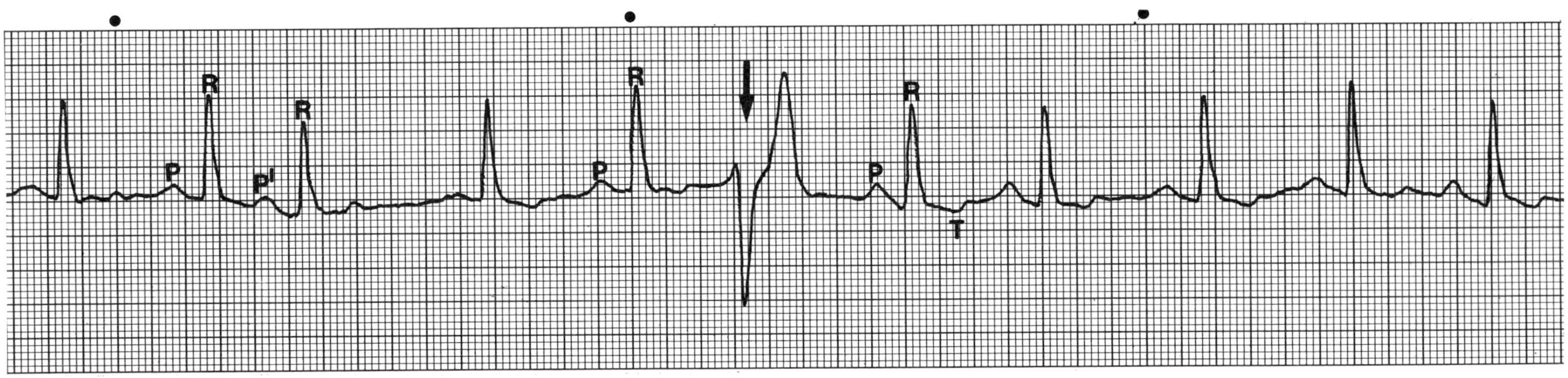

Answer: Sinus rhythm with one atrial premature complex (P′-R-T) and one ventricular premature complex (arrow). Heart rate is 140 beats/min. Progressive mitral valvular insufficiency with left atrial dilation and ventricular myocardial disease are the most likely underlying disorders. Administration of a diuretic and a vasodilator is the best therapeutic approach if congestive heart failure is confirmed on radiography. Antiarrhythmic therapy is not indicated because of the heart rate and low frequency of premature complexes. Atrial premature complexes are characterized by premature P′ waves followed by QRS complexes that resemble the sinus beats. Ventricular premature complexes are typified by premature QRS complexes that are bizarre when compared with the sinus complexes. No relationship exists between atrial depolarization (P waves) and ventricular premature complexes.

Case 123

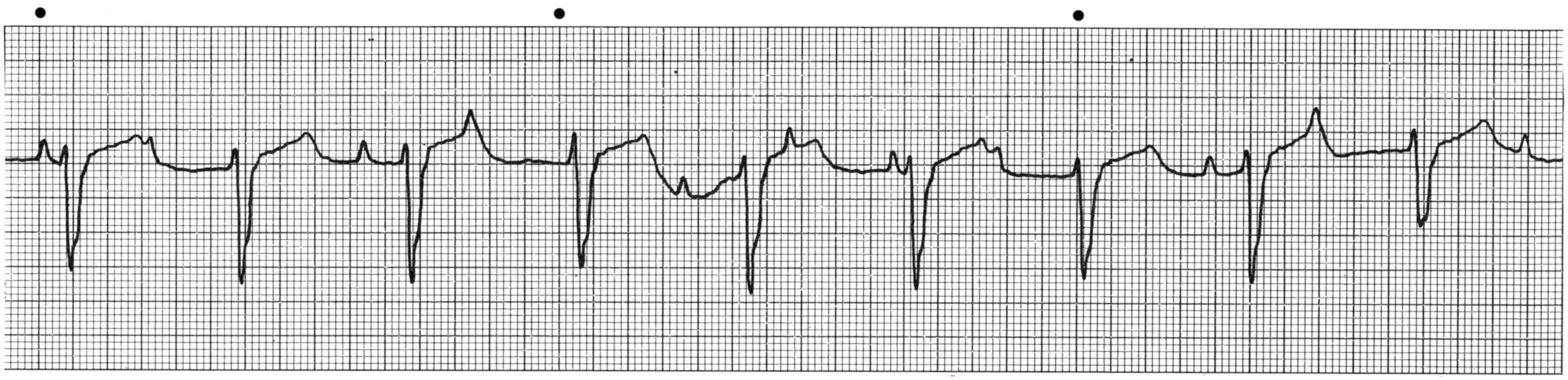

Question: This lead II ECG was obtained from a 14-year-old mixed-breed dog with no clinical signs. The dog had intermittent jugular venous pulsations and a variable intensity first heart sound.

1. What is the rhythm diagnosis?
2. What is the most likely underlying disorder?
3. What is the best therapeutic approach?

Case 124

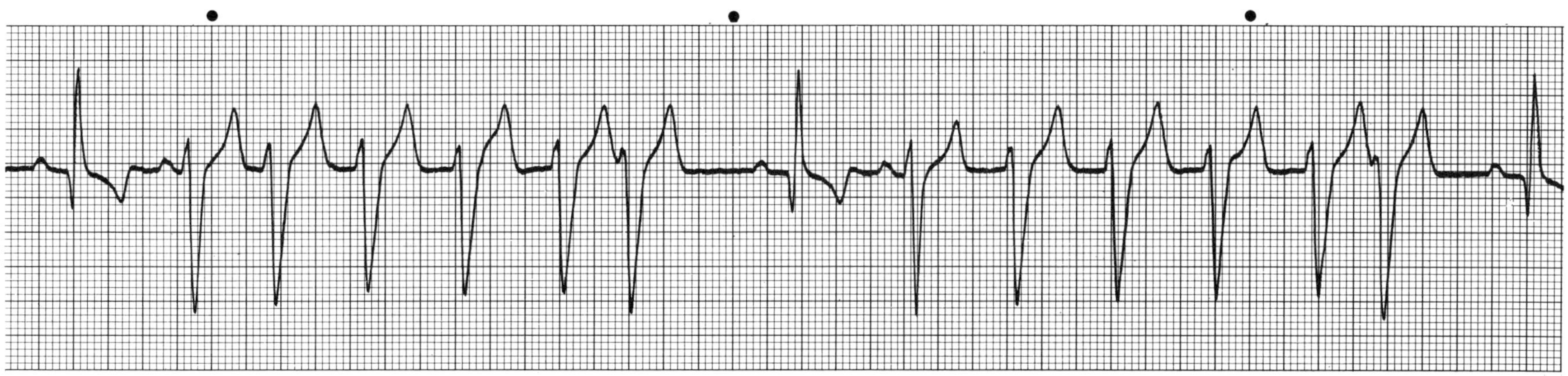

Question: This rhythm strip was recorded from a 6-year-old German Shepherd with a history of collapse. A splenic mass was seen on radiographs.

1. What is the rhythm diagnosis?
2. What are common causes of this arrhythmia?
3. What is the most likely underlying disorder?
4. What is the best therapeutic approach?

Case 123

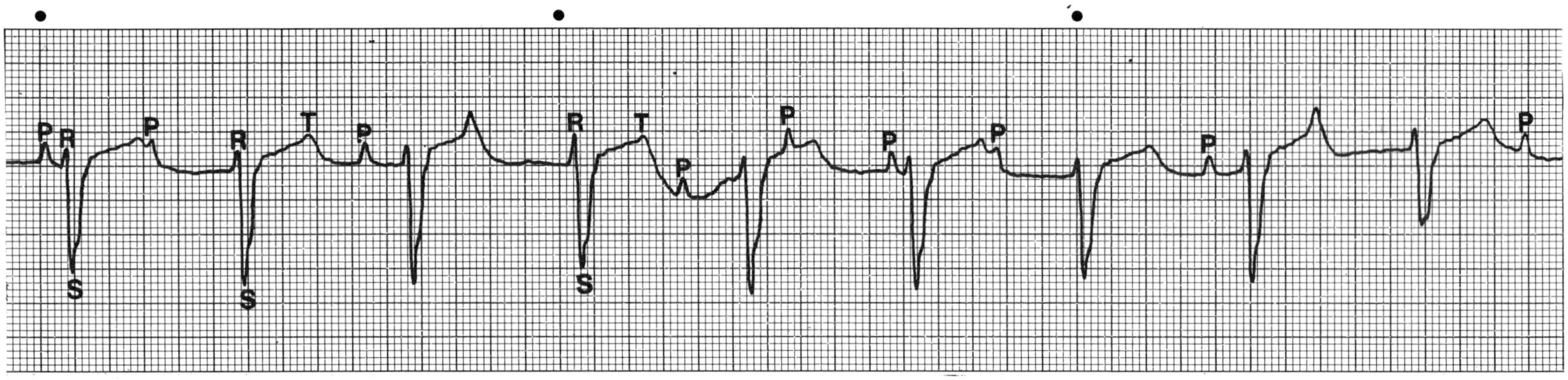

Answer: Sinus rhythm with complete (third-degree) AV block. Heart rate is 120 beats/min. Idiopathic fibrosis of the AV conduction system is the most likely underlying disorder. Hypertrophic cardiomyopathy, infectious endocarditis, and Lyme myocarditis should also be considered. Because the dog has no clinical signs, treatment is not needed. If a slower escape rhythm and subsequent clinical signs of weakness or syncope develop, a permanent cardiac pacemaker will be required to maintain adequate heart rate and cardiac output. Jugular venous pulsations and variable intensity first heart sounds are physical examination indicators of AV dissociation caused by complete heart block or ventricular arrhythmias.

Case 124

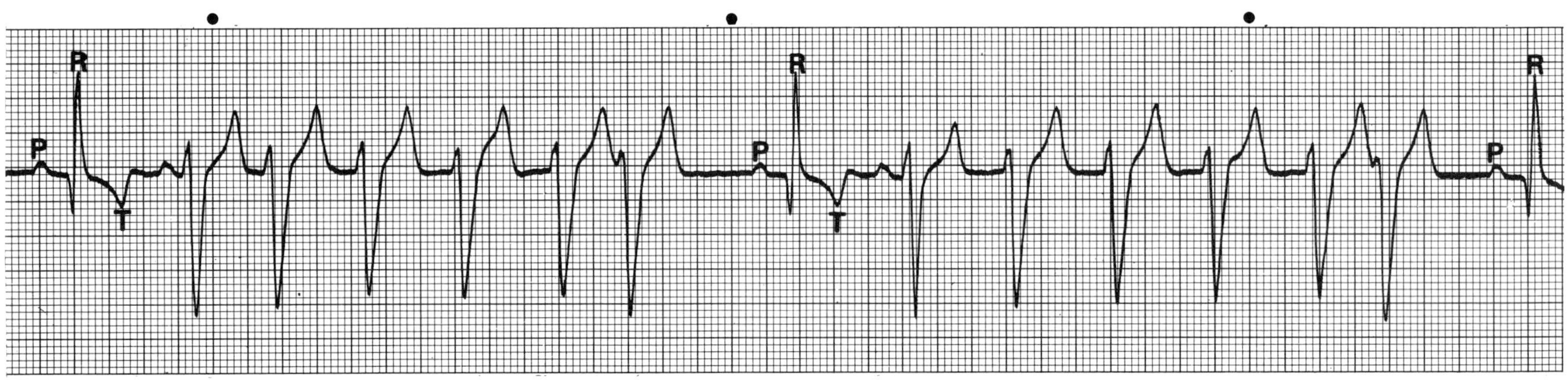

Answer: Sinus rhythm with paroxysmal ventricular tachycardia. Heart rate is approximately 200 beats/min. Ventricular tachycardia is associated with numerous diseases of the myocardium. The differential diagnosis includes dilated cardiomyopathy, myocarditis, trauma, toxin ingestion, and neoplasia. The mass seen on abdominal radiographs raises concern about a neoplastic cause for this arrhythmia. Hemangiosarcoma is common in this breed. The tumor may be a primary cardiac tumor or may be secondary to metastasis from the spleen. Dilated cardiomyopathy is also common in this breed. Collapse may have been caused by the arrhythmia or by rupture of the spleen. Thoracic radiographs were normal. The arrhythmia was controlled with lidocaine and a splenic hemangiosarcoma was removed. Long-term antiarrhythmic control was maintained with procainamide.

Case 125

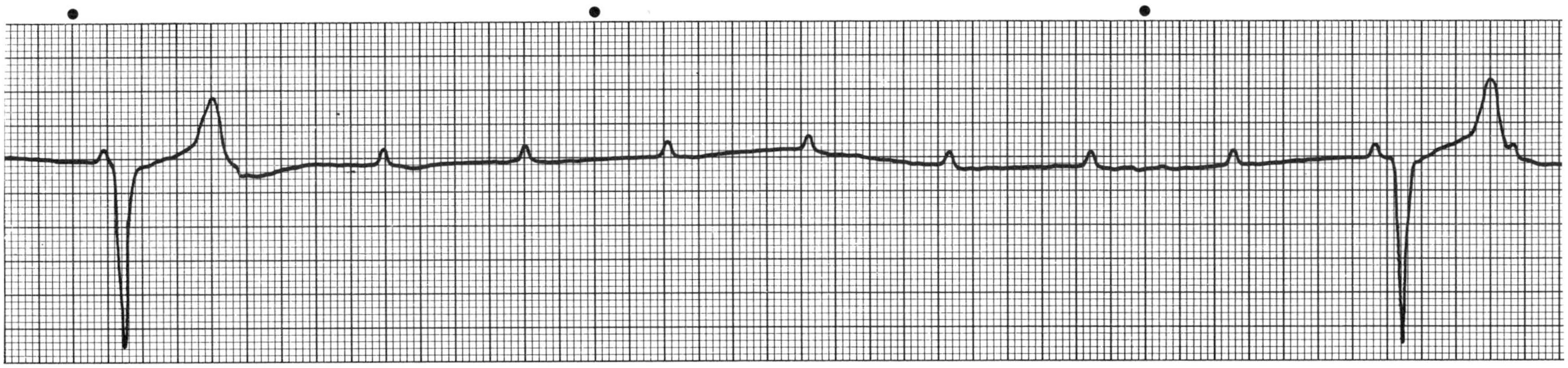

Question: This lead II ECG was obtained from a 3-year-old German Shepherd with a recent history of forelimb lameness and progressive weakness. Laboratory testing revealed a positive titer for antibodies to *Borrelia burgdorferi*.

1. What is the rhythm diagnosis?
2. What is the most likely underlying disorder?
3. What is the best therapeutic approach?

Case 126

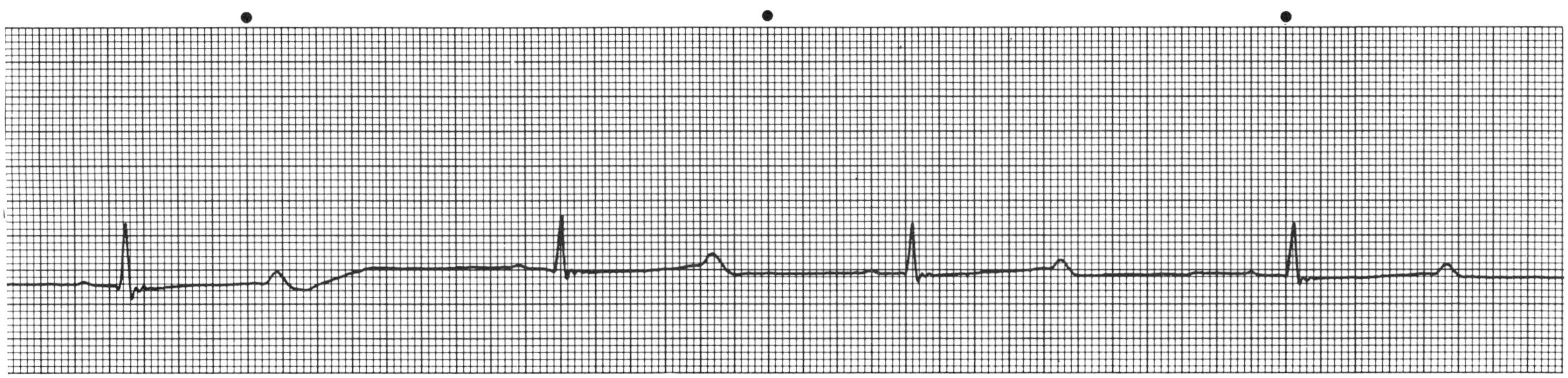

Question: This tracing was recorded from a 7-year-old Great Dane with severe vomiting and diarrhea secondary to pancreatitis.

1. What is the rhythm diagnosis?
2. To what serious arrhythmia is the animal prone?
3. What is the most likely underlying disorder?

Case 125

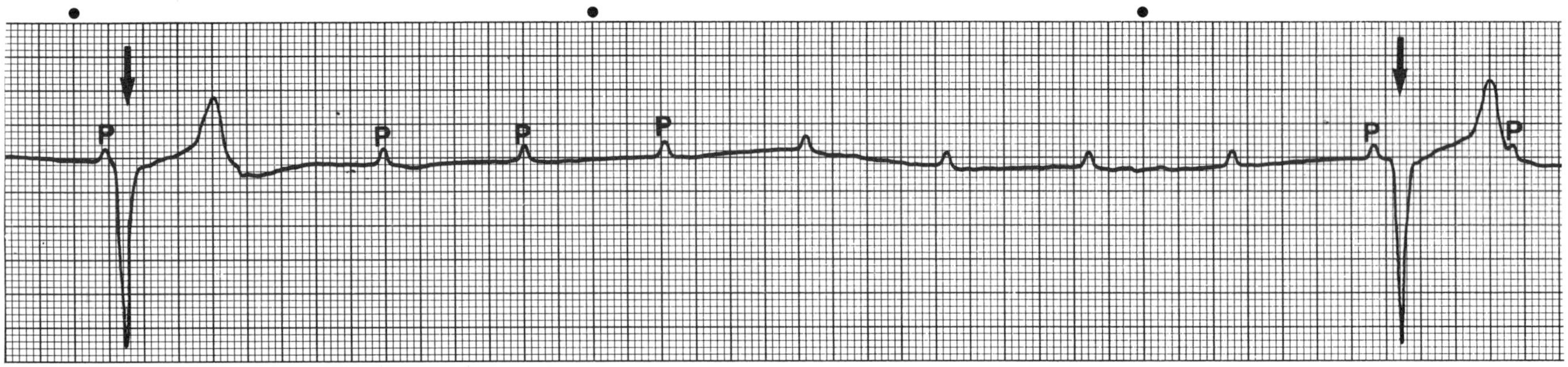

Answer: Sinus rhythm with complete (third-degree) AV block. Ventricular heart rate is 16 beats/min; atrial heart rate is 145 beats/min. Lyme carditis should first be considered as the underlying disorder. Hypertrophic cardiomyopathy should be ruled out by echocardiography. If an anticholinergic drug (e.g., atropine) does not cause a marked increase in heart rate, a temporary or permanent cardiac pacemaker is the best therapeutic approach. The location of the heart block may be the AV node, His bundle, or bundle-branch fascicles. The heart block location is important, because AV nodal block often responds to anticholinergics and sympathomimetics. Conversely, AV block in the His bundle or below does not respond to cardiac drugs. The ventricular escape impulse rate (arrows) may increase with intravenously administered sympathomimetics (e.g., isoproterenol and dobutamine). The AV block associated with Lyme carditis in human beings is often reversible with appropriate antibiotic therapy, but the success of such therapy has not been determined in dogs. A His bundle electrogram with measurement of the A-H and H-V intervals is of great value in determining the location of advanced AV block.

Case 126

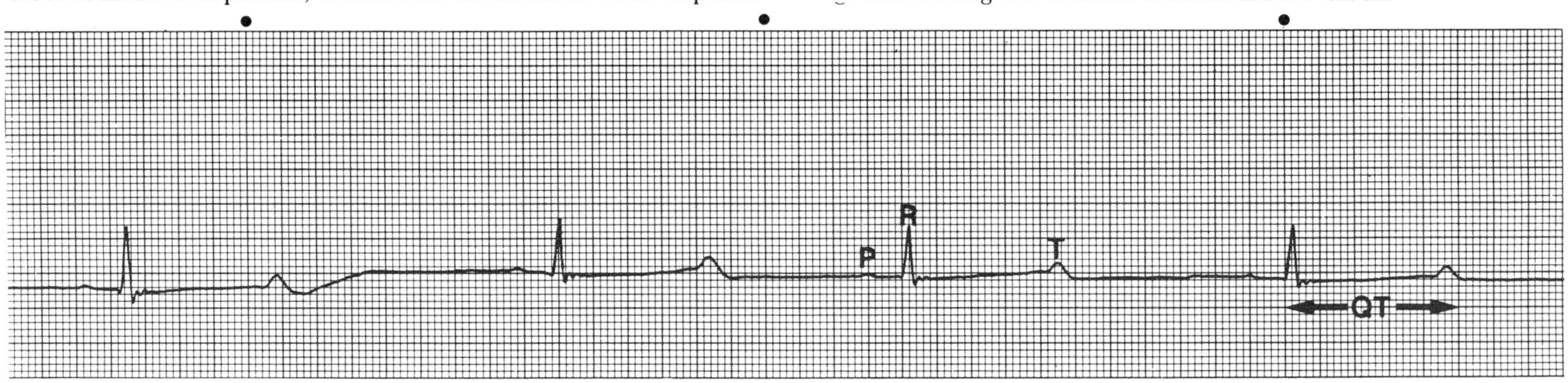

Answer: Sinus bradycardia and prolongation of the Q-T interval (0.50 sec or 25 boxes). Heart rate is 50 beats/min. The Q-T interval varies with the heart rate; the faster the heart rate, the shorter the interval. Various formulas and tables define the relationship of the Q-T interval to heart rate, age, and sex. A sometimes useful rule states that the Q-T interval should be less than half the preceding R-R interval for normal sinus heart rates. Severe hypocalcemia (serum calcium: 1.9 mg/dl) was present. Potential causes of hypocalcemia in pancreatitis include hypoalbuminemia, saponification of calcium salts in necrotic peripancreatic fat, hyperglucagonemia causing hypercalcitoninism, and decreased parathormone release or activity resulting from hypomagnesemia. Some other causes of a prolonged Q-T interval are ethylene glycol poisoning, hypokalemia hypothermia, and central nervous system disorders, and drugs (e.g., quinidine). The vulnerable period of the ventricles is increased so that ventricular premature complexes falling within that period can result in ventricular fibrillation. The Q-T interval returns to normal when the underlying disorder has been controlled.

Case 127

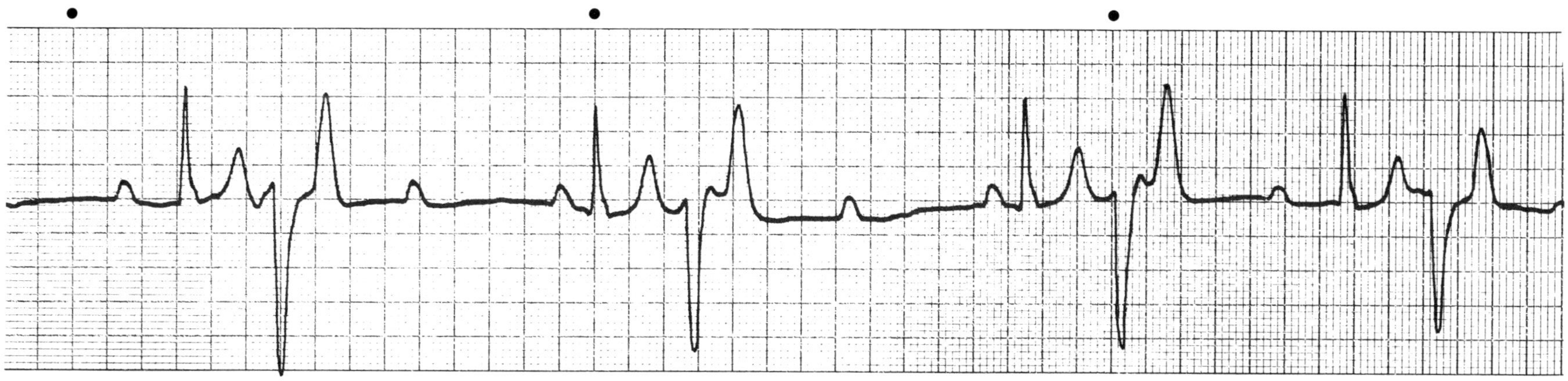

Question: This lead II ECG was obtained from a 9-year-old male Wirehaired Fox Terrier after 2 years of digoxin and furosemide administration for treatment of congestive heart failure.

1. What is the rhythm diagnosis?
2. What is the most likely underlying disorder?
3. What is the best therapeutic approach?

Case 128

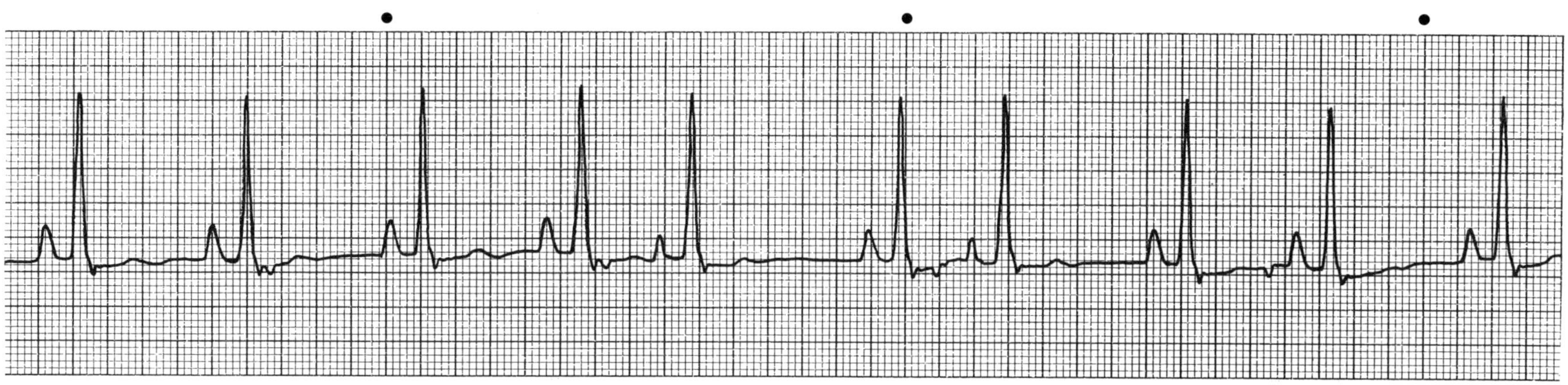

Question: This lead II ECG was obtained from a 9-year-old female Miniature Poodle examined because of a worsening cough.

1. What is the rhythm diagnosis?
2. What is the most likely underlying disorder?
3. What is the best therapeutic approach?

Case 127

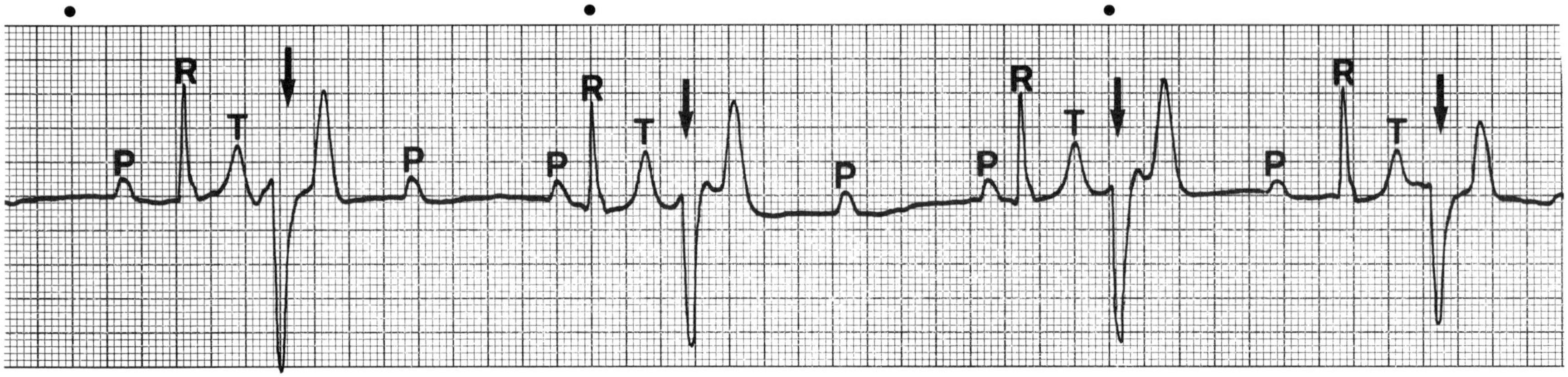

Answer: Sinus rhythm with ventricular premature complexes (arrows) and second-degree AV block. Heart rate is 100 beats/min. The digoxin should be stopped for 48 to 72 hours followed by a repeat ECG. The administration of antiarrhythmic drugs should be delayed until the results of the follow-up ECG are assessed. The bizarre, negative QRS complexes that are not associated with P waves typify ventricular premature complexes. Ventricular bigeminy is present, with every other complex a ventricular premature complex. The P waves not followed by QRS complexes represent second-degree AV block secondary to concealed conduction and possible primary AV nodal conduction disease associated with digitalis toxicity. The ventricular premature complex impulses conduct retrograde to the area of the AV node and depolarize this area. The sinus beats following the ventricular premature complex either do not conduct to the ventricles (P wave following the first ventricular premature complex) or conduct slower than normal (P-R interval following the third ventricular premature complex is longer than the normal P-R interval in front of the third ventricular premature complex). The elimination of the ventricular premature complexes probably will allow the nonconducted or poorly conducted sinus beats to resolve.

Case 128

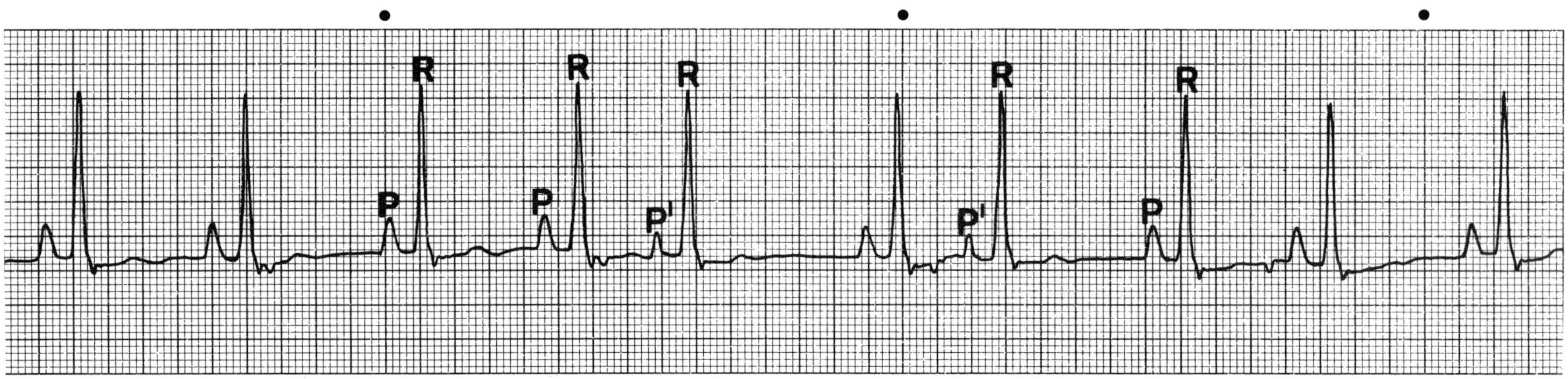

Answer: Sinus rhythm with atrial premature complexes. Heart rate is 130 beats/min. Mitral valvular insufficiency with a dilated left atrium is the most likely underlying disorder, provided a prominent heart murmur is heard over the left hemithorax. Digoxin is the preferred drug for treating the atrial premature complexes, along with a diuretic and vasodilator if congestive heart failure is confirmed on thoracic radiographs. High-amplitude P waves suggest right atrial enlargement and possible bronchial disease or tracheal collapse. The atrial premature complexes could be caused by cardiac or pulmonary disease. The premature P′ waves followed by QRS complexes that resemble those of the sinus beat are the hallmark of atrial premature complexes. The change in P′ wave morphology also supports a diagnosis of atrial premature complexes.

Case 129

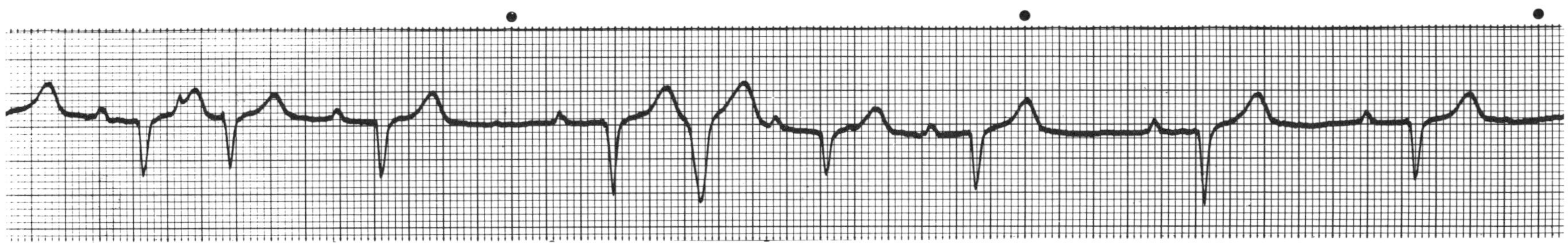

Question: This lead II ECG was obtained from a 12-year-old cat with pleural effusion and an echocardiographic diagnosis of dilated cardiomyopathy.

1. What is the rhythm diagnosis?
2. What is the best therapeutic approach?

Case 130

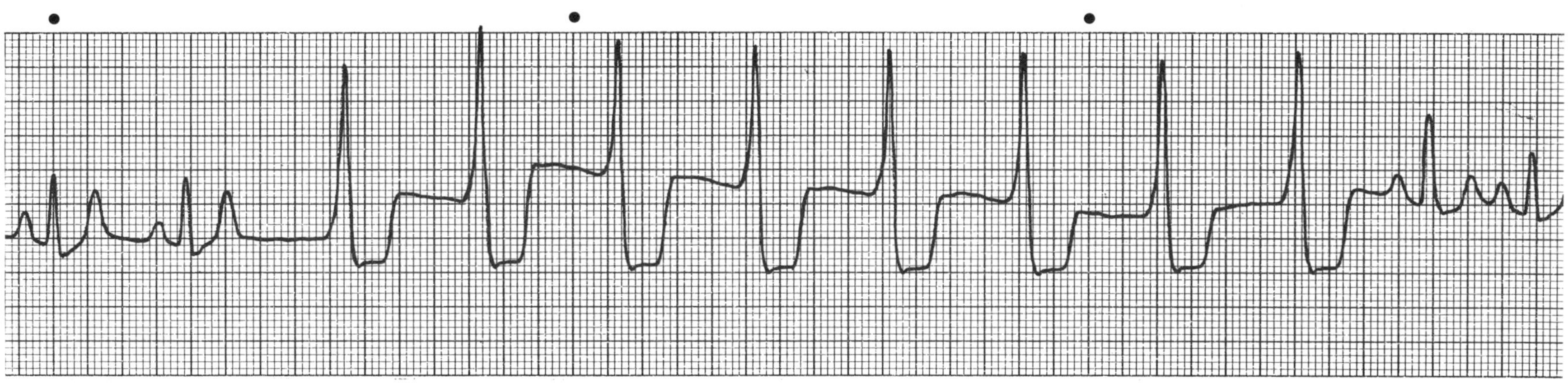

Question: This rhythm strip was recorded from a 10-year-old Poodle with a grade III/VI holosystolic mitral murmur. The dog was being treated with furosemide for congestive heart failure and had no clinical signs.

1. What is the rhythm diagnosis?
2. What are common causes of this arrhythmia?
3. What is the best therapeutic approach?

Case 129

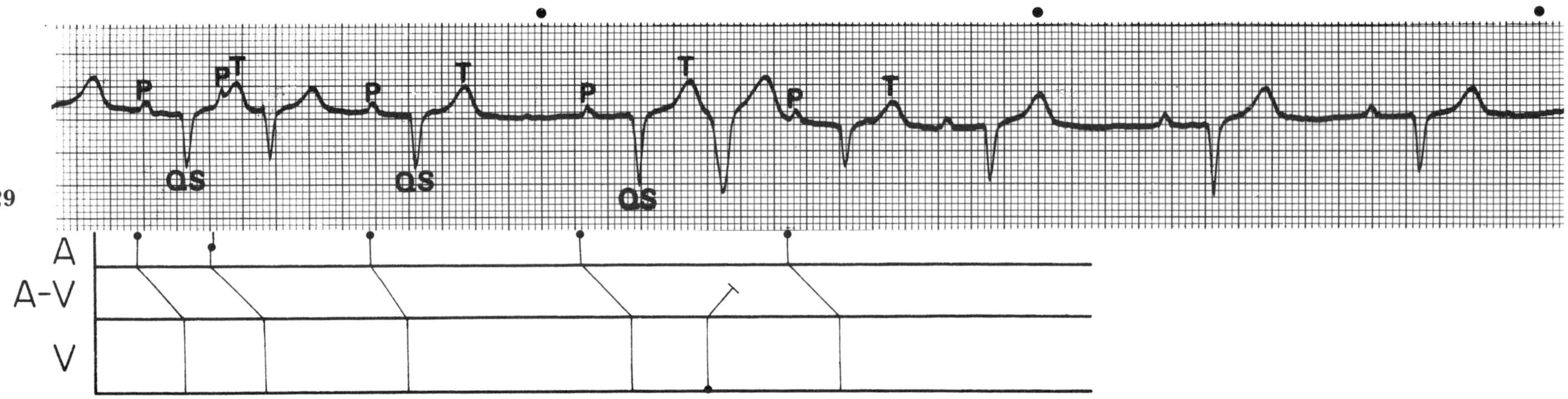

Answer: Sinus arrhythmia and bradycardia with first-degree AV block, one atrial premature complex, and ventricular premature complexes. Heart rate is variable. The best therapeutic approach for treating dilated cardiomyopathy includes the administration of dobutamine, diuretics, taurine, and vasodilators and the intake of fluids. Therapeutic goals include improving cardiac output, increasing heart rate, and controlling pulmonary edema and pleural effusion. The ladder diagram is a tiered schematic representation of the cardiac conduction system that helps to differentiate atrial premature complexes from ventricular premature complexes. The first sinus beat with first-degree AV block (prolonged P-R interval) is followed by an atrial premature complex (P on T) that travels retrograde, resets the sinus node, and is followed by another sinus beat at the expected P wave-to-P wave interval. The ventricular premature complex (fifth QS) is interpolated between two sinus beats. Notice that the P-R interval following the ventricular premature complex is prolonged when compared with other sinus beats. This prolongation is caused by retrograde conduction of the ventricular premature complex into the AV node area, thus affecting AV conduction of the following sinus beat. No direct measurement of the AV conduction system is on the ECG. Only the atrial and the ventricular myocardium are represented by the P wave and QRS complex. The influence of the ventricular premature complex on AV conduction is deduced by its effect on the following P-R interval, and is termed concealed conduction. Most ventricular premature complexes are not interpolated and do not reset the sinus node because of a block in retrograde conduction of the ventricular premature complex in the AV junctional area. Accordingly, the interval from sinus beat to ventricular premature complex to sinus beat is usually fully compensatory, a concept that can aid in identifying ventricular premature complexes.

Case 130

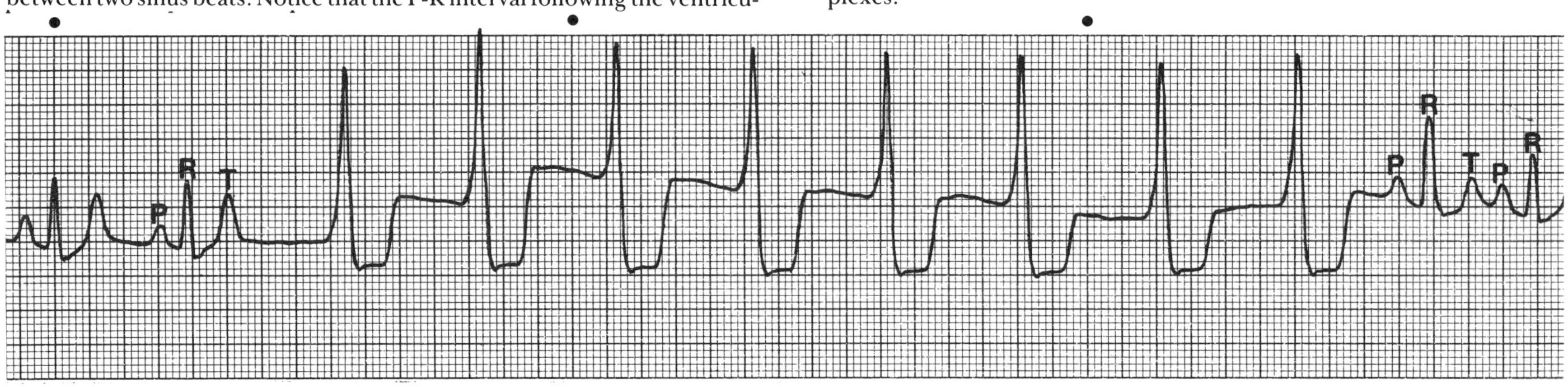

Answer: Sinus rhythm with periods of accelerated idioventricular rhythm. Heart rate is approximately 150 beats/min. The run of abnormal-appearing complexes in the center of the strip represents an accelerated idioventricular rhythm, also known as idioventricular tachycardia. An accelerated idioventricular rhythm is a form of ventricular tachycardia in which the rate is generally within 10 beats/min of the sinus rate. When ventricular escape impulses control the rhythm, the term "idioventricular tachycardia" is used. The term may be a misconception, because the ventricular rhythm may not be caused by an accelerated normal ventricular pacemaker. (Purkinje fibers) Fusion beats (second-to-last complex) occur frequently at the transition zones between idioventricular and sinus rhythm. The onset of the arrhythmia is generally gradual and reflects an increase in the ventricular rate or a slowing of the sinus rate or AV block. In this dog, the onset of the arrhythmia is associated with the slowing of the sinus rate. The arrhythmia generally accompanies structural heart disease or digitalis toxicity. The rhythm disturbance rarely requires treatment, because the rate is usually not rapid and the hemodynamic consequences are few. If the rate is rapid enough to cause clinical signs, suppressive therapy with lidocaine or procainamide is recommended. Atropine administered to increase the sinus rate is an alternative treatment. This will often overdrive suppress the accelerated idioventricular rhythm.

Case 131

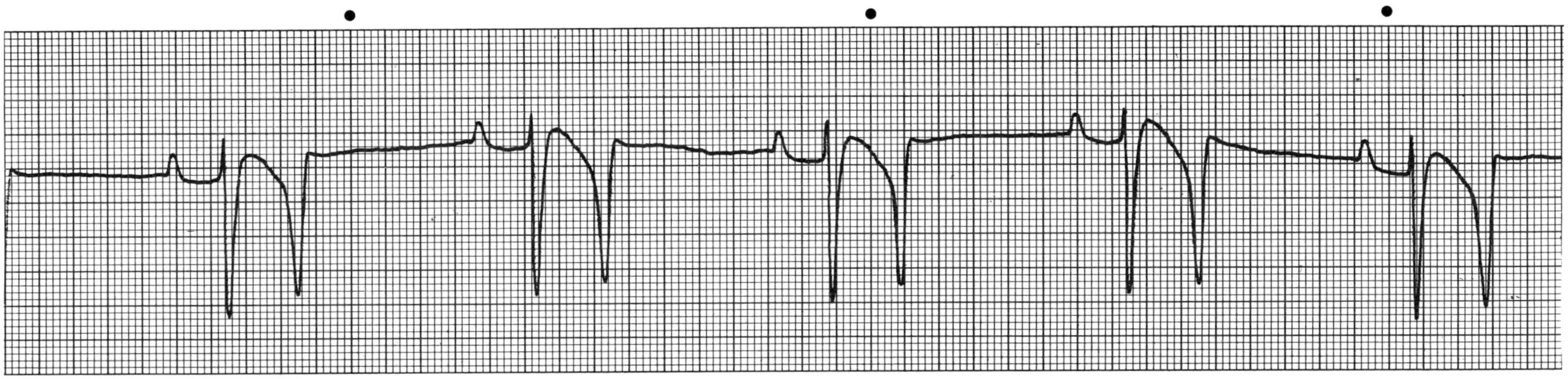

Question: This rhythm strip was recorded from a Springer Spaniel with heartworm disease and ascites.

1. What is the rhythm diagnosis?
2. What is the most likely underlying disorder?
3. What is the best therapeutic approach?

Case 132

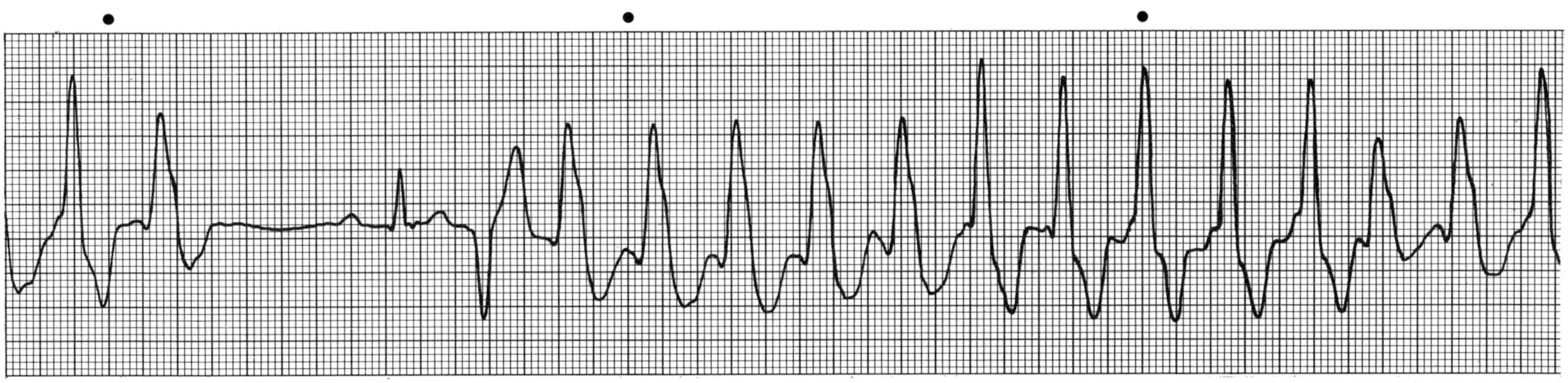

Question: This rhythm strip was recorded from a Brittany Spaniel that had been hit by a truck 24 hours before the ECG was recorded.

1. What is the rhythm diagnosis?
2. What are common causes of this arrhythmia?
3. What is the most likely underlying disorder?
4. What is the best therapeutic approach?

Case 131

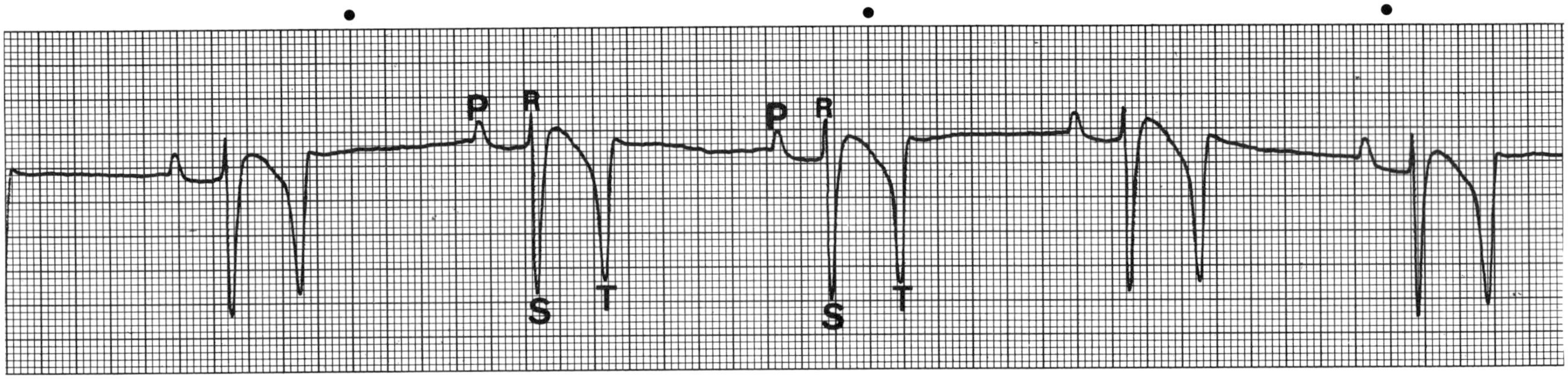

Answer: Sinus rhythm with first-degree AV block. Heart rate is 70 beats/min. The P-R interval is prolonged. First-degree AV block may be secondary to increased vagal tone or structural disease involving the AV node. The QRS complexes (RS) are negative and wide (also seen in leads I and III), thus suggesting right bundle-branch block and right ventricular enlargement. Large T waves often accompany conduction disturbances. They can also occur in animals with hyperkalemia and myocardial hypoxia. Evaluation of serum electrolytes should be part of the diagnostic work-up. No treatment is indicated for the first-degree AV block and possible intraventricular conduction disturbance.

Case 132

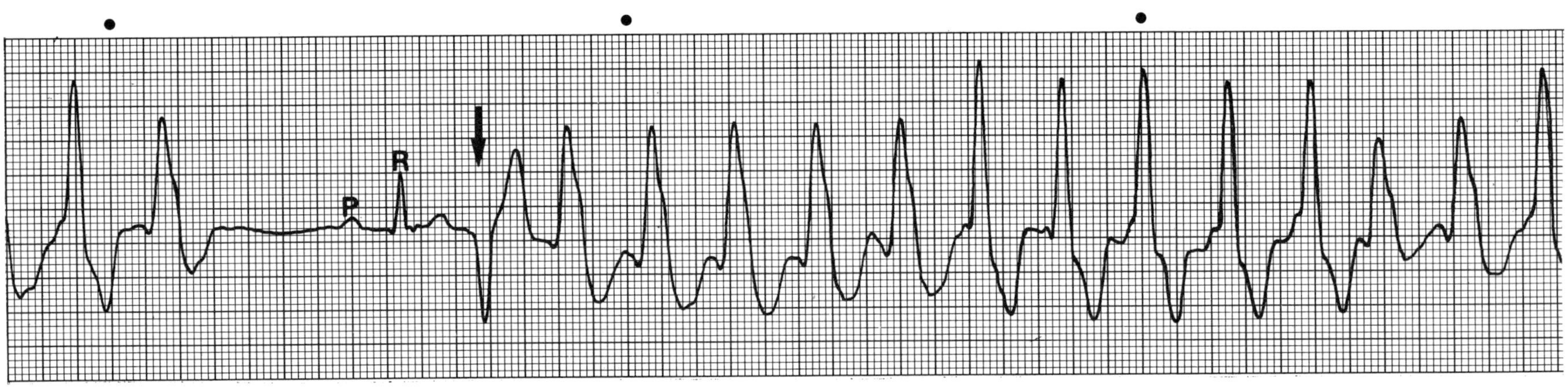

Answer: Sinus rhythm with first-degree AV block and paroxysmal ventricular tachycardia. Heart rate is approximately 240 beats/min during periods of tachycardia. The predominant rhythm is ventricular tachycardia. The sinus complex (third complex) is conducted with first-degree AV block. The block may be associated with traumatic injury or, if the block preceded the trauma, may be associated with degeneration or fibrosis of the AV node. The QRS complexes of the ventricular tachycardia exhibit several different morphologies, thus possibly representing multifocal ventricular tachycardia or re-entrant tachycardia with variations in conduction. The first premature complex (arrow) after the sinus complex may be an atrial premature complex with aberrant ventricular conduction. The atrial premature complex then is followed by a paroxysmal ventricular tachycardia. The ventricular tachycardia in this instance is probably associated with trauma. Cardiomyopathy, neoplasia, and infectious myocarditis are less likely explanations for the arrhythmia in this dog. The arrhythmia should be controlled with boluses of lidocaine, and a lidocaine infusion should be instituted. Oral antiarrhythmic therapy with procainamide, quinidine, tocainide, or mexiletine then can be administered.

Case 133

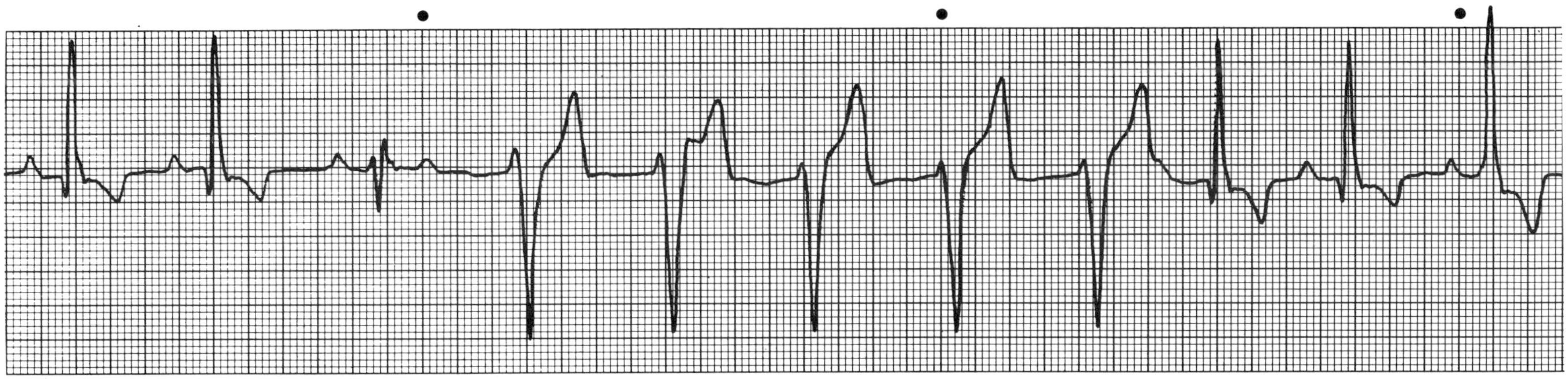

Question: This lead II ECG was obtained from an 8-year-old Labrador Retriever examined because of severe exercise intolerance. Thoracic radiographs and an echocardiographic study were normal.

1. What is the rhythm diagnosis?
2. What is the most likely underlying disorder?
3. What is the best therapeutic approach?

Case 134

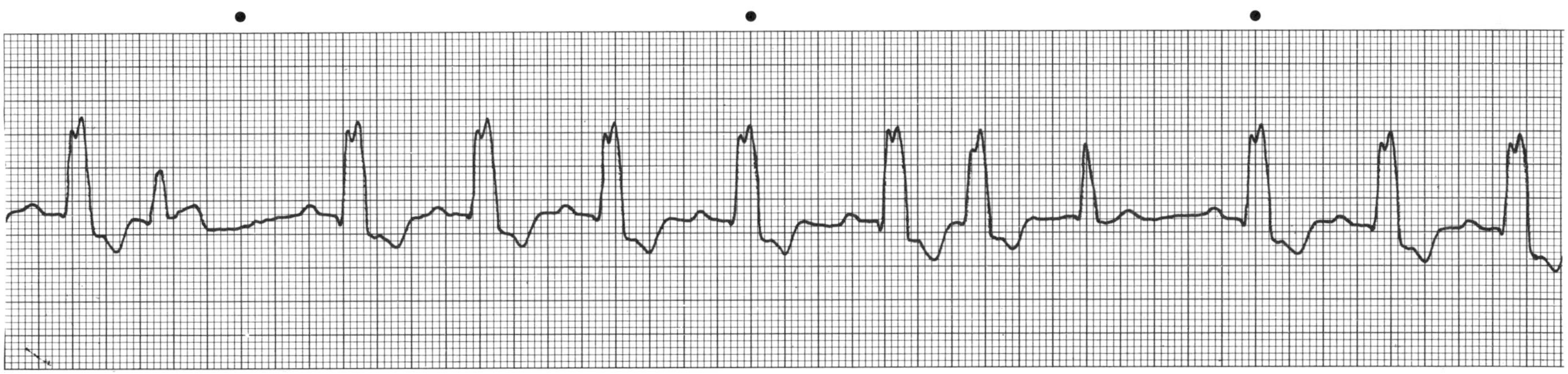

Question: This rhythm strip was recorded from a 5-year-old Boxer with a history of syncope.

1. What is the rhythm diagnosis?
2. What is the most likely underlying disorder?
3. What is the best therapeutic approach?

Case 133

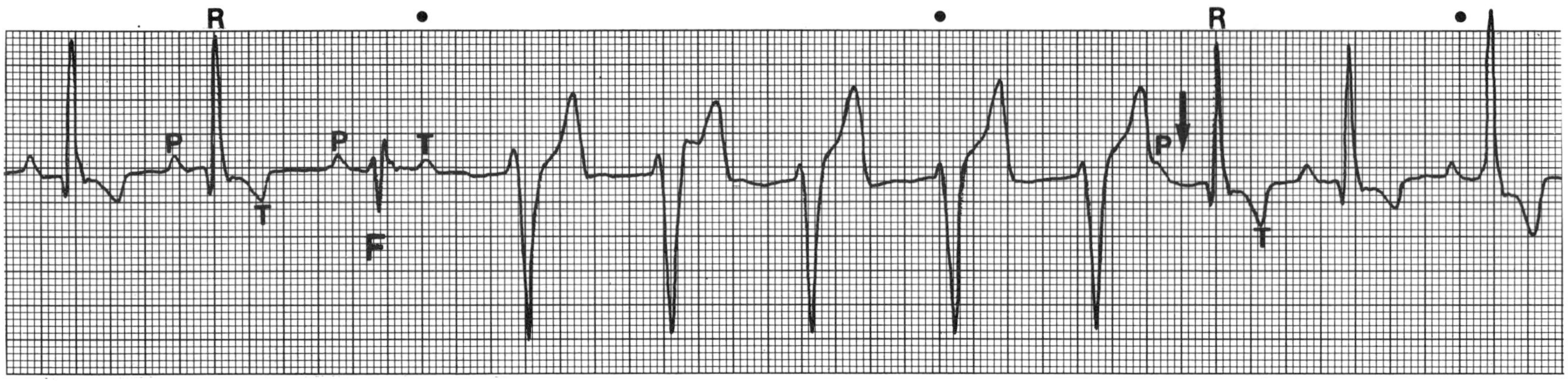

Answer: Sinus rhythm with paroxysmal ventricular tachycardia. Heart rate is 150 beats/min. Myocarditis associated with numerous conditions (e.g., infection, trauma, neoplasia, autoimmune disease, and idiopathic disease) is the most likely underlying disorder. Administration of ventricular antiarrhythmic drugs (e.g., procainamide, quinidine, and propranolol) is the best therapeutic approach. A diagnostic work-up, including history, physical examination, complete blood count, and biochemical profile, is needed to detect the cause of the myocarditis. Premature, wide, and bizarre QRS complexes that are not associated with P waves are the hallmark of ventricular premature complexes. The appearance of three or more ventricular premature complexes in succession among sinus beats (P-R-T) is termed paroxysmal ventricular tachycardia. Another important finding typical of ventricular arrhythmias is fusion beats. A fusion beat is a QRS complex (F) caused by a combination of the sinus beat meeting the ventricular premature complex in the ventricles. The P-R interval of the fusion beat is similar to that of the sinus beats. The prolonged P-R interval (arrow), when compared with the P-R interval of the other sinus beats, is caused by concealed conduction of the last ventricular premature complex into the AV junction. Concealed conduction affects the refractory period and conduction speed of the following sinus beat.

Case 134

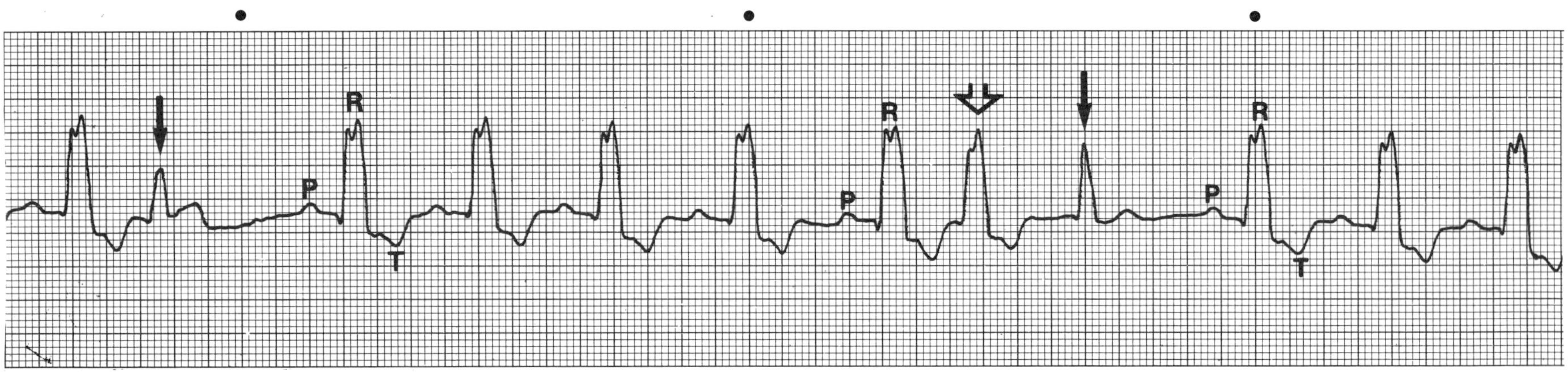

Answer: Sinus rhythm with one supraventricular premature complex and two ventricular premature complexes. Heart rate is approximately 140 beats/min. The sinus complexes are extremely wide and notched. These changes are probably caused by left heart enlargement or left bundle-branch block. One probable supraventricular premature complex (open arrow) is labelled near the center of the strip. This QRS complex and the sinus QRS complexes share the same morphology. Two ventricular premature complexes are designated by solid arrows. These ventricular premature complexes are narrower and look more like a normal sinus complex than this dog's sinus complexes. The ventricular premature complex allows for earlier activation of the left ventricle than would occur with a sinus complex and left bundle-branch block. The combination of supraventricular and ventricular arrhythmias in this breed suggests dilated cardiomyopathy. Procainamide, quinidine, tocainide, or mexiletine may be needed to treat the ventricular arrhythmia, especially if the arrhythmia increases in severity. Periods of ventricular tachycardia may account for the syncope.

Case 135

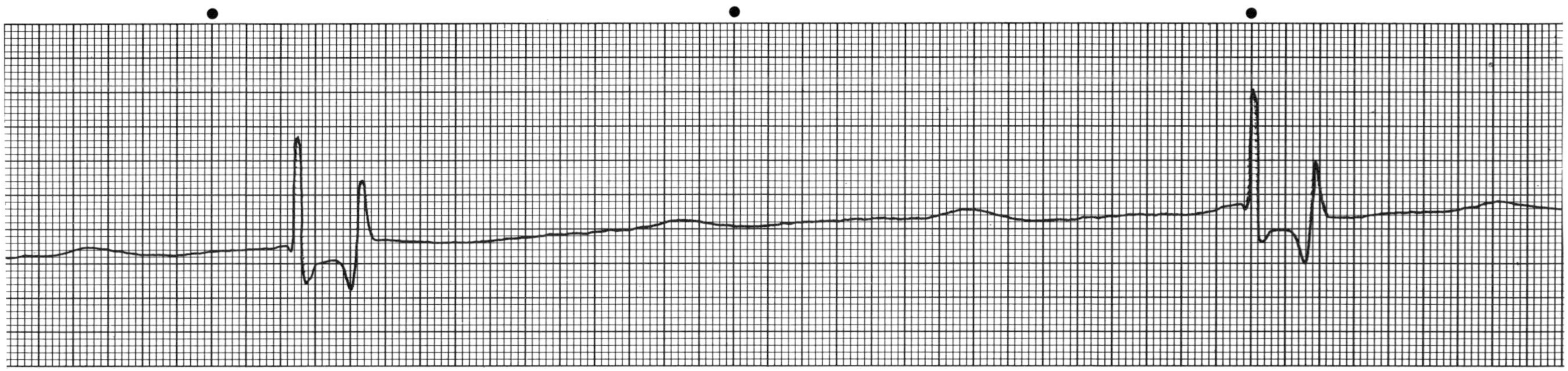

Question: This lead II ECG was obtained from a 2-year-old English Springer Spaniel with a history of marked lethargy and episodic collapse. A marked bradycardia was heard on auscultation.

1. What is the rhythm diagnosis?
2. What is the most likely underlying disorder?
3. What is the best therapeutic approach?

Case 136

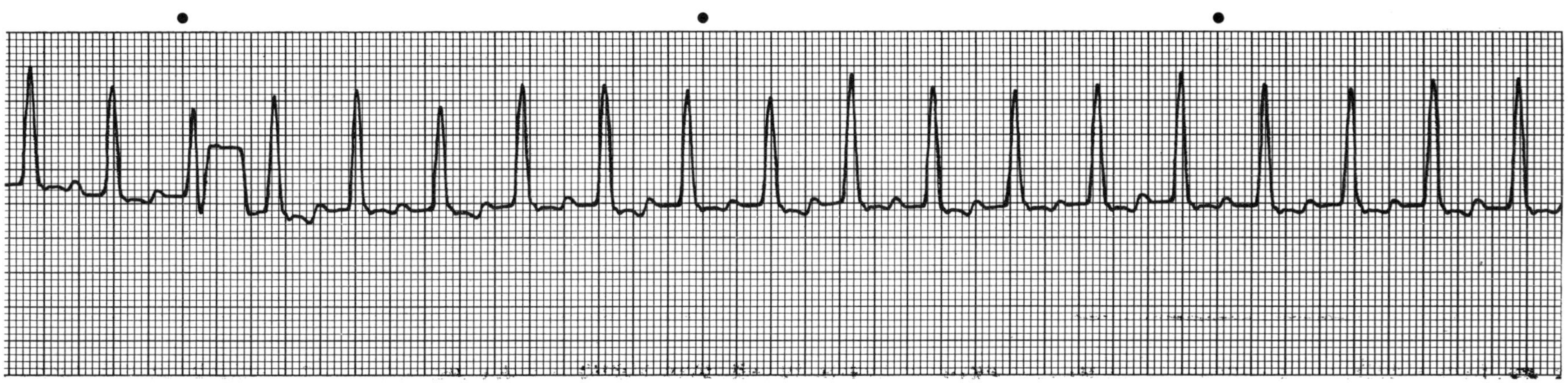

Question: This lead II ECG was obtained from a 5-year-old German Shepherd examined because of frequent episodes of collapse.

1. What is the rhythm diagnosis?
2. What is the best therapeutic approach?

Case 135

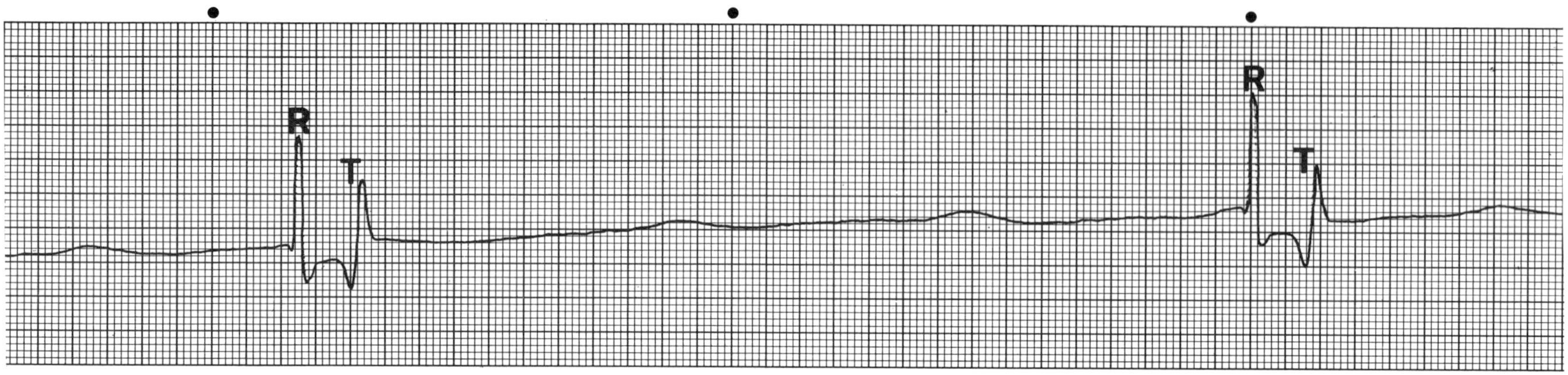

Answer: Persistent atrial standstill. Baseline artifact. Heart rate is approximately 30 beats/min. Persistent atrial standstill is part of a muscular dystrophy syndrome reported in the English Springer Spaniel and other dog and cat breeds. A permanent cardiac pacemaker is the best therapeutic approach. The heart failure also must be treated. Cardiomyopathy combined with persistent atrial standstill has a guarded prognosis. Severe hyperkalemia should also be considered as the cause of atrial standstill. Clinical signs of persistent atrial standstill (not related to hyperkalemia) include weakness, fainting, and dyspnea. Radiographs may reveal pleural effusion and ascites. Extreme enlargement of the atria is evident on radiographic, angiocardiographic, and echocardiographic studies. The atria are immobile when viewed with fluoroscopy or echocardiography. Electrocardiographic features of persistent atrial standstill include a heart rate of less than 60 beats/min in the dog and no P waves observed in any lead, including intracardiac electrograms. Small P waves may be associated with atrial standstill involving only one atrium. The QRS complex may be of normal configuration with supraventricular-type escape QRS complexes, or of increased duration typical of bundle-branch block, ventricular enlargement, or ventricular escape complexes. Atropine sulfate has no effect on the rate or rhythm, and the atria cannot be stimulated electrically or mechanically.

Case 136

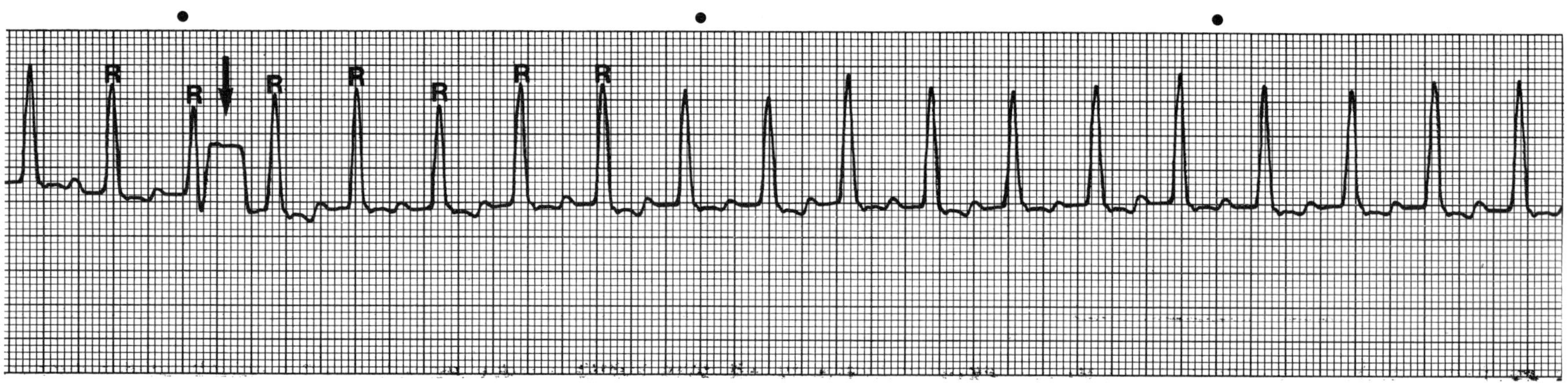

Answer: Supraventricular tachycardia. Heart rate is 250 beats/min. A vagal maneuver (ocular or carotid sinus pressure) can be performed in an attempt to terminate this tachyarrhythmia. The vagal maneuver may also provide a way to establish the mechanism of the supraventricular tachycardia (e.g., atrial ectopic tachycardia, atrial flutter, AV nodal re-entrant tachycardia, and Wolff-Parkinson-White syndrome). The narrow QRS complexes support a diagnosis of supraventricular, instead of ventricular, tachyarrhythmia. The P waves are hidden in the preceding T waves or in the QRS complexes. The regular R wave-to-R wave intervals eliminate atrial fibrillation from the ECG differential diagnosis. The tachyarrhythmia must be terminated and the QRS complexes of the sinus beats examined (they should be similar to the QRS complexes during the tachycardia) to prove the supraventricular origin of this tachyarrhythmia. Atrial arrhythmic drugs (i.e., digoxin, diltiazem, propranolol, or a combination) then can be administered. The slight difference in QRS complex amplitudes is commonly seen in dogs with supraventricular tachyarrhythmias. The complex labelled with an arrow is a 1-mv standardization impulse (1 mv = 1 cm).

Case 137

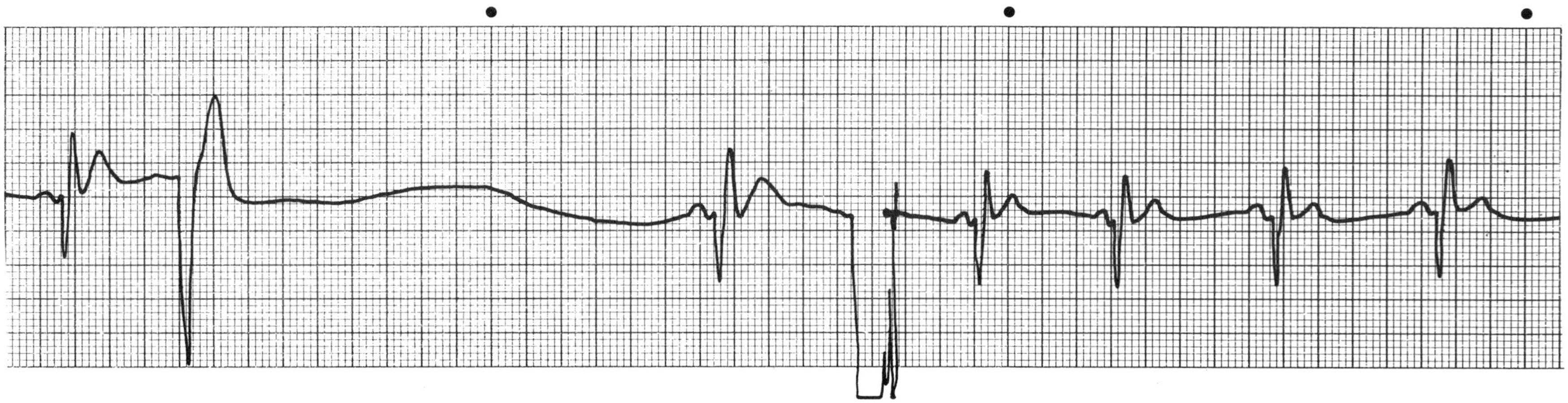

Question: This rhythm strip was recorded from a 7-year-old German Shorthaired Pointer.

1. What is the rhythm diagnosis?

Case 138

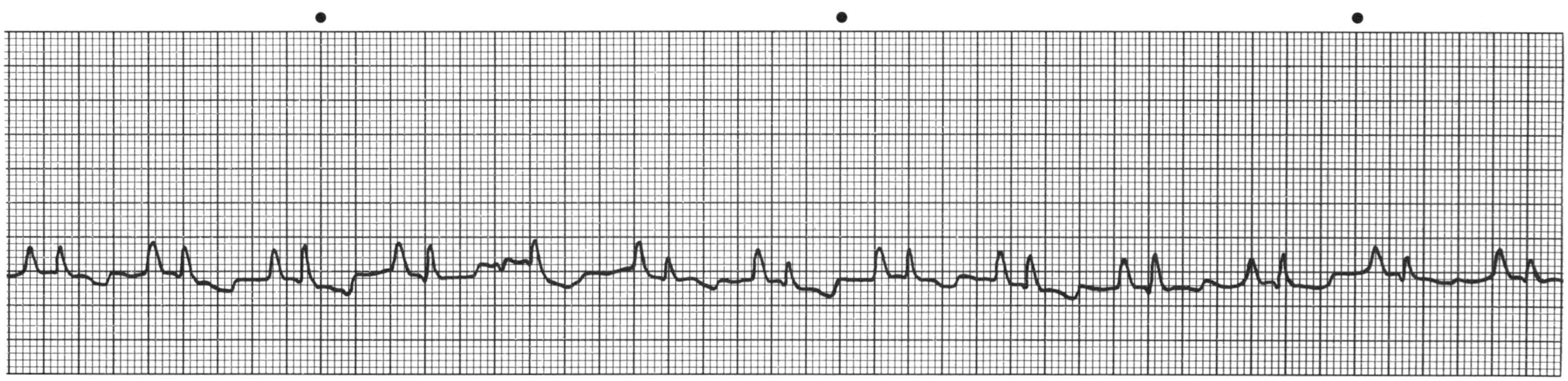

Question: This rhythm strip was obtained from a 9-year-old Yorkshire Terrier with a history of chronic coughing and no audible murmur.

1. What is the rhythm diagnosis?
2. What is the most likely underlying disorder?
3. What is the best therapeutic approach?

Case 137

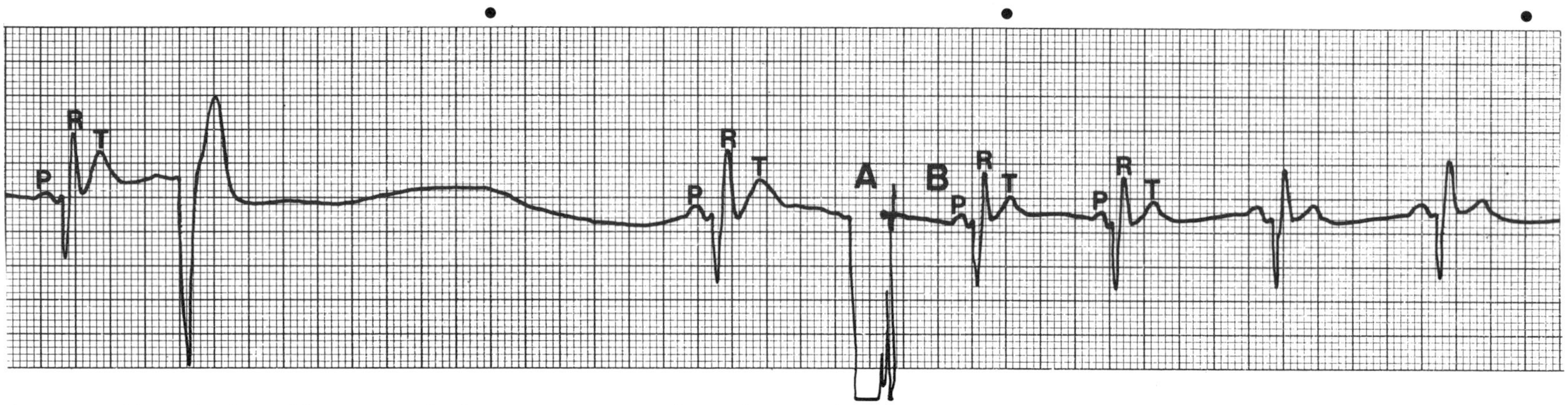

Answer: Sinus rhythm with one ventricular premature complex and a period of sinus arrest or sinoatrial block. The second complex is a ventricular premature complex, which is followed by a long period of sinus arrest or sinoatrial block. In the center of the strip is an artifact labelled "A." A lead change, which occurs at "B," accounts for the slight change in the morphology of the complexes.

Case 138

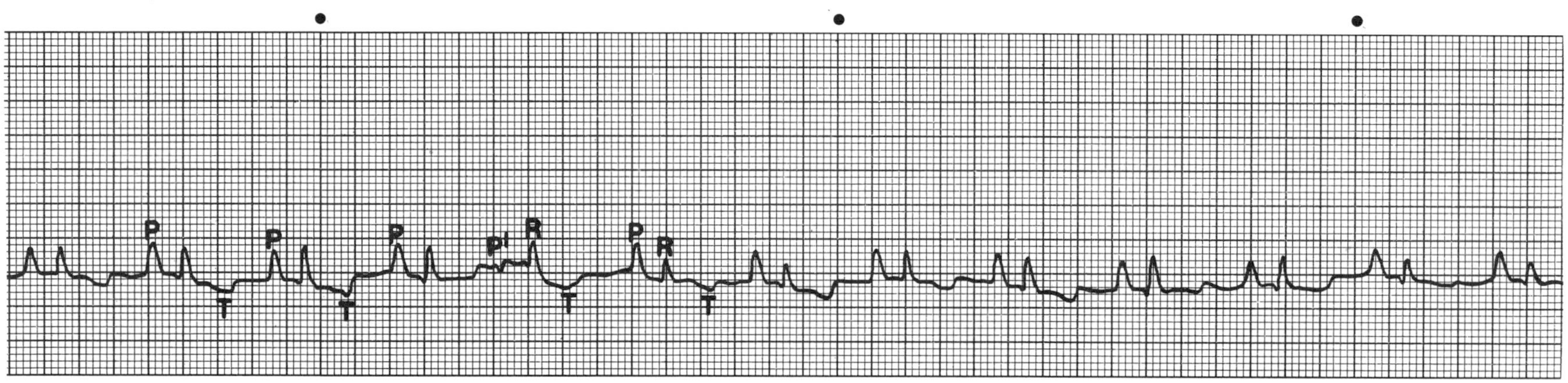

Answer: Sinus rhythm with one atrial premature complex. Heart rate is approximately 170 beats/min. The tall P waves (P pulmonale) suggest right atrial enlargement, which frequently accompanies pulmonary hypertension. Atrial premature complexes are usually caused by atrial distention. Notice that the QRS complex associated with the premature P′ wave is similar in morphology to the sinus QRS complexes. In this dog, the atrial premature complexes probably originate in the right atrium as a result of atrial enlargement caused by chronic airway disease. Atrial premature complexes can also originate in the left atrium. Remarkable left atrial enlargement, however, is uncommon in small-breed dogs without an audible murmur. The atrial premature complexes occur infrequently in this dog and are not associated with clinical signs of weakness. Therefore, antiarrhythmic therapy is not indicated at this time.

Case 139

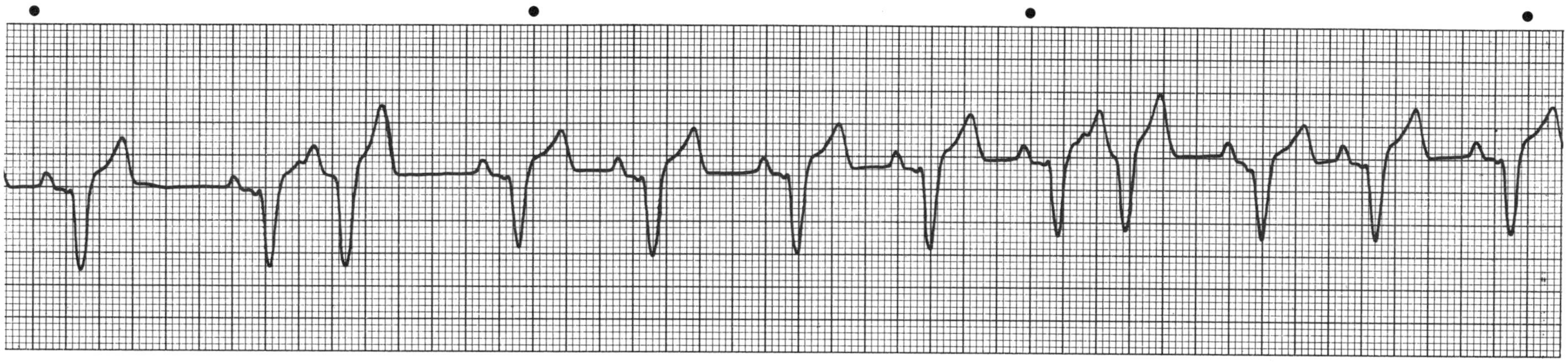

Question: This lead II ECG was obtained from a 6-year-old mixed-breed dog in which occult heartworm disease was diagnosed. Lead I had negative QRS complexes.

1. What is the rhythm diagnosis?
2. What is the best therapeutic approach?

Case 140

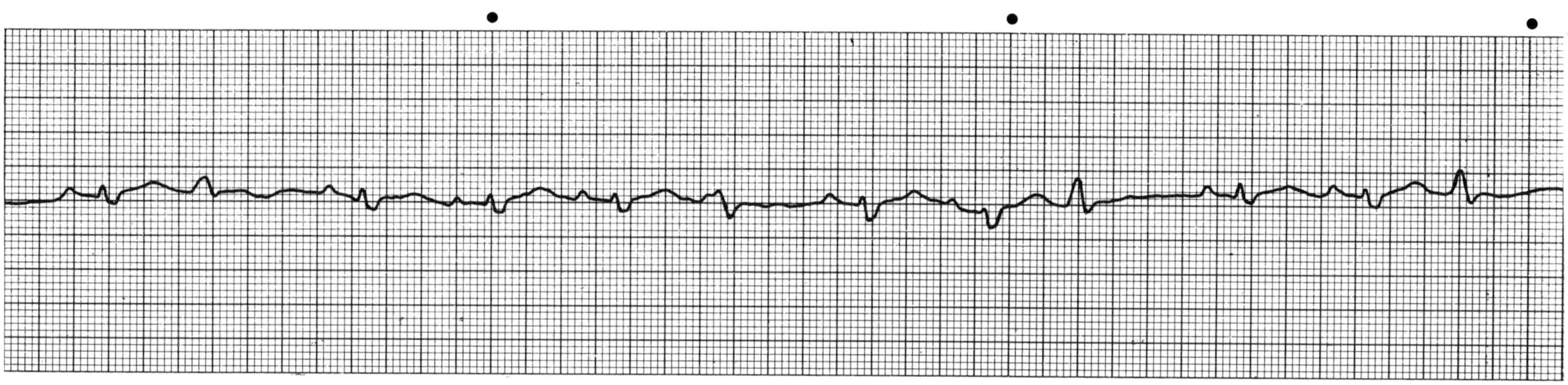

Question: This lead II rhythm strip was obtained from a geriatric cat that was being examined because of vague signs of lethargy and anorexia. Physical examination revealed a high respiratory rate, gallop rhythm, and pulse deficits.

1. What is the rhythm diagnosis?
2. What is the most likely underlying disorder?
3. What is the best therapeutic approach?

Case 139

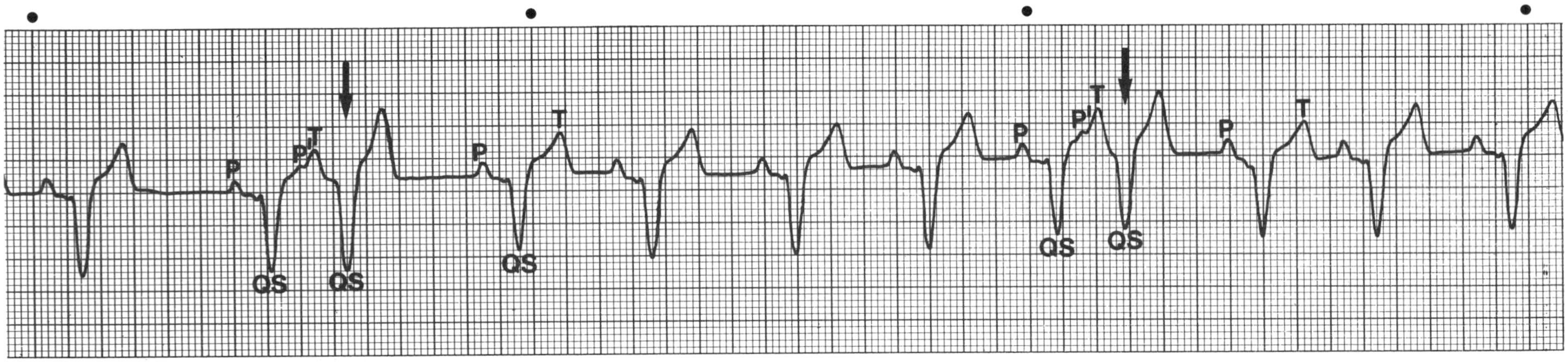

Answer: Sinus rhythm with possible right ventricular enlargement and atrial premature complexes. Heart rate is approximately 140 beats/min. Treating the heartworms with adulticide is the best therapeutic approach. If the atrial arrhythmia persists and syncope or dyspnea occurs, digoxin or diltiazem may be needed. Treatment of the heartworms usually causes the various arrhythmias to disappear. Propranolol is a beta 1 and beta 2 sympathetic blocker that may cause bronchoconstriction and therefore should not be administered. The negative in leads I and II QRS complexes denote right axis deviation and may be caused by expected right ventricular enlargement. The consistent P-R interval of the sinus beats eliminates ventricular premature complexes from the ECG differential diagnosis. The premature QRS complexes (arrows) resemble the sinus beat QRS complexes, typical of atrial premature complexes. The premature P′ waves of the atrial premature complexes are hidden in the preceding T waves. The T wave following the atrial premature complexes appears larger than the other T waves because of aberrant ventricular conduction, or may contain premature P′ waves (nonconducted atrial premature complexes).

Case 140

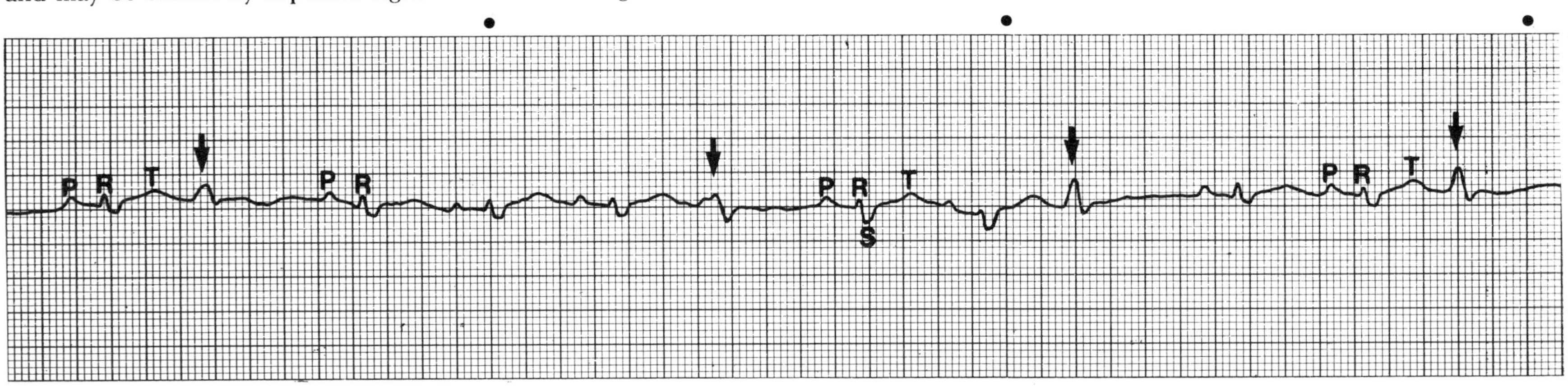

Answer: Sinus rhythm with frequent ventricular premature complexes. Heart rate is approximately 150 beats/min. The QRS complexes are wide (0.06 sec) because of the prolongation of the S wave. The ventricular premature complexes (arrows) support underlying myocardial disease. The QRS complexes of the ventricular premature complexes are of different morphology than that of the sinus QRS complexes and are not associated with P waves. The gallop rhythm supports the finding of heart enlargement. These findings suggest cardiomyopathy or hyperthyroidism. S wave prolongation can be associated with right ventricular enlargement or an intraventricular conduction disturbance. The slightly prolonged P-R interval (0.10 sec) can be a normal variation in geriatric cats. The rest of the cardiovascular data base needs to be completed to determine the underlying cause. The antiarrhythmic drug of choice for this arrhythmia may be propranolol. A follow-up ECG is of paramount importance in this cat. Propranolol decreases AV nodal conduction and could worsen the conduction disturbance and reduce the heart rate.

Case 141

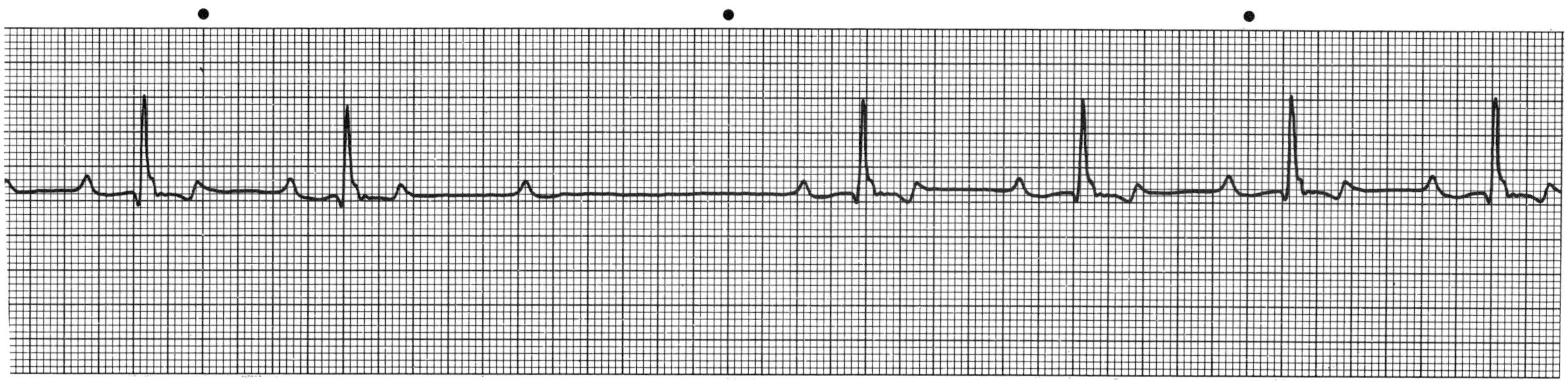

Question: This rhythm strip was recorded from a 9-year-old Pug that had an ECG performed as part of a preanesthetic screen.

1. What is the rhythm diagnosis?
2. What are common causes of this arrhythmia?
3. What is the best therapeutic approach?

Case 142

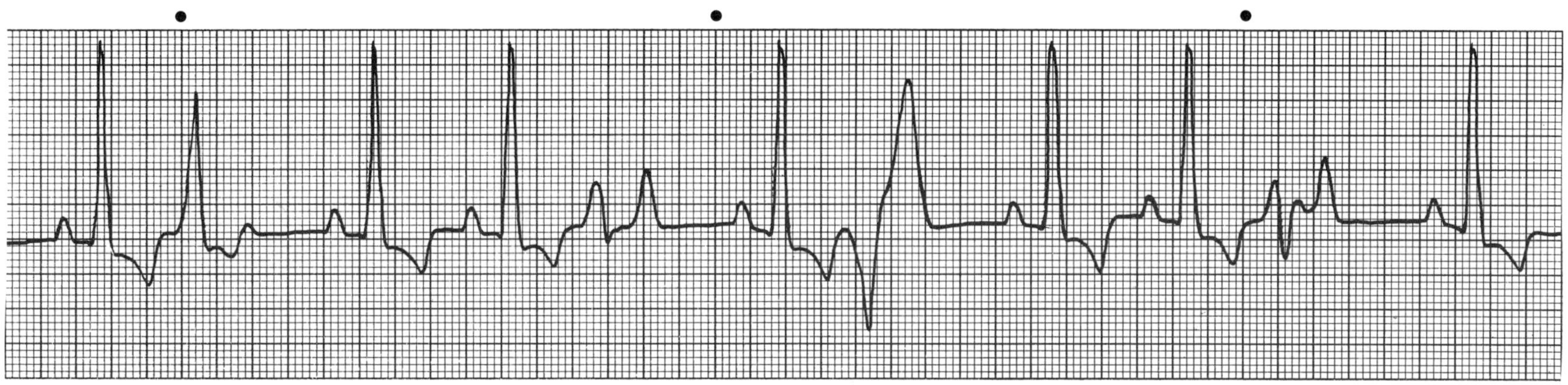

Question: This lead II rhythm strip was obtained from a large mixed-breed dog that had been hit by a car 48 hours before the ECG was recorded.

1. What is the rhythm diagnosis?
2. What is the most likely underlying disorder?
3. What is the best therapeutic approach?

Case 141

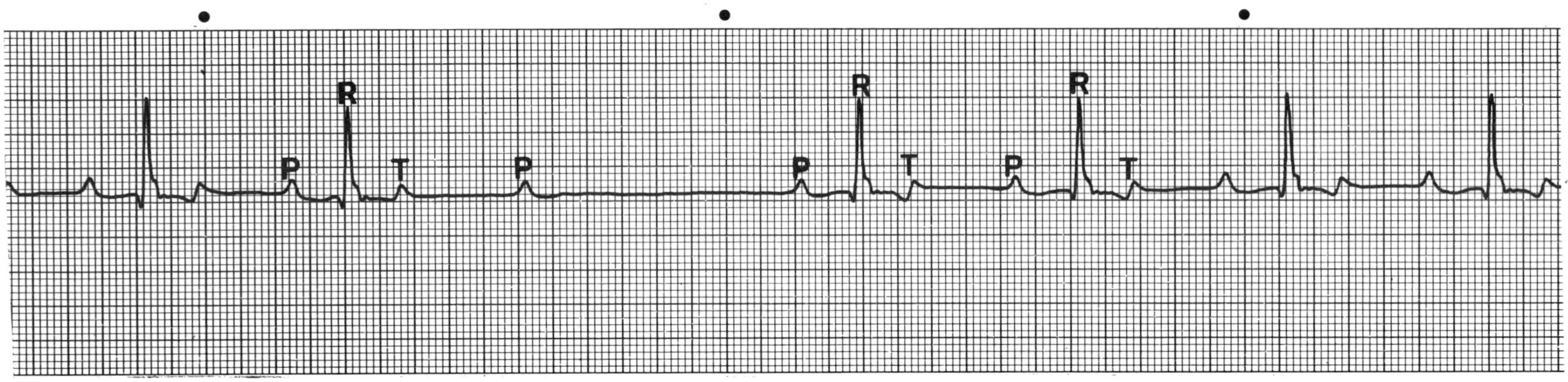

Answer: Sinus rhythm with first- and second-degree (Mobitz type II) AV block. Heart rate is 60 to 80 beats/min. The P-R interval is prolonged (0.18 sec) and constant. One P wave is not conducted. The constant P-R interval of the conducted complexes is characteristic of Mobitz type II second-degree AV block. The presence of first-degree and Mobitz type II second-degree AV block supports underlying AV nodal disease or, more likely, His-Purkinje system disease. Hereditary stenosis of the bundle of His has been documented in Pugs. Degeneration, fibrosis, and neoplastic infiltration of the AV node can also develop. The dog has no clinical signs of a conduction disturbance and does not require treatment. Atropine should be administered 30 minutes before induction of general anesthesia to increase the heart rate and minimize the risk of intraoperative bradycardia. If signs of exercise intolerance or collapse develop, the rhythm should be reassessed.

Case 142

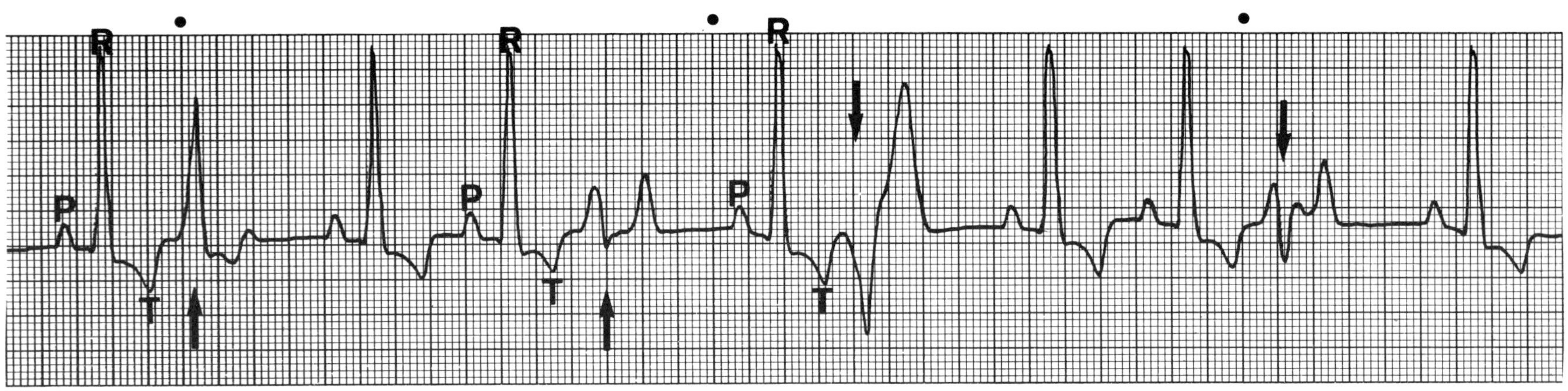

Answer: Sinus tachycardia with frequent multiform ventricular premature complexes (arrows). Heart rate is approximately 160 beats/min. Traumatic myocarditis is the most likely cause of this arrhythmia. Traumatic myocarditis usually causes ventricular arrhythmias, but atrial arrhythmias are sometimes seen. Arrhythmias develop within 72 hours after the traumatic episode. They result from either blunt trauma to the heart or increased sympathetic tone to the heart. The multiform nature of the arrhythmia suggests injury to both ventricles. Treatment should be initiated with lidocaine for short-term correction. Procainamide should be administered concurrently. The addition of a beta-blocker, such as propranolol, to the regimen may be necessary. Drug therapy is usually only necessary for 7 to 10 days.

Case 143

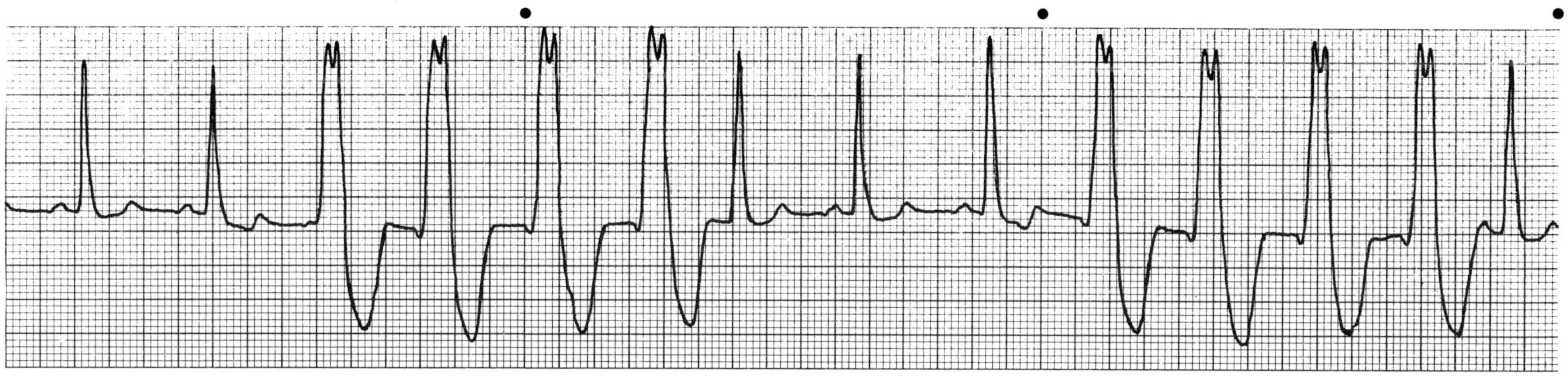

Question: This rhythm strip was recorded from a 10-year-old German Shepherd with a history of acute collapse. The dog had no history of cardiac disease. A midabdominal mass was palpated.

1. What is the rhythm diagnosis?
2. What is the most likely underlying disorder?
3. What is the best therapeutic approach?
4. What is the prognosis?

Case 144

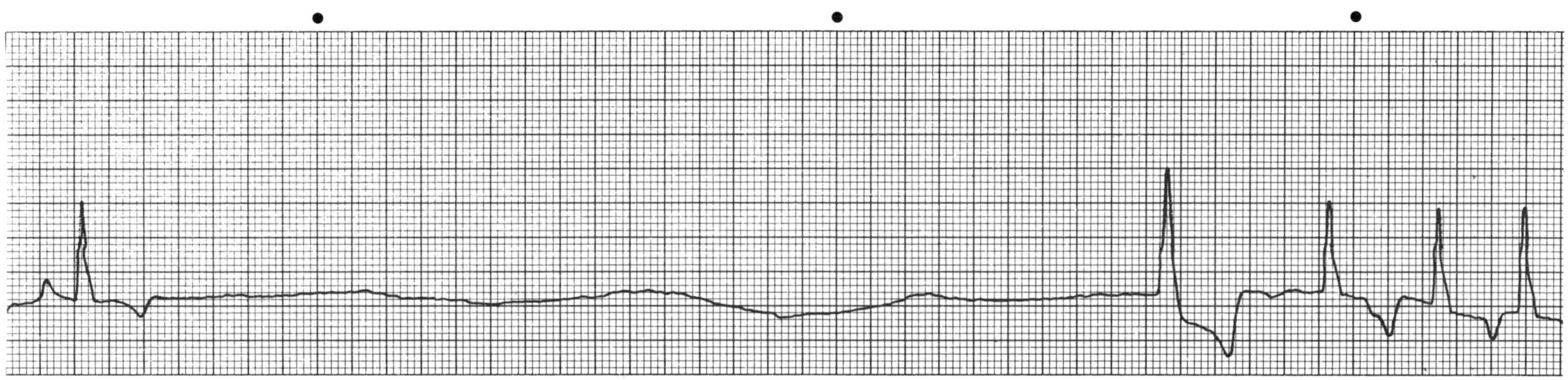

Question: This rhythm strip was recorded from a 9-year-old Miniature Schnauzer with a history of syncope.

1. What is the rhythm diagnosis?
2. What is the most likely underlying disorder?
3. What is the best therapeutic approach?

Case 143

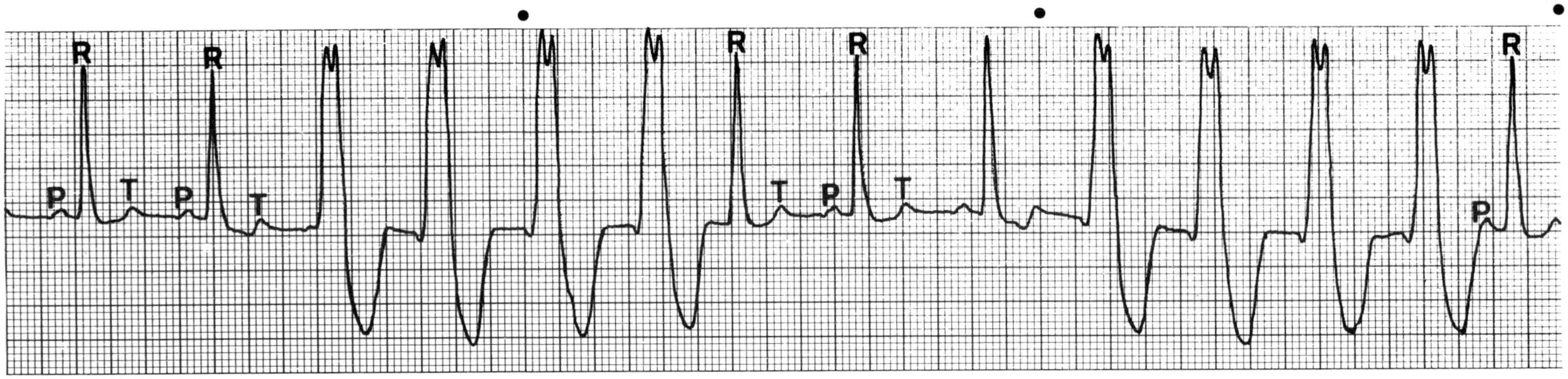

Answer: Sinus tachycardia with paroxysmal ventricular tachycardia. Heart rate is approximately 190 beats/min. The ventricular arrhythmia may originate from the right ventricle, because the R waves are positive in lead II. The QRS complexes of the ventricular tachycardia are wide and bizarre when compared with the sinus QRS complexes. Sinus tachycardia may be the result of either hypotension caused by the arrhythmia or acute rupture of the abdominal mass (suspected splenic tumor). The ventricular arrhythmia may be caused by cardiomyopathy, myocarditis, neoplastic infiltration of the myocardium, or hypoxia caused by acute hypotension and low coronary artery perfusion. Metastatic infiltration of hemangiosarcoma into the myocardium would have to be considered in this dog. Lidocaine boluses should be administered to control the arrhythmia, and then the dog should be put on a lidocaine infusion. Procainamide should also be initiated for long-term management. A poor prognosis must be given.

Case 144

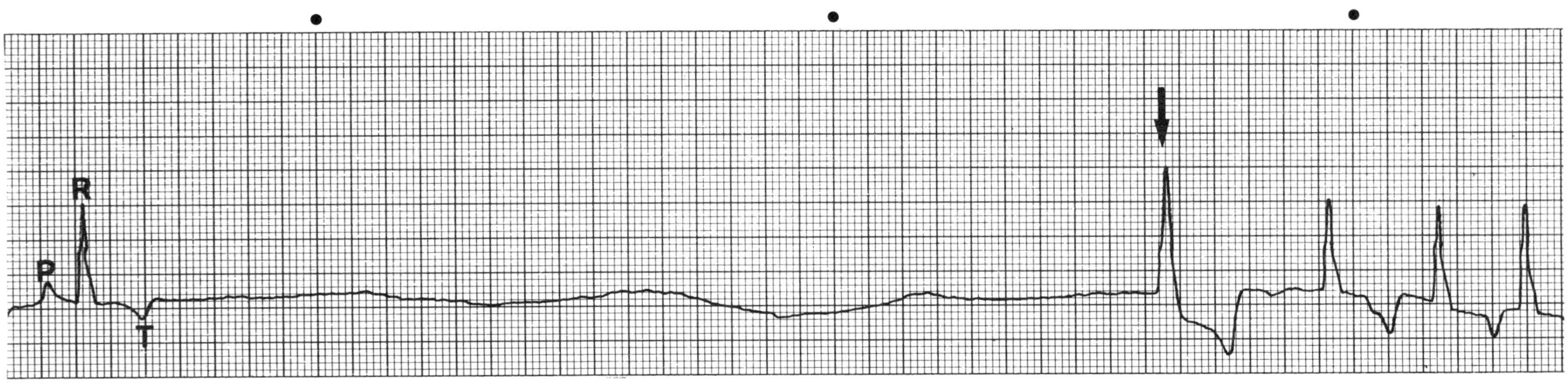

Answer: Sick sinus syndrome (bradycardia-tachycardia syndrome). Heart rate is variable. The first sinus complex is followed by a period of sinus arrest or sinoatrial block and then a ventricular escape beat or junctional escape beat with aberrant conduction (arrow). This complex is followed by a sinus complex and supraventricular premature complexes. These findings are typical of a variant of sick sinus syndrome referred to as bradycardia-tachycardia syndrome. Sick sinus syndrome is commonly seen in old, female, small-breed dogs. Affected breeds include Miniature Schnauzers, Cocker Spaniels, Dachshunds, Pugs, and Poodles. Treatment of dogs with bradycardia and tachycardia is difficult. Ideal management involves implanting a pacemaker to treat the bradycardia and administering digoxin, propranolol, or diltiazem for any persistent supraventricular arrhythmias. An atropine response test would be recommended. If the bradycardia improves without causing severe tachycardia, a trial course of treatment with propantheline or isopropamide would be recommended.

Case 145

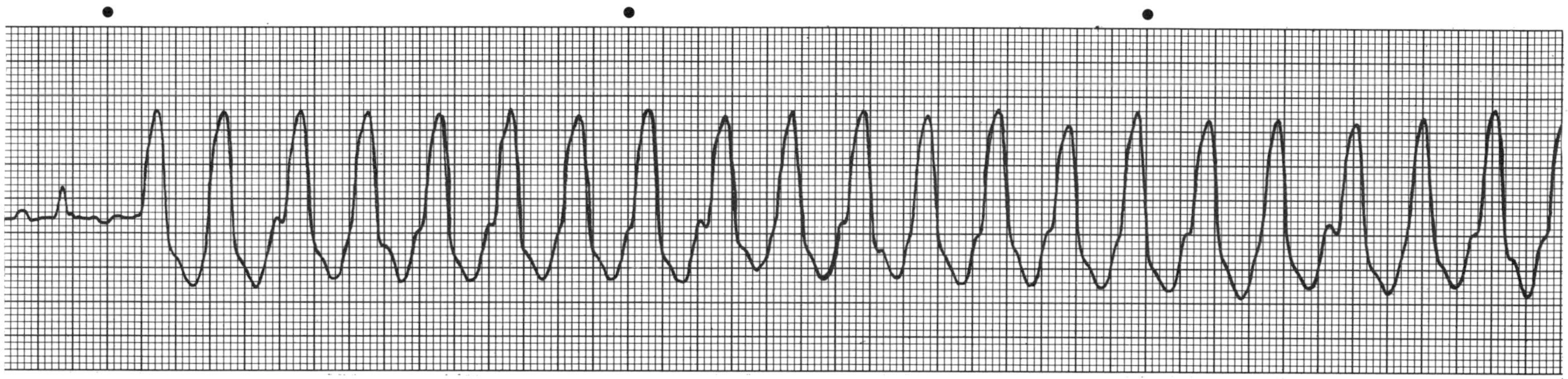

Question: This tracing was obtained from a 5-year-old Boxer with a history of syncope.

1. What is the rhythm diagnosis?
2. What is the most likely underlying disorder?
3. What is the best therapeutic approach?
4. What cautions should be given to the owners?

Case 146

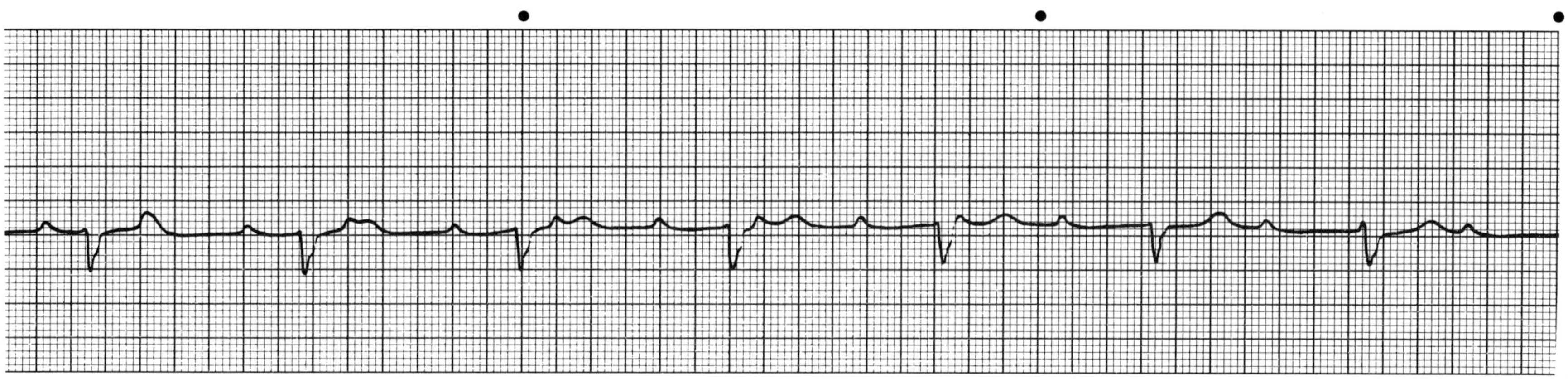

Question: This lead II rhythm strip was obtained from a 15-year-old domestic shorthair cat during routine examination. Bradycardia was heard on auscultation.

1. What is the rhythm diagnosis?
2. What are common causes of this arrhythmia?
3. What is the best therapeutic approach?

Case 145

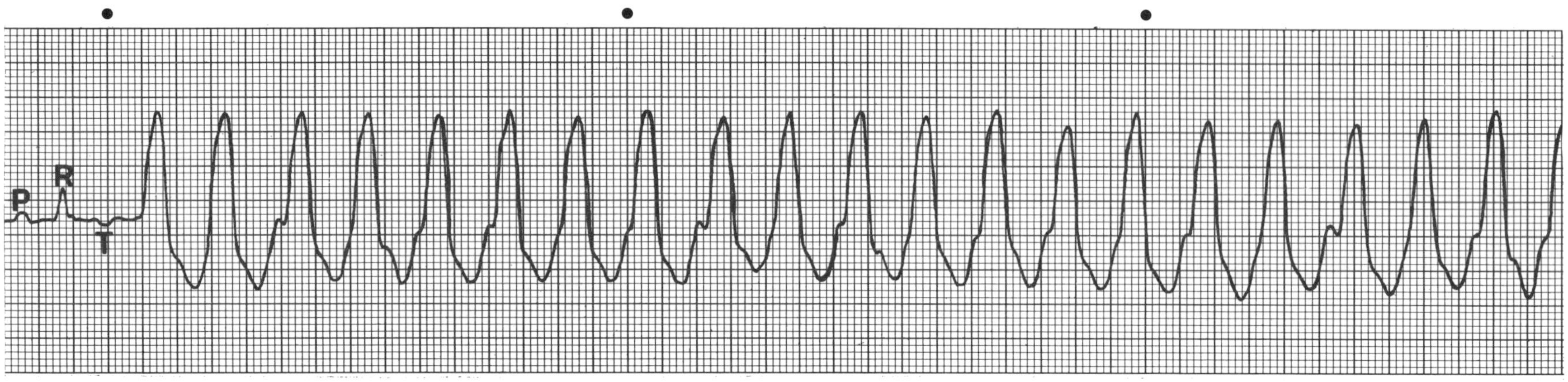

Answer: Sinus rhythm (one sinus complex) with paroxysmal ventricular tachycardia. Heart rate is 300 beats/min. Ventricular tachycardia is identified by the rapid heart rate, wide and bizarre appearance of the complexes, and the presence of P waves that are not associated with the QRS complexes. The origin of the impulses could be the right ventricle (QRS positive in lead II). This characteristic is typical of Boxers with myocarditis or cardiomyopathy. This arrhythmia should be treated with lidocaine. A lidocaine infusion should be administered and procainamide used for long-term management. Ventricular tachycardia associated with myocarditis and cardiomyopathy in the Boxer is often relatively refractory to treatment. Propranolol often needs to be added to a class Ia or Ib antiarrhythmic drug. Propranolol also increases the threshold for ventricular fibrillation and may decrease the risk of sudden death. The owners should be warned about the possibility of sudden death and the potential for the dog to develop congestive heart failure.

Case 146

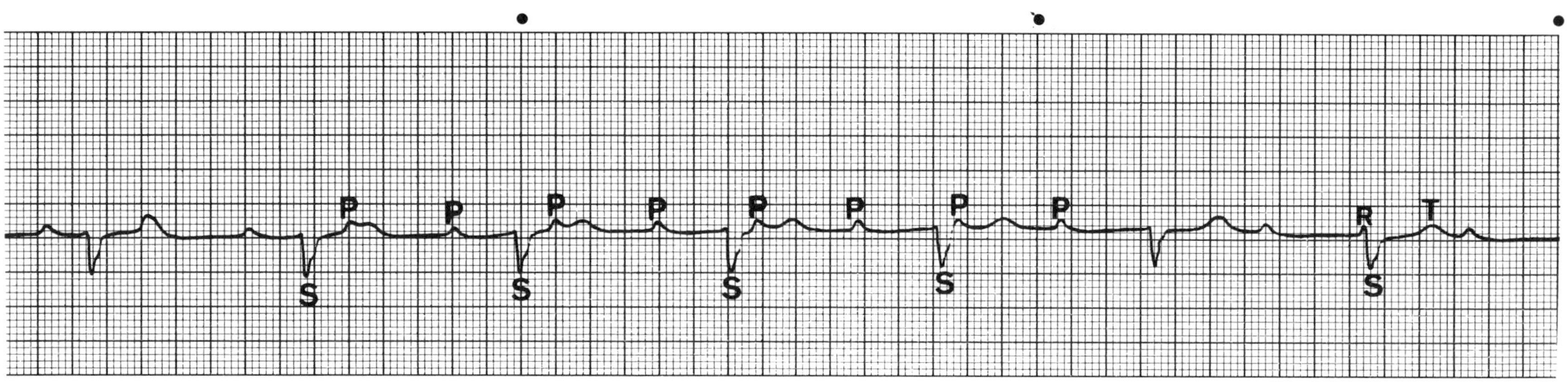

Answer: Complete AV block. Atrial heart rate is 200 beats/min; ventricular heart rate is 95 beats/min. P waves occurring between the RS complexes and T waves are definitely not conducted. The P waves occurring before the R waves are probably blocked, and the QRS complexes represent a ventricular escape rhythm. Some P-R intervals are consistent with conducted complexes. However, the absence of capture complexes rules out penetration of the sinus impulse to the ventricle. A capture complex would alter the ventricular rhythm and have a different QRS morphology to reflect the different origin and conduction path of the ventricular impulse. Conduction disturbances are not unusual in old cats, and they often reflect degeneration or fibrosis in the area of the AV node. Most of these cats have no clinical signs. AV nodal disease is also associated with cardiomyopathy and, less commonly, with hyperthyroidism. Cats with cardiomyopathy and complete AV block are more likely to have signs, because their cardiac output is limited not only by the bradycardia but also by structural heart disease. Animals with no clinical signs do not require treatment. If signs are present, propantheline or a trial course of bronchodilator therapy may be effective. Xanthines (e.g., aminophylline and theophylline) and B_2 agonists (e.g., terbutaline and albuterol) increase sympathetic tone and indirectly increase the ventricular response rate. If signs persist, pacemaker implantation should be considered.

Case 147

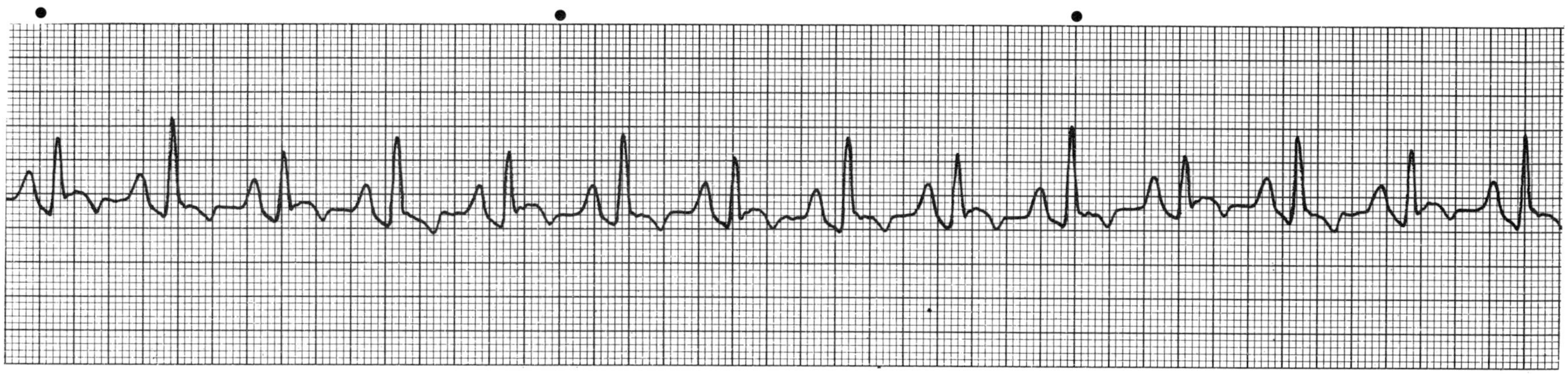

Question: This tracing was taken from an 8-year-old German Shepherd with a history of sudden onset of weakness and ascites.

1. What is the rhythm diagnosis?
2. What is the likely cause of this arrhythmia?
3. What is the most likely underlying disorder?
4. What is the best therapeutic approach?

Case 148

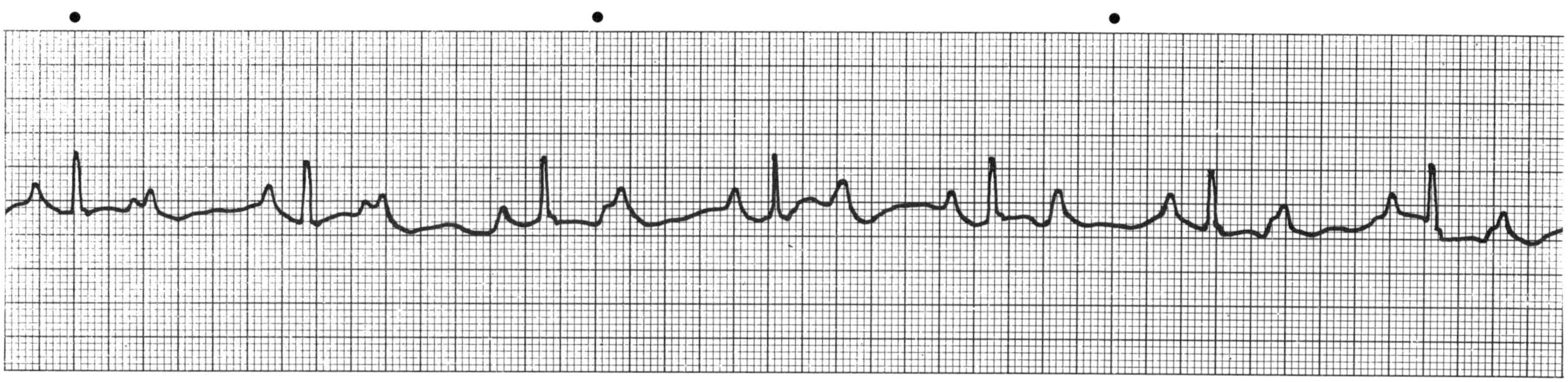

Question: This lead II ECG was obtained from a 16-year-old Basset Hound examined because of coughing. Thoracic radiographs revealed bronchial thickening.

1. What is the rhythm diagnosis?
2. What is the most likely underlying disorder?
3. What is the best therapeutic approach?

Case 147

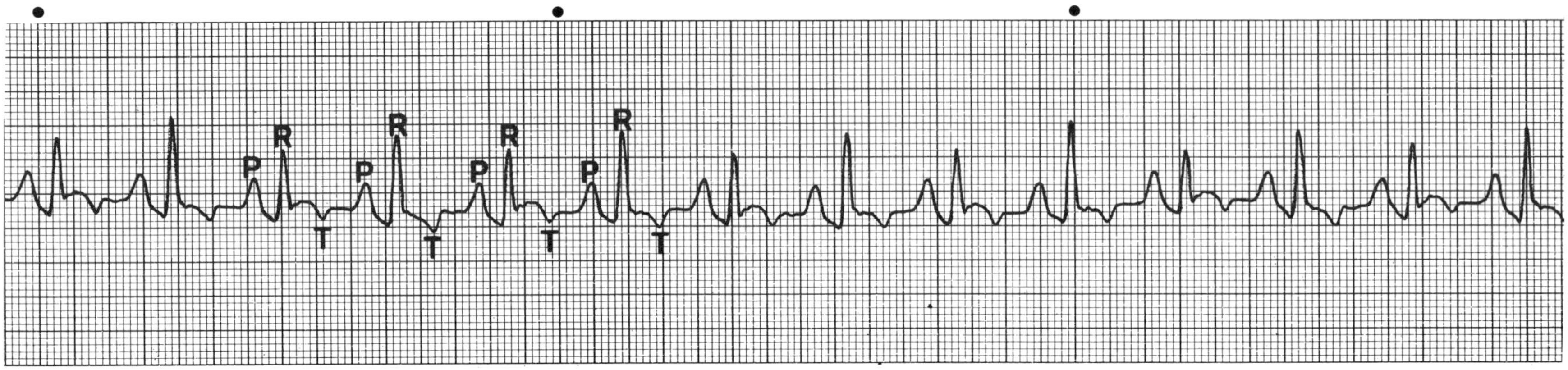

Answer: Sinus tachycardia with electrical alternans. Heart rate is 180 beats/min. Sinus tachycardia is a nonspecific finding that is often associated with stress, fever, pain, anemia, hypotension, and heart failure. The history of this dog suggests heart failure as a cause for the tachycardia. Electrical alternans is characterized by an alternation in the height of the QRS complexes. Causes include pericardial effusion, pleural effusion, and atrial tachycardia. In this instance, the breed and sudden onset of weakness and heart failure suggest pericardial effusion secondary to right atrial hemangiosarcoma. The P waves are large, thus suggesting biatrial enlargement and raising the possibility of dilated cardiomyopathy. Pericardial effusion can also occur secondary to cardiomyopathy. Thoracic and abdominal radiographs are needed. Echocardiography may be necessary to differentiate pericardial effusion from dilated cardiomyopathy. Electrical alternans is not an arrhythmia and does not require treatment. Therapy should be directed at the underlying cause. Sinus tachycardia caused by cardiomyopathy should be treated with digoxin. Sinus tachycardia caused by pericardial effusion-induced hypotension should be treated by pericardiocentesis.

Case 148

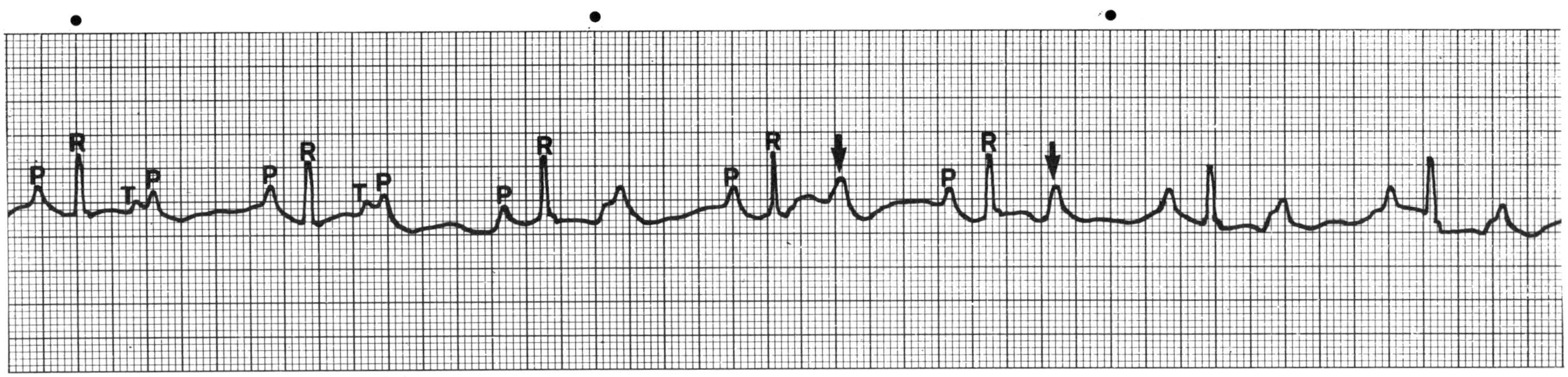

Answer: Sinus rhythm with second-degree AV block. Ventricular heart rate is 90 beats/min; atrial heart rate is 170 beats/min. Fibrosis of the AV node or His bundle tissue may account for this conduction disorder. Treatment of the cough with an antibiotic and bronchodilator is the best therapeutic approach. Pulmonary hypoxia causing increased levels of vagal tone can be reversed. If signs of weakness or syncope occur, anticholinergics or a permanent cardiac pacemaker may be required. Sinus beats (P-R-T) along with intermittent P waves not followed by QRS complexes are the hallmark of second-degree AV block. Notice how the P waves can be hidden in the preceding T waves (arrows), thereby confusing the diagnosis. The second and fourth P waves are separated from the preceding T waves, thus allowing their identification. Also, the P wave-to-P wave interval remains consistent throughout the ECG strip.

Case 149

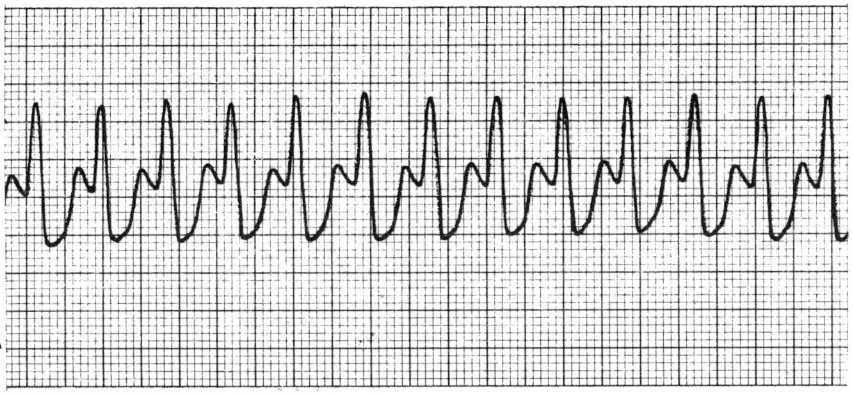

A

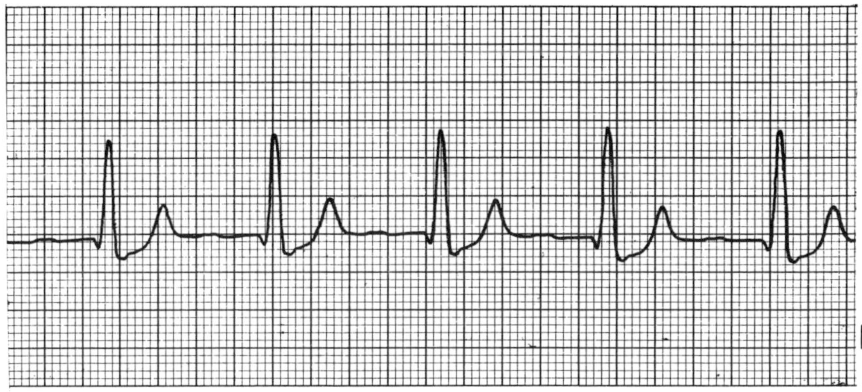

B

Question: Strip A was obtained from a 5-year-old male Great Dane that was examined in a state of collapse. Strip B was taken after treatment.

1. What is the rhythm diagnosis in strips A and B?
2. What is the best therapeutic approach?

Case 150

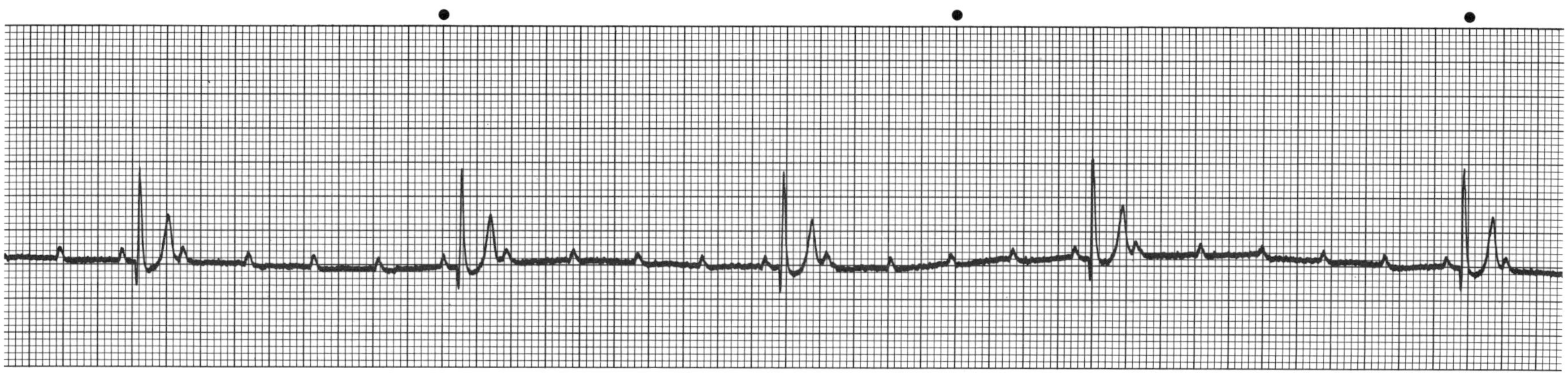

Question: This lead II rhythm strip was recorded from a dog with weakness and one episode of fainting. Paper speed: 25 mm/sec.

1. What is the rhythm diagnosis?
2. What is the best therapeutic approach?

Case 149

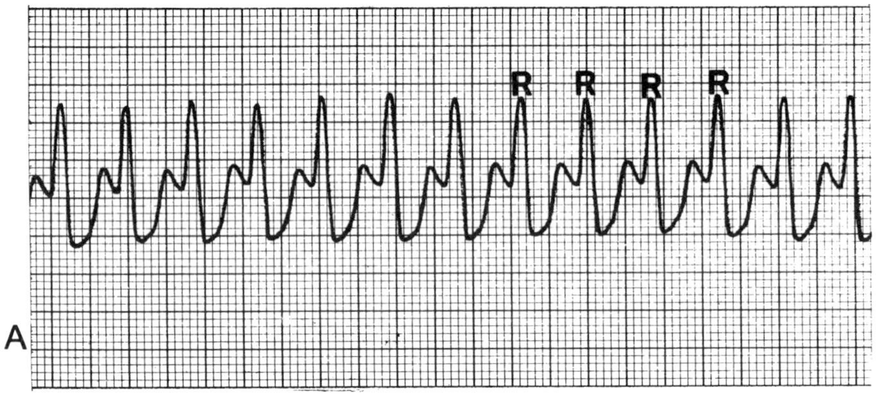

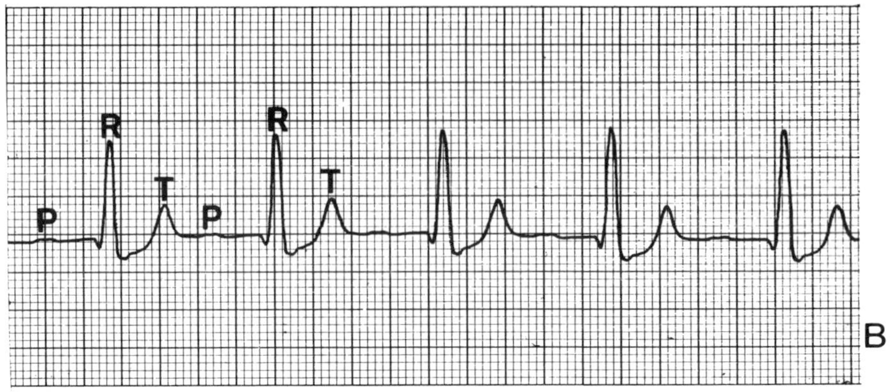

Answer: A. Atrial tachycardia. Heart rate is approximately 350 beats/min. B. Sinus rhythm with first-degree AV block. Heart rate is 140 beats/min. The extremely rapid tachycardia coupled with the positive QRS complexes of normal width in lead II suggest atrial tachycardia. At this rapid heart rate, the possibility of ventricular tachycardia is difficult to completely rule out on the basis of the ECG alone. Vagal maneuvers are often effective in breaking atrial tachycardia. Carotid sinus massage and ocular pressure were not effective in this dog. If uncertain whether the rhythm is supraventricular or ventricular, drug therapy for ventricular tachycardia should be initiated first, because this arrhythmia is more life threatening. Lidocaine boluses were not effective in breaking the tachycardia. A combination of procainamide and propranolol was then administered. Procainamide has both atrial and ventricular antiarrhythmic properties. Propranolol was chosen for its combination of atrial and ventricular antiarrhythmic properties. The tachycardia resolved. The morphology of the complexes in the sinus rhythm is similar to that of the tachycardia complexes, thus suggesting that the original rhythm was atrial tachycardia. The first-degree AV block may be the effect of propranolol on AV nodal conduction.

Case 150

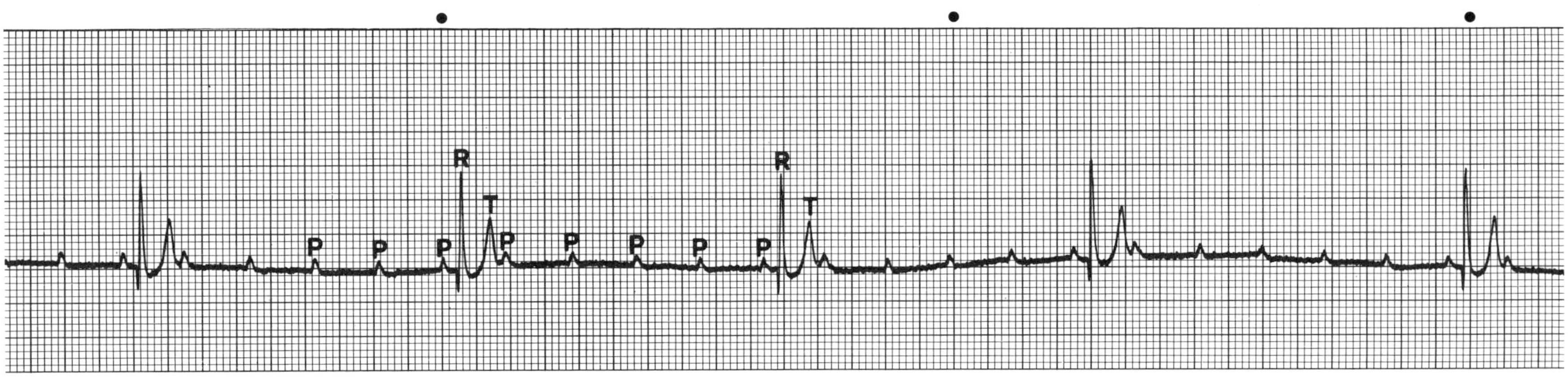

Answer: Advanced second-degree AV block (Mobitz type II). Heart rate is approximately 60 beats/min (atrial rate, 160 beats/min). Advanced second-degree AV block is characterized by a frequent intermittent failure of AV conduction. Many of the P waves are not followed by QRS-T complexes. The P-R interval is constant on conducted P-QRS complexes. The normal duration of the QRS complex indicates that the conduction failure is most likely in the AV node or proximal His bundle. The term "advanced" or "high-grade" AV block is used when the AV conduction ratio equals or exceeds 3 : 1 and no preceding P-R interval prolongation is evident. Advanced or high-grade Mobitz type II AV block frequently progresses to complete heart block. This high-grade or advanced form of AV block usually requires treatment with a permanent pacemaker because of the poor prognosis if left untreated. Drug therapy may include beta-agonists, such as isoproterenol.

Case 151

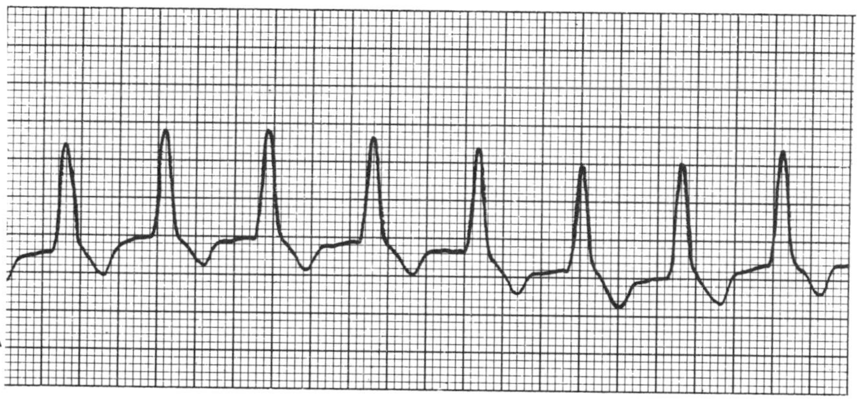

A

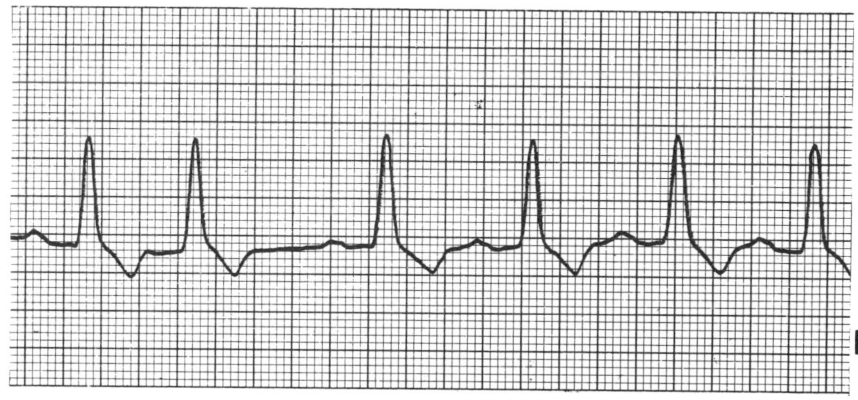

B

Question: These lead II ECGs were obtained from a small 14-year-old mixed-breed dog with a history of coughing. A grade V/VI holosystolic murmur was auscultated.

1. What are the rhythm diagnoses?
2. What is the most likely underlying disorder?
3. What is the best therapeutic approach?

Case 152

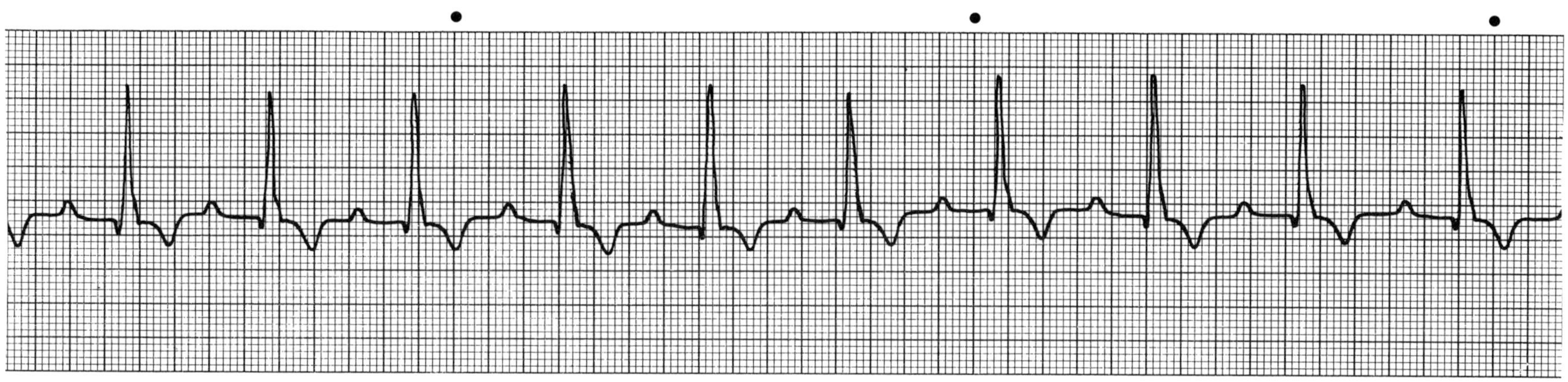

Question: This lead II ECG was obtained from a 5-year-old male Newfoundland with no clinical signs. A low-grade (I/VI) left-sided heart murmur was heard on auscultation.

1. What is the rhythm diagnosis?
2. What is the most likely underlying disorder?
3. What is the best therapeutic approach?

Case 151

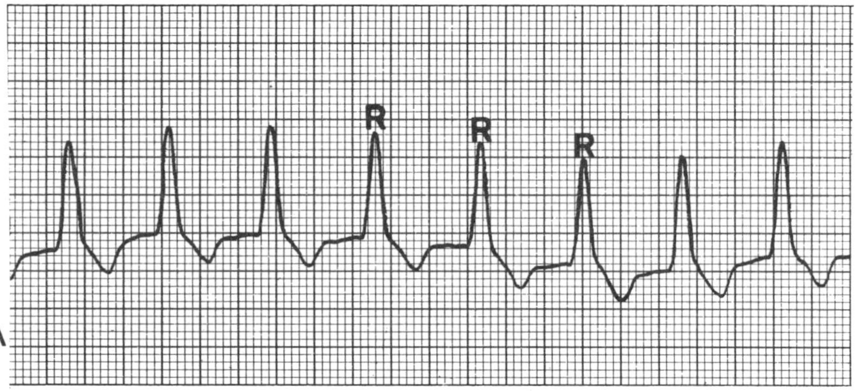

A

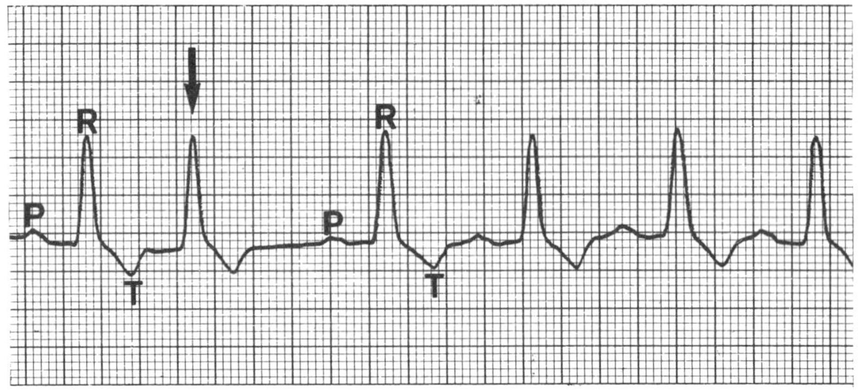

B

Answer: A. Atrial tachycardia. Heart rate is 220 beats/min. B. Sinus rhythm with one atrial premature complex. The initial rhythm is atrial tachycardia. This rhythm is characterized by supraventricular-appearing complexes occurring at a rapid rate and regular rhythm. The P waves are often superimposed on the T waves of the preceding complexes, as in this dog. The QRS complexes in strip A are relatively wide; therefore, ventricular tachycardia should also be considered. The atrial tachycardia was temporarily eliminated by a vagal maneuver (carotid sinus massage). The one atrial premature complex (arrow) helps to support the diagnosis of atrial tachycardia in strip A, because "company attracts company." The P waves of the sinus complexes in strip B are wide, thus suggesting left atrial enlargement. The arrhythmia and atrial distention are probably the result of mitral valve cardosis in this small-breed dog. Thoracic radiographs should be obtained to determine the cause of the coughing and to further assess heart size. The arrhythmia should be treated with digoxin. Propranolol and diltiazem are also effective in controlling atrial arrhythmias, but digoxin is preferred in animals with congestive heart failure. Diuretics are indicated if the dog has pulmonary edema.

Case 152

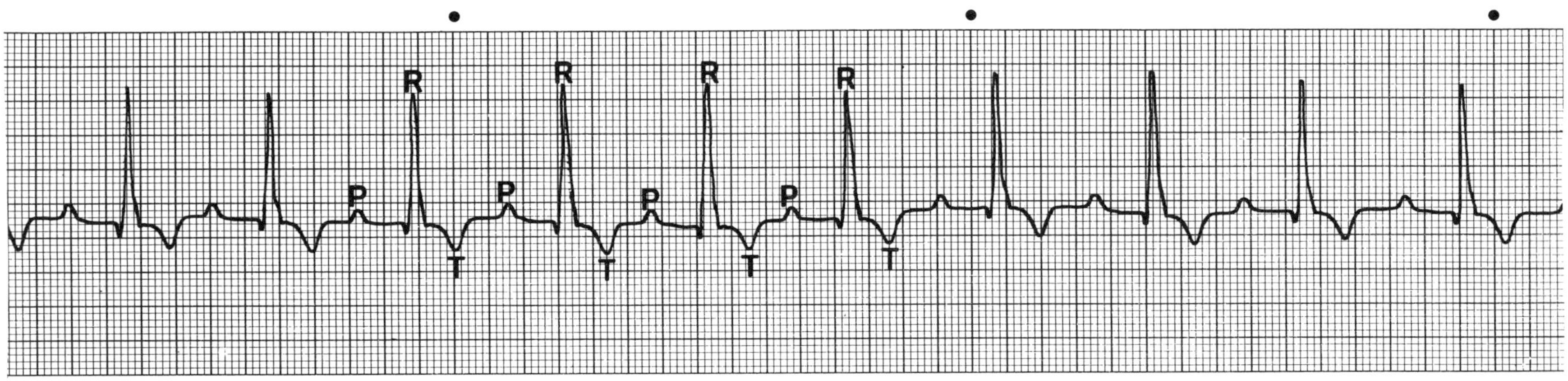

Answer: Sinus rhythm with first-degree AV block. Heart rate is 140 beats/min. First-degree AV block (P-R interval, > 0.13 sec) may be a physiologic variation in a large-breed dog caused by large heart size or high levels of vagal tone rather than by actual cardiac disease. No treatment is required. The P-R interval represents AV conduction time. Conduction delay may occur in the atria, AV junction, or His-Purkinje system. A low-grade heart murmur is often physiologic (flow murmur) and not caused by cardiac disease. The murmur of a significant subaortic stenosis should be a loud (grade III/VI or higher) systolic ejection murmur, loudest over the aortic area at left base or cranial right thorax. An echocardiogram should be performed if subaortic stenosis is a major consideration. The Newfoundland breed is prone to subaortic stenosis. The ECG should be repeated in the near future to monitor any progression of the AV block.

Case 153

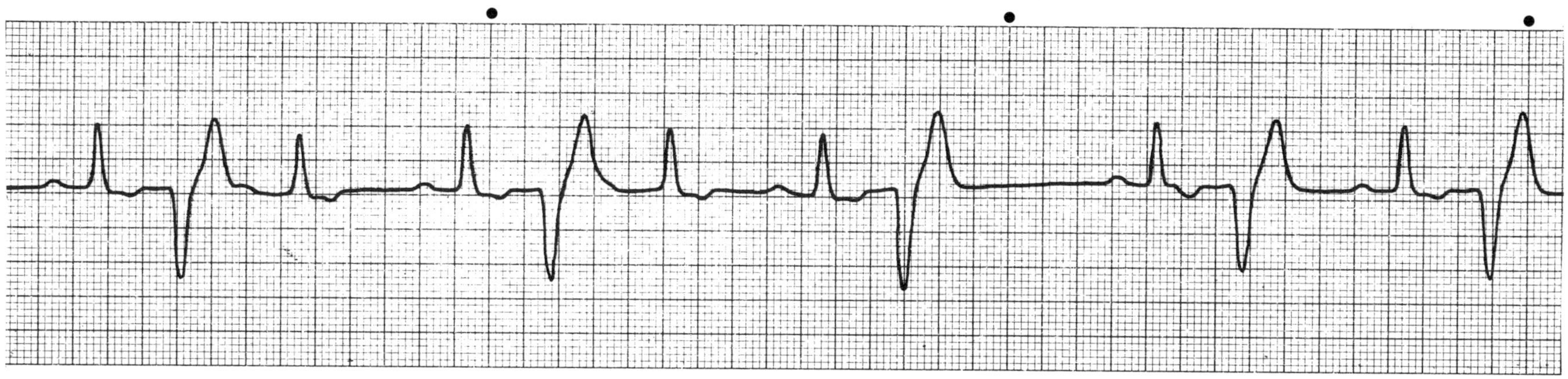

Question: This lead-II rhythm strip was recorded from a 2-year-old Golden Retriever that had collapsed after exercise. A II/VI crescendo-decrescendo systolic murmur loudest at the left heart base was detected on auscultation.

1. What is the rhythm diagnosis?
2. What is the most likely underlying disorder?
3. What is the most likely mechanism for this arrhythmia?
4. What is the best therapeutic approach?
5. What warning should be given to the owners?

Case 154

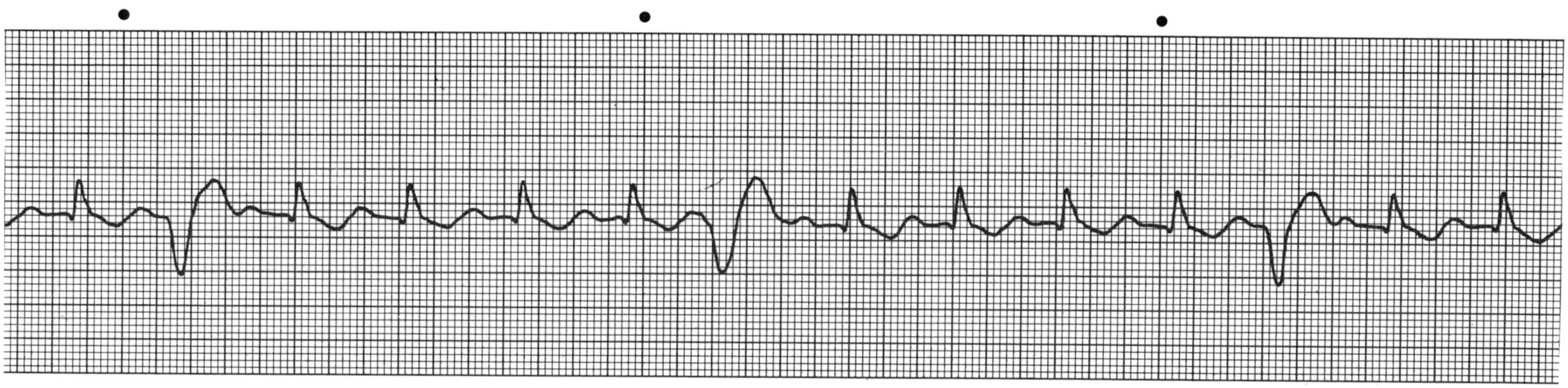

Question: This lead II ECG was recorded from a 6-year-old Boxer with a history of dyspnea, ascites, and syncope. The dog was being treated with digoxin and furosemide at the time the ECG was recorded.

1. What is the rhythm diagnosis?
2. What is the most likely cause of this arrhythmia?
3. What is the most likely underlying disorder?
4. What is the best therapeutic approach?

Case 153

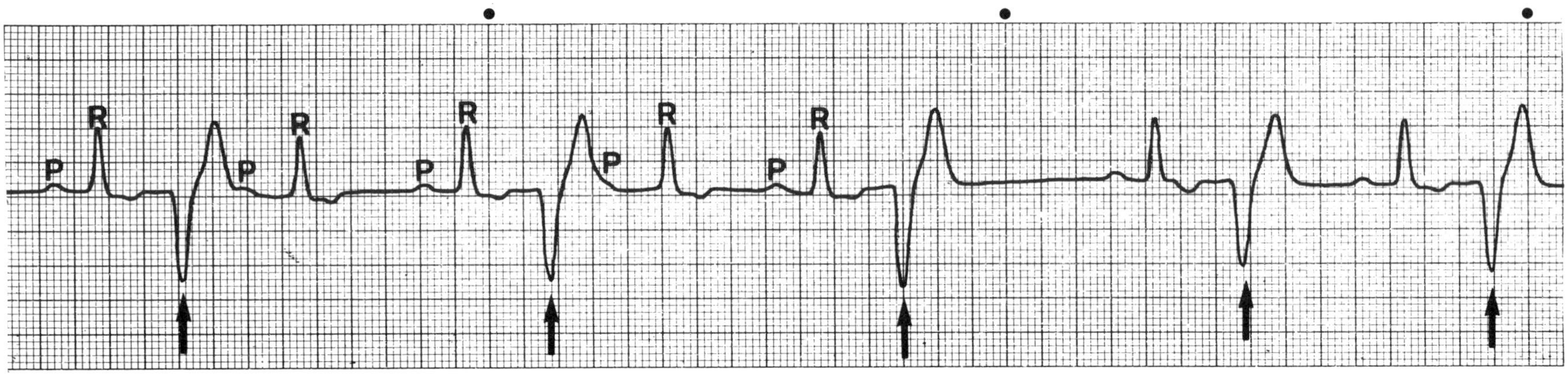

Answer: Sinus rhythm with frequent ventricular premature complexes. Heart rate is approximately 140 beats/min. Frequent ventricular premature complexes (arrows) are present. The coupling interval between the sinus complexes and ventricular premature complexes is identical for each pair. This consistency suggests re-entry as the mechanism for the arrhythmia. Notice the prolonged P-R interval following the first and second ventricular premature complexes. This prolongation is caused by concealed conduction of the ventricular premature complex into the AV node, thus affecting its refractory period and the conduction speed of the following sinus complex. The history of collapse suggests that the dog had experienced a run of ventricular tachycardia. The signalment and description of the murmur are strongly suggestive of subaortic stenosis. Ventricular arrhythmias are commonly associated with this congenital defect. Dilated cardiomyopathy must also be considered, but the murmur is usually louder at the left apex in dogs with this disease. Thoracic radiography and echocardiography are recommended. Treatment with procainamide was instituted while awaiting results of the echocardiogram. Subaortic stenosis was diagnosed, and propranolol was added to the treatment regimen. The dog was eventually taken off procainamide, and the arrhythmia was controlled with propranolol. The owners should be warned that dogs with subaortic stenosis and ventricular arrhythmias are at high risk for sudden death.

Case 154

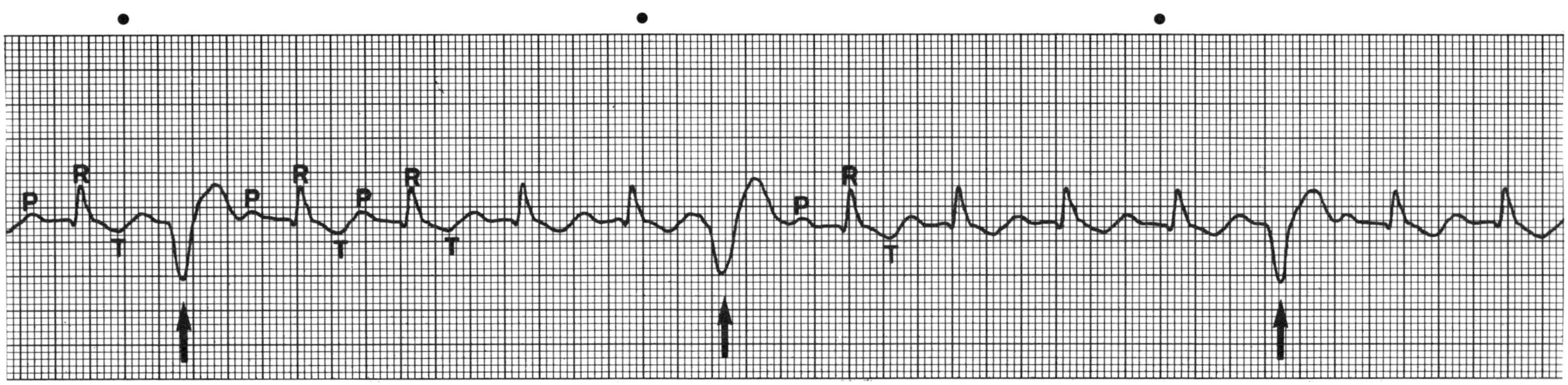

Answer: Sinus tachycardia with ventricular premature complexes (arrows). Heart rate is 190 beats/min. Sinus tachycardia would be consistent with heart failure in this dog. Ventricular premature complexes are common in Boxers with cardiomyopathy. Syncope may be caused by periods of ventricular tachycardia or low-output cardiac failure associated with myocardial failure. The small QRS complexes of the sinus complexes may indicate pleural or pericardial effusion. Serum digoxin concentrations should be assessed and thoracic radiographs obtained. Because of the history of collapse and ventricular premature complexes, antiarrhythmic therapy with procainamide, quinidine, tocainide, or mexiletine should be instituted. Diuretics and vasodilators should be continued for congestive heart failure. The ECG should be rechecked 2 to 3 days after modifying treatment.

Case 155

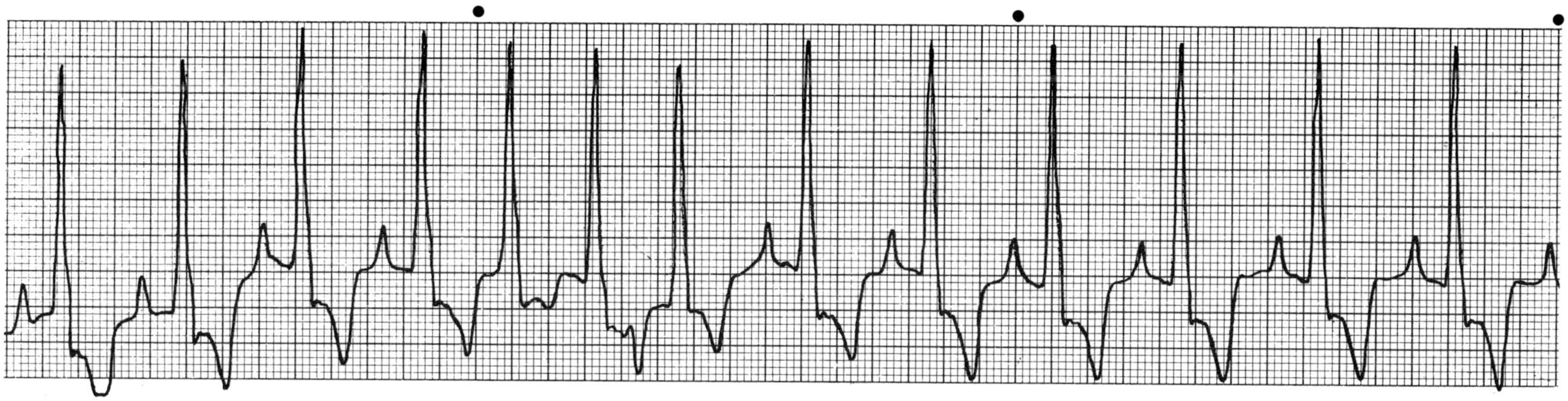

Question: This lead II ECG was obtained from a 3-year-old dyspneic Poodle with patent ductus arteriosus.

1. What is the rhythm diagnosis?
2. What is the best therapeutic approach?

Case 156

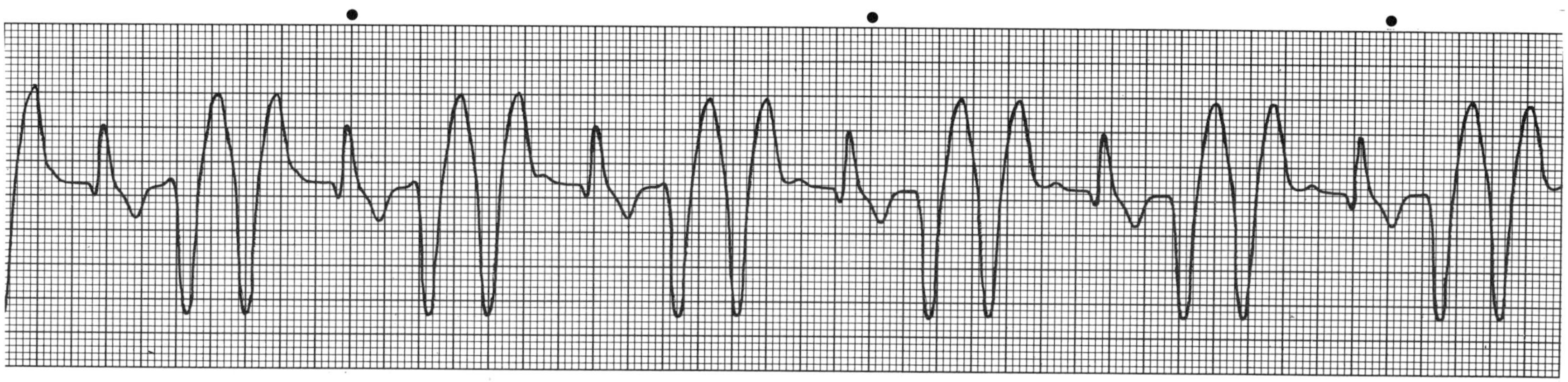

Question: This lead II rhythm strip was recorded from a 7-year-old Great Dane with gastric torsion. The dog requires surgery to correct the torsion.

1. What is the rhythm diagnosis?
2. What is the likely cause of this arrhythmia?
3. What is the best therapeutic approach?

Case 155

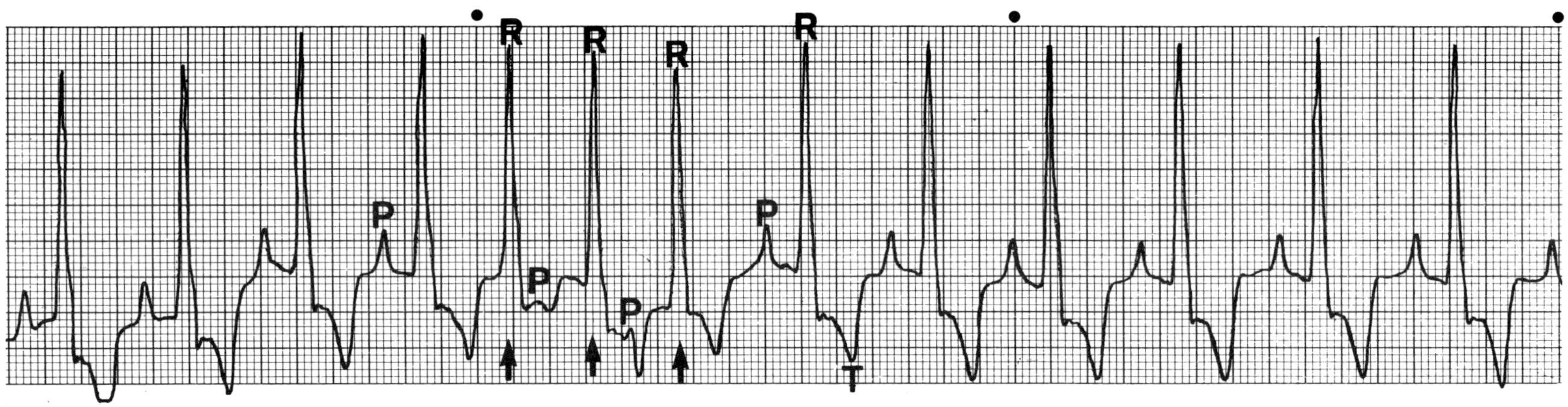

Answer: Sinus rhythm with atrial premature complexes. Heart rate is 160 beats/min. Digoxin is the preferred drug for treating this arrhythmia. The three QRS complexes labelled with arrows are premature, with their preceding P′ waves hidden in the QRS-T complexes. The QRS complexes of the atrial premature complexes resemble the sinus beats, an important criterion. The large P-QRS complexes support a diagnosis of possible atrial and left ventricular enlargement.

Case 156

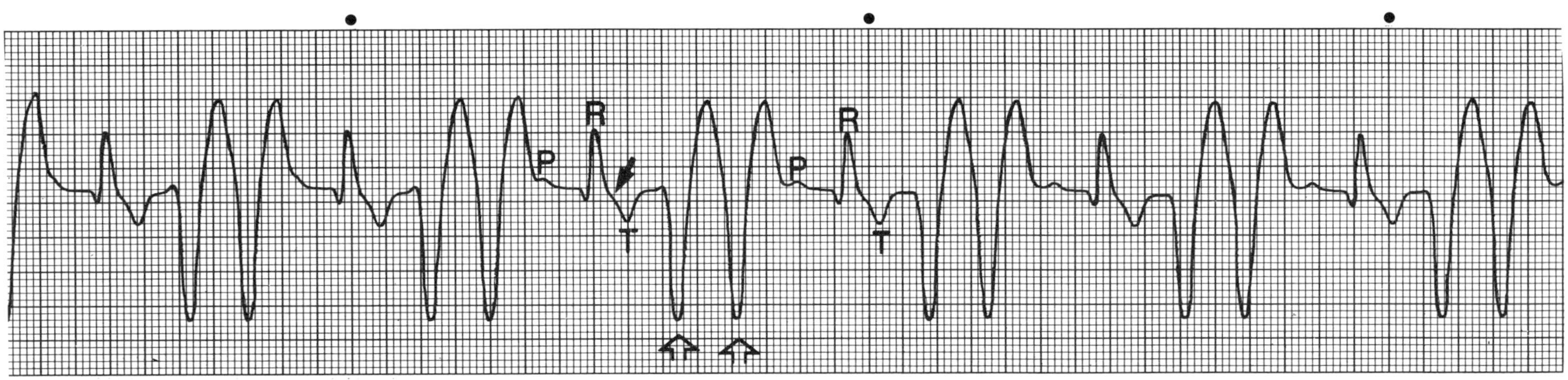

Answer: Sinus rhythm with couplets (open arrows) of ventricular premature complexes. Heart rate is 250 beats/min. Ventricular arrhythmias are frequently associated with gastric dilatation and volvulus. Causes include myocardial hypoxia, low perfusion of the coronary arteries, acid-base disturbances, and release of myocardial depressant factors after correction of the torsion. The presence of wide QRS complexes and slurring or coving of the S-T segment (closed arrow) of the sinus beats in this breed suggests left ventricular enlargement and possible dilated cardiomyopathy. This arrhythmia is also seen in dogs with dilated cardiomyopathy. Thoracic radiographs are indicated. The dog should receive fluids to control hypotension. The arrhythmia must be controlled before anesthesia can be induced. Boluses of lidocaine should be administered to correct the arrhythmia and a lidocaine infusion should be maintained during surgery. The infusion should be continued after surgery while instituting treatment with procainamide. If the dog responds well to treatment, lidocaine usually can be tapered off in 1 to 2 days and procainamide usually can be discontinued in 7 to 10 days.

Case 157

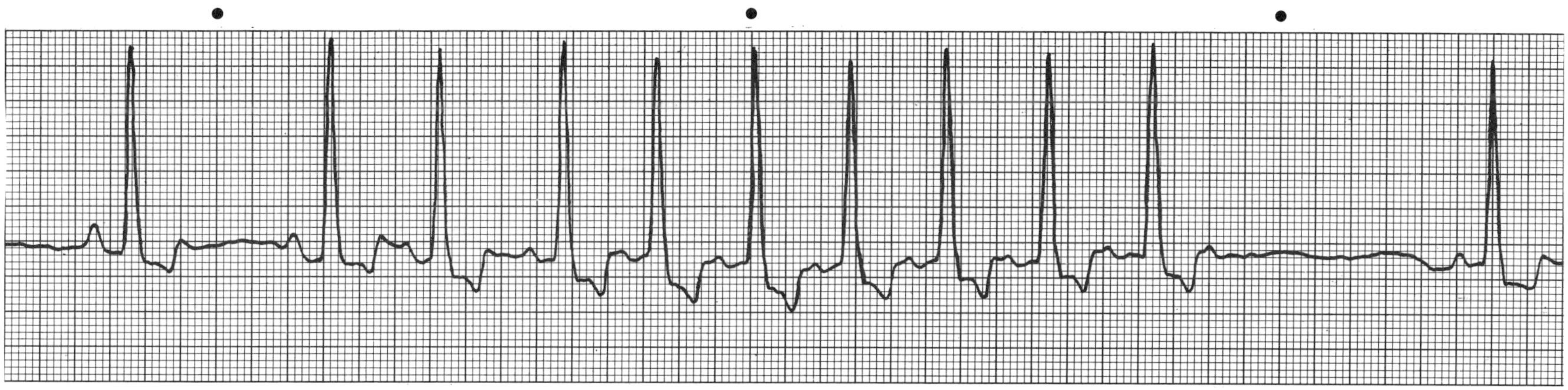

Question: This lead II ECG was obtained from a 9-year-old female Dalmatian examined because of dyspnea and periodic collapsing episodes.

1. What is the rhythm diagnosis?
2. What is the most likely underlying disorder?
3. What is the best therapeutic approach?

Case 158

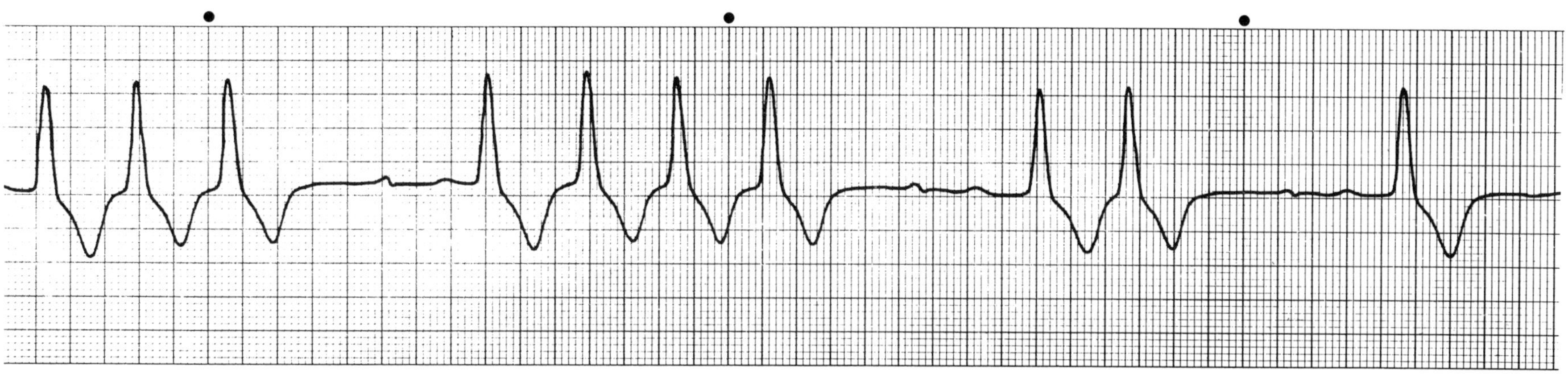

Question: This lead II ECG was obtained from a 10-year-old dyspneic female cat. Pleural effusion was seen on thoracic radiographs.

1. What is the rhythm diagnosis?
2. What is the best therapeutic approach?

Case 157

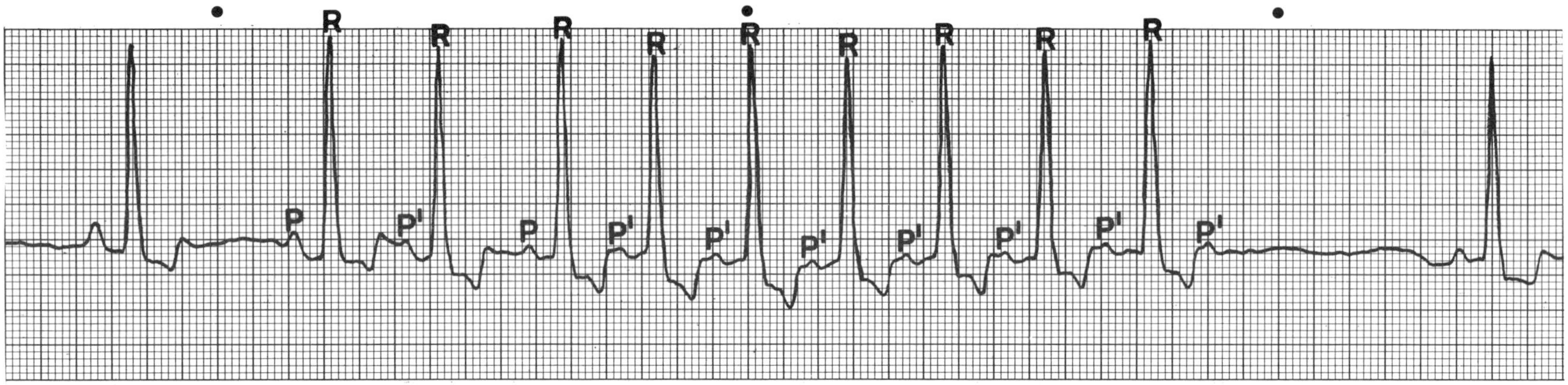

Answer: Sinus rhythm with paroxysmal supraventricular tachycardia. Heart rate is 160 beats/min. Dilated cardiomyopathy is the most likely disorder causing the arrhythmia, but chronic mitral valvular insufficiency is another possible consideration. The QRS complexes are of increased amplitude and duration, thus indicating possible left ventricular enlargement. The premature QRS complexes (between the P′ waves) resemble the basic QRS complexes, one of the criteria for atrial premature complexes. The appearance of three or more consecutive atrial premature complexes is termed paroxysmal atria tachycardia. The last P′ wave is not conducted to the ventricles. The conduction delay most likely occurs in the AV node and correlates with the termination of the arrhythmia. Digoxin or a combination of digoxin and diltiazem is the best therapeutic approach to control and prevent atrial tachycardia.

Case 158

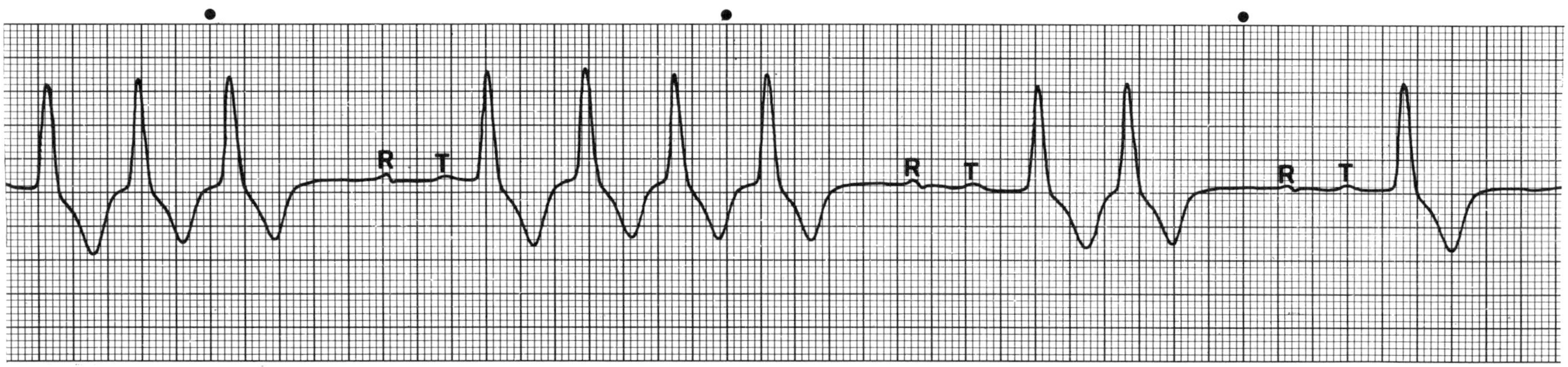

Answer: Ventricular premature complexes and paroxysmal ventricular tachycardia. Heart rate is 170 beats/min. Thoracocentesis and treatment of the underlying disorder comprise the best therapeutic approach. The sinus beats (R-T) are easy to miss because of their low amplitudes. The P waves also are not visible. Precordial chest leads can be used to amplify the complexes. The pleural effusion is probably attenuating the voltages of the sinus complexes. The high-amplitude and wide QRS complexes are the ventricular premature complexes. Antiarrhythmic drugs, such as propranolol, are not advised initially, because the overall heart rate is slow and a further reduction in heart rate may reduce cardiac output. The use of lidocaine also should be carefully considered.

Case 159

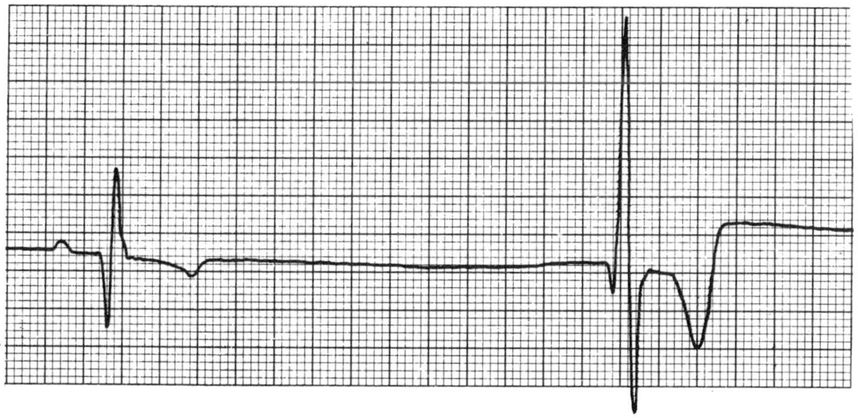

A

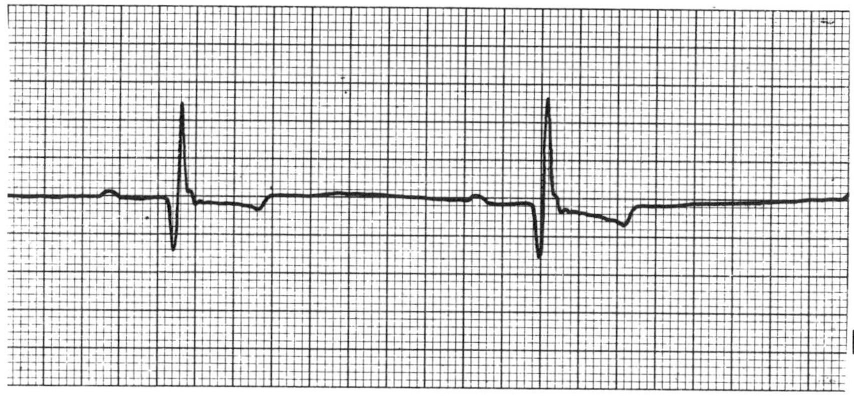

B

Question: These ECG strips were recorded from a 12-year-old female Pug. The dog was examined because of syncope, and bradycardia was noticed on physical examination. Strip A was taken initially, and strip B was taken after atropine had been administered.

1. What is the rhythm diagnosis?
2. What is the explanation for the changes that occurred after atropine administration?
3. What is the most likely underlying disorder?
4. What is the best therapeutic approach?

Case 160

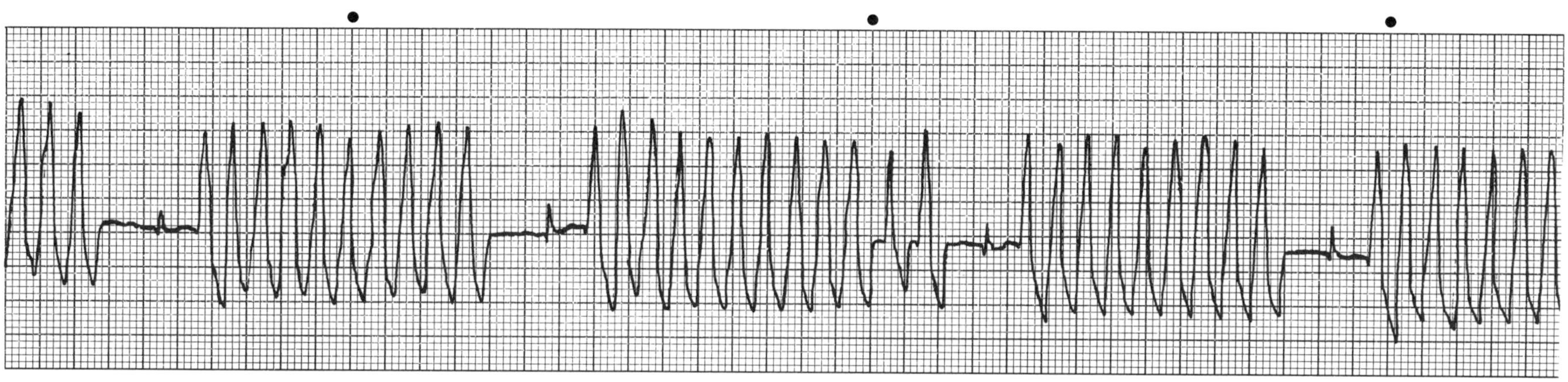

Question: This lead II ECG was obtained from a 3-year-old Boxer with syncopal episodes. Paper speed: 25 mm/sec, 0.5 gain.

1. What is the rhythm diagnosis?
2. What is the most likely underlying disorder?
3. What is the best therapeutic approach?

Case 159

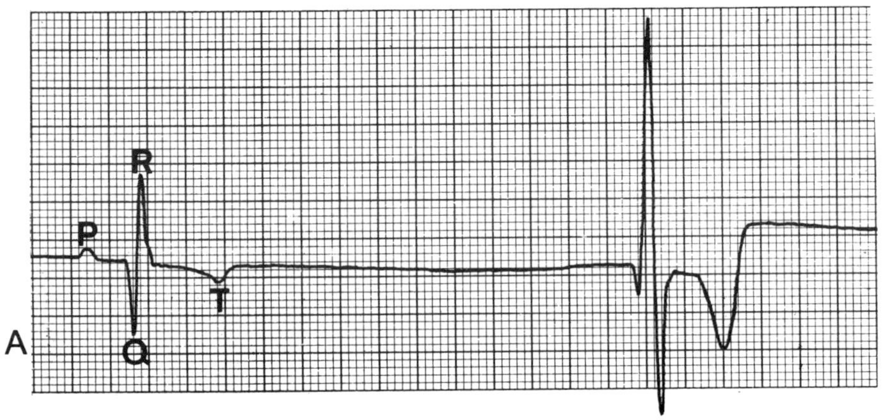

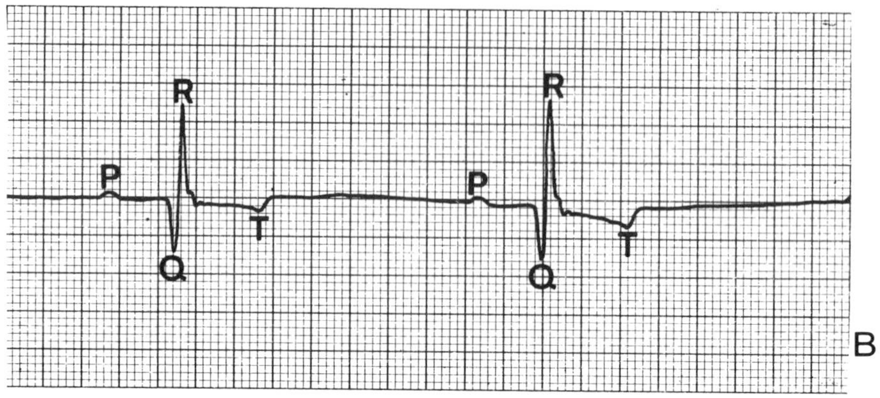

Answer: A. Sinus complex followed by a ventricular escape beat. B. Sinus rhythm with first-degree AV block. The initial ECG shows sinus rhythm and a ventricular escape beat. Sinus bradycardia and ventricular escape complexes in an old female Pug are generally associated with sick sinus syndrome and/or increased vagal tone. Atropine increases the sinus rate and, therefore, abolishes the escape complexes. The interesting finding is that first-degree AV block developed after atropine administration. This development is surprising because atropine also enhances AV nodal conduction and the block had not been present before atropine administration. The block can be attributed to underlying AV nodal or His-Purkinje disease or to the dosage of atropine. Atropine dosages of less than 0.015 mg/kg may cause AV block. Before atropine administration, the slow heart rate allowed for complete repolarization of the diseased AV conduction tissue, and therefore, AV block was not present. Because atropine increases the sinus rate, however, impulses arrived at the diseased AV node before repolarization was complete. This sequence of events delayed conduction, and a first-degree AV block developed. Despite the development of the first-degree AV block, the overall heart rate increased with atropine, and the dog should be treated with propantheline or isopropamide.

Case 160

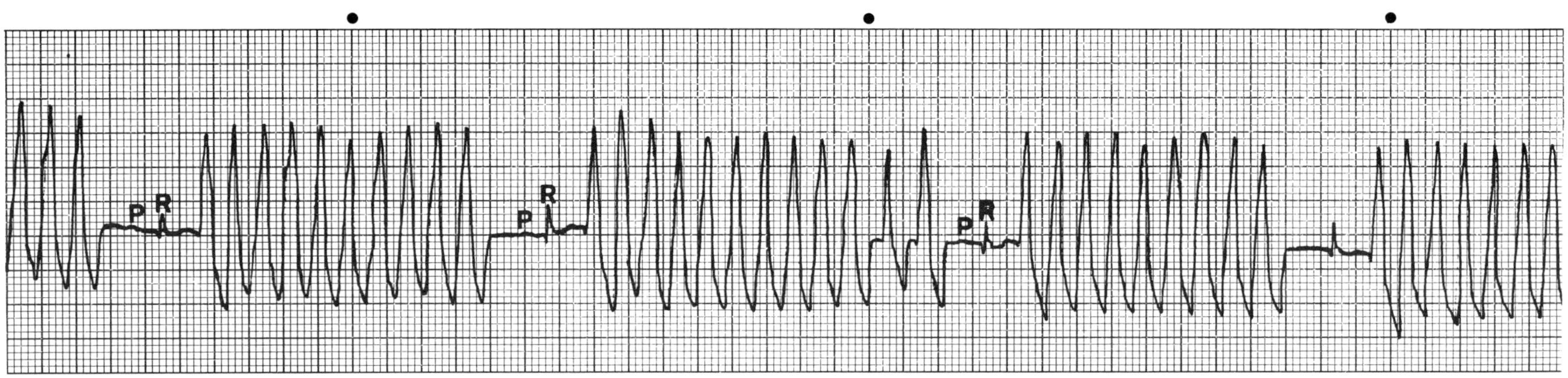

Answer: Sinus rhythm with paroxysmal ventricular tachycardia-flutter. Heart rate is approximately 280 beats/min. Cardiomyopathy is the most likely underlying disorder. Intravenous administration of lidocaine followed by procainamide and propranolol given orally is the best therapeutic approach. The morphology of the wide QRS complexes in tachycardia differs markedly from that of the sinus beats and is characteristic of ventricular tachycardia. During the tachycardia, the QRS is difficult to distinguish from the T waves (no S-T segment), a characteristic typical of ventricular flutter. This arrhythmia is electrically unstable and may proceed to ventricular fibrillation. Propranolol is antifibrillatory and may help to prevent such an outcome.

Case 161

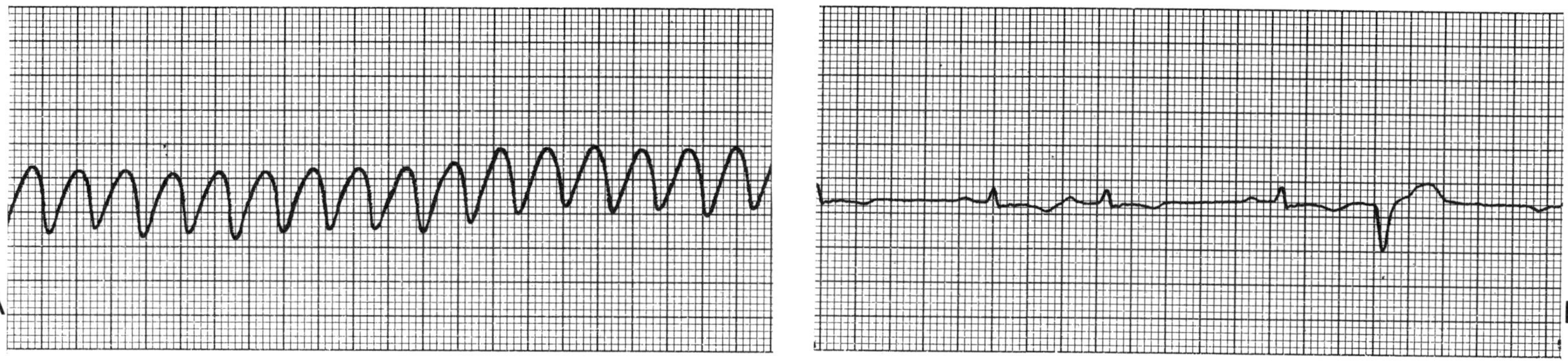

A B

Question: This lead II ECG was obtained from a 10-year-old cat examined because of severe dyspnea. ECG strips A and B were recorded before and after treatment, respectively.

1. What is the rhythm diagnosis?
2. What is the most likely underlying disorder?
3. What is the best therapeutic approach?

Case 162

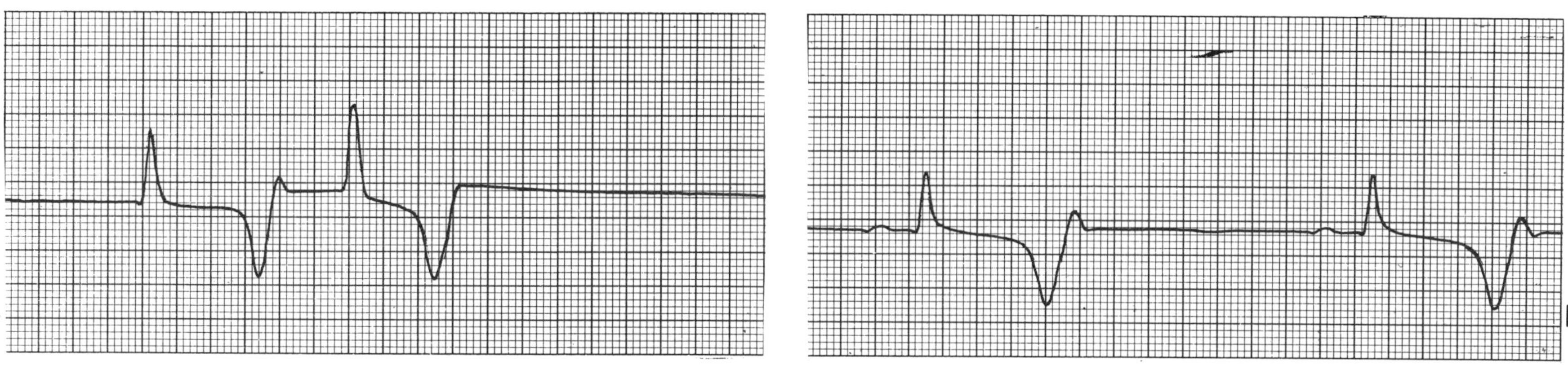

A B

Question: The lead II ECG in strip A was obtained from a 3-year-old Miniature Poodle examined because of severe weakness, vomiting, and diarrhea. The ECG in strip B was recorded after treatment.

1. What is the rhythm diagnosis?
2. What is the most likely underlying disorder?
3. What is the best therapeutic approach?

Case 161

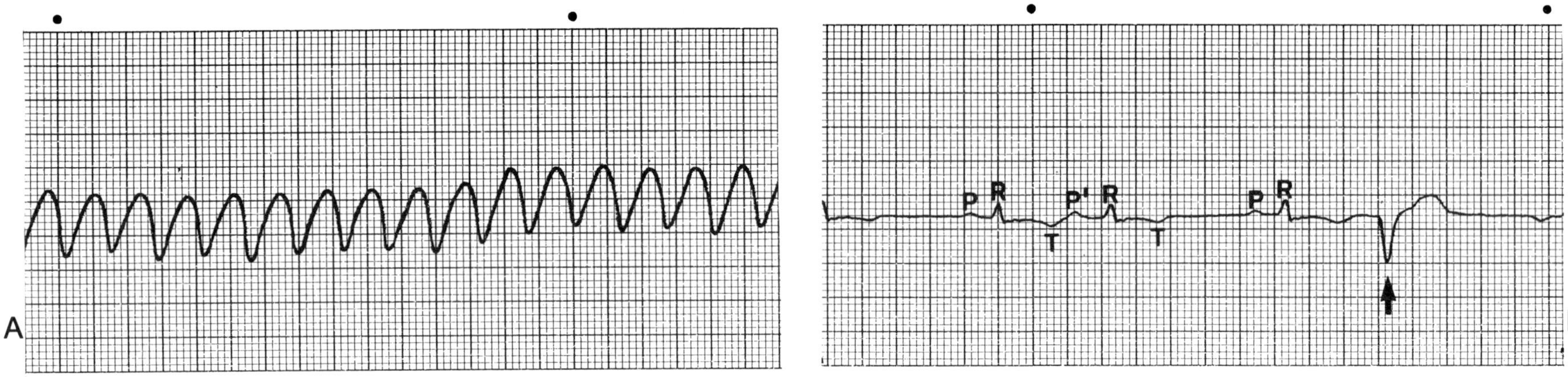

A
B

Answer: A. Ventricular tachycardia. Heart rate is 400 beats/min. B. Sinus rhythm with an atrial premature complex (P′-R-T) and a ventricular premature complex (arrow). Heart rate is approximately 150 beats/min. Feline cardiomyopathy, hyperthyroidism, and myocarditis (associated with infection, neoplasia, uremia, trauma, or other condition) are the most common causes of this arrhythmia. Administration of beta-blocker (e.g., propranolol or atenolol) or lidocaine is the best therapeutic approach. Ventricular tachycardia should be considered first because of the wide complex tachycardia in strip A. Also, in strip B, the QRS complex of the isolated ventricular premature complex resembles the QRS complex during the tachycardia. Supraventricular tachycardia with right bundle-branch block is another possibility for the wide-complex tachycardia in strip A. The lack of a right bundle-branch block pattern in the sinus beats in strip B helps to rule out this diagnosis.

Case 162

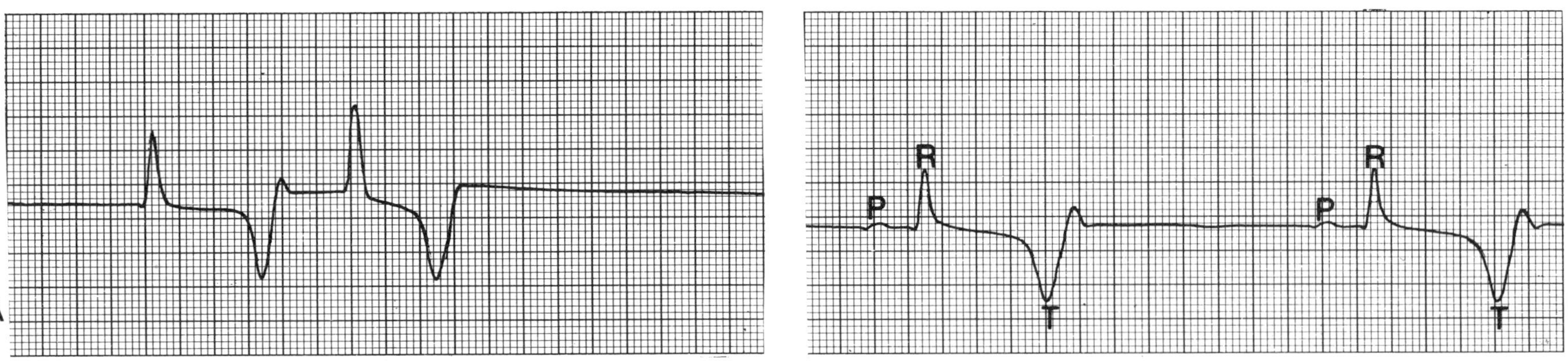

A
B

Answer: A. Atrial standstill. B. Sinus rhythm. Hyperkalemia associated with Addison's disease is the most likely underlying disorder. Treatment for hyperkalemia includes the administration of 0.9% sodium chloride, sodium bicarbonate, or dextrose and regular insulin given intravenously. Corticosteroids are used to correct hypoadrenocorticism in dogs with Addison's disease. Atrial standstill is typified by bradycardia, no readily visible P waves, and, often, bizarre QRS complexes and T waves. The wide and bizarre QRS complexes in strip A simulate an idioventricular rhythm. Experimental studies indicate, however, that the SA node continues to fire, and its impulses are transmitted by the internodal pathways. Atrial standstill caused by hyperkalemia may be rapidly converted to sinus rhythm by the previously described treatment. Given the abnormal-appearing T waves and flattened P waves, the dog was probably still hyperkalemic at the time strip B was obtained. Persistent atrial standstill caused by a hereditary form of muscular dystrophy occurs in English Springer Spaniels.

Case 163

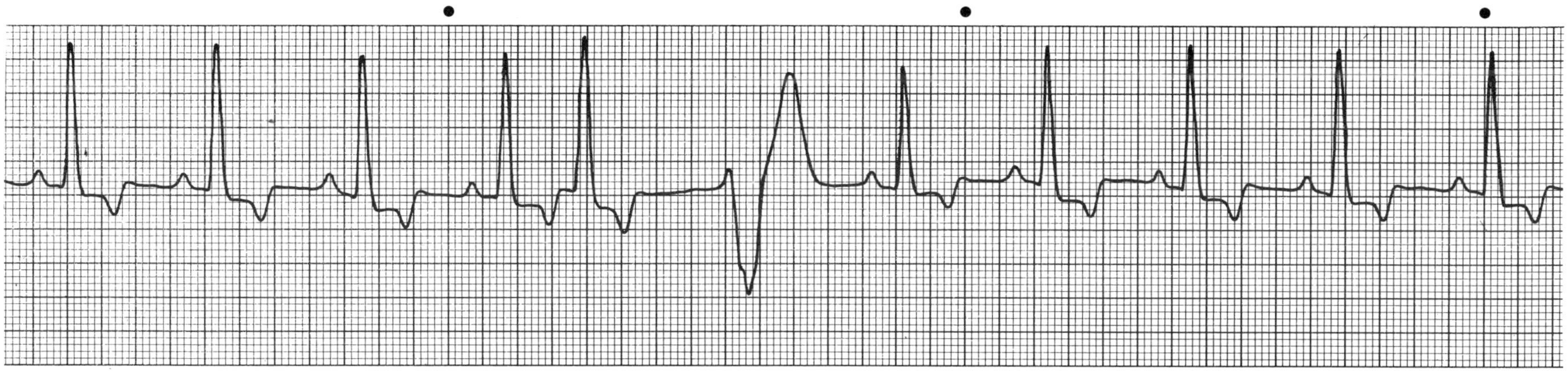

Question: This lead II ECG was obtained from a 10-year-old Golden Retriever with no clinical signs. An irregular heart rhythm was heard on auscultation during routine physical examination.

1. What is the rhythm diagnosis?
2. What is the most likely underlying disorder?
3. What is the best therapeutic approach?

Case 164

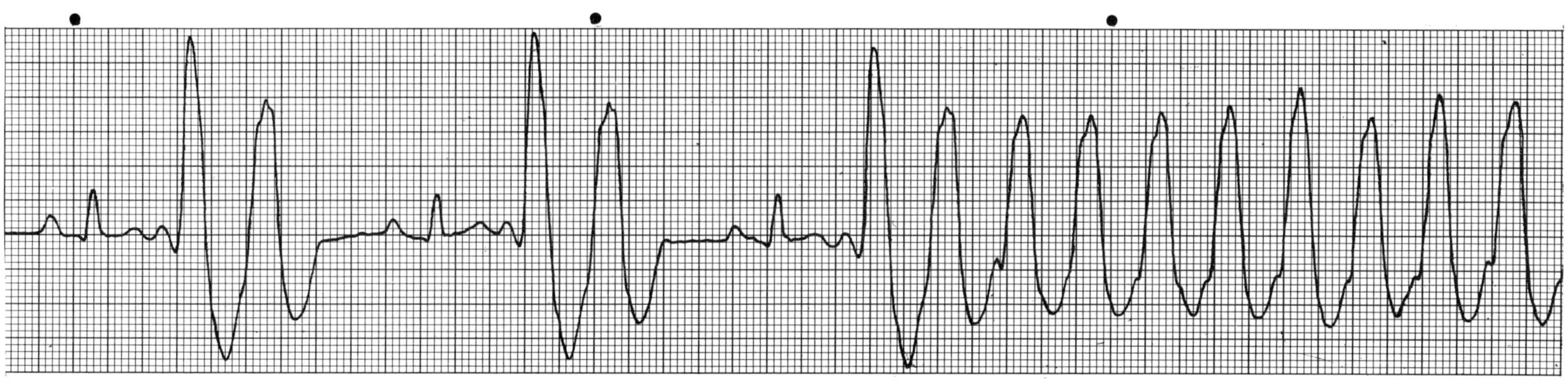

Question: This lead II ECG was obtained from a 6-year-old Boxer examined because of collapsing episodes during exercise.

1. What is the rhythm diagnosis?
2. What is the best therapeutic approach?

Case 163

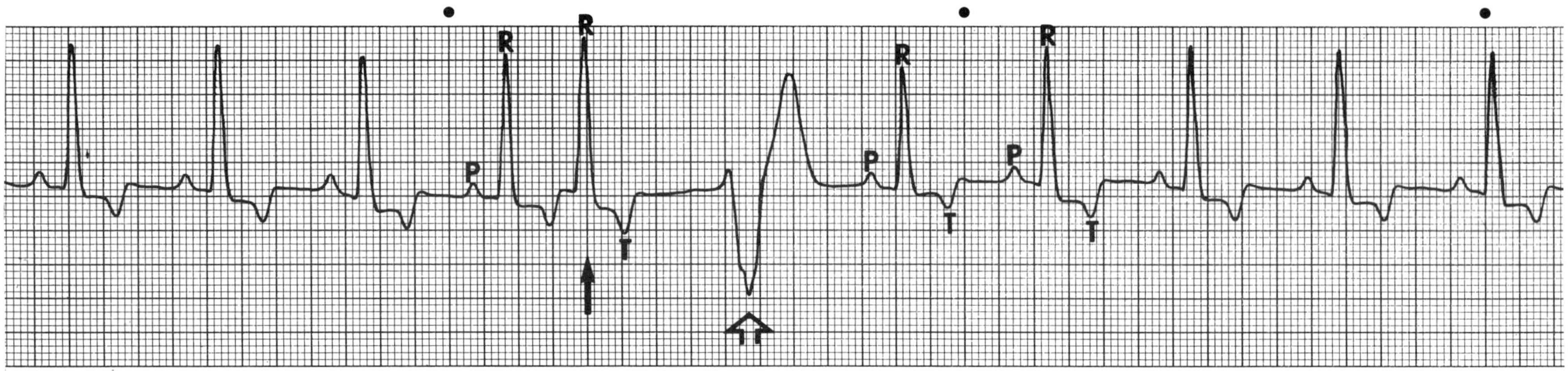

Answer: Sinus rhythm with an atrial premature complex (closed arrow) and ventricular escape beat (open arrow). Heart rate is 140 beats/min. Chronic AV valvular endocardiosis, cardiomyopathy, and myocarditis are common causes of this arrhythmia. Thoracic radiographs, blood tests, and, possibly, an echocardiogram are useful. The dog should be monitored for the development of clinical signs (e.g., dyspnea, weakness, and syncope), and if they develop, the ECG should be repeated. Antiarrhythmic drugs are not advised. The premature QRS complex (closed arrow) that resembles the sinus beats (P-R-T) is typical of atrial premature complexes. The P wave of the atrial premature complex is probably hidden in the preceding T wave. The wide and bizarre QRS complex (open arrow) resembles a beat originating in the ventricle, but it occurs late rather than prematurely and is a probable escape beat.

Case 164

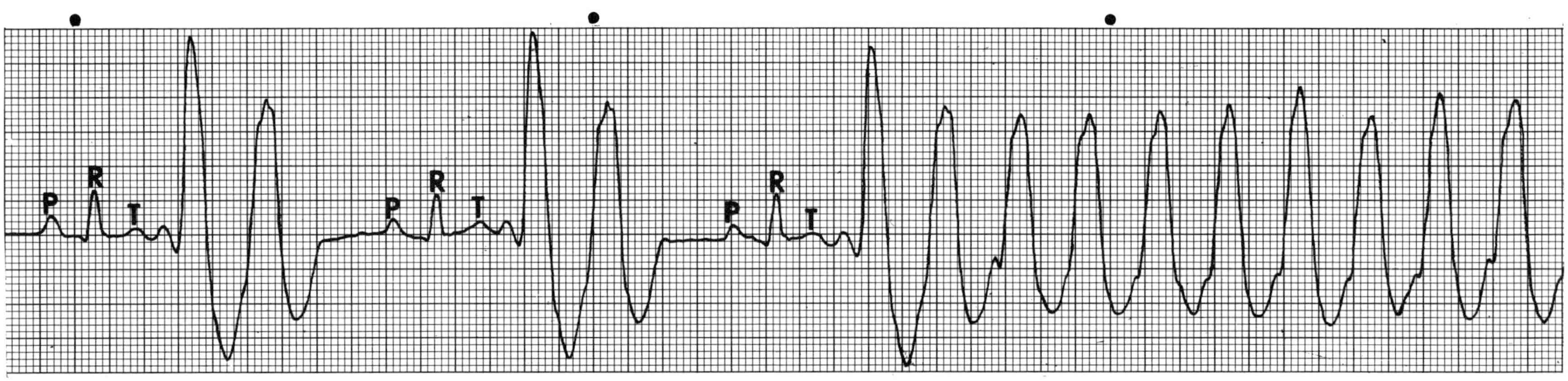

Answer: Sinus rhythm with repetitive ventricular premature complexes and paroxysmal ventricular tachycardia. Heart rate during the tachycardia is approximately 300 beats/min. A bolus of lidocaine without epinephrine should be administered, followed by a lidocaine infusion if the arrhythmia has stopped. Parenteral procainamide is an alternative to lidocaine. Oral therapy with procainamide and propranolol can also be initiated, followed by a slow reduction of the lidocaine infusion. The wide and bizarre QRS complexes that are not associated with P waves are typical of ventricular premature complexes. The appearance of three or more ventricular premature complexes in succession is ventricular tachycardia. Notice that the first ventricular premature complex after each sinus beat (P-R-T) has a greater amplitude than that of the second ventricular premature complex or of other ventricular premature complexes in the ventricular tachycardia sequence. The reason for the change in ventricular premature complex morphology is not clear. The change is probably related to a resetting of the Purkinje fiber and ventricular myocardial fiber transmembrane potential refractory period that occurs with the sinus beat and the first ventricular premature complex cycle.

Case 165

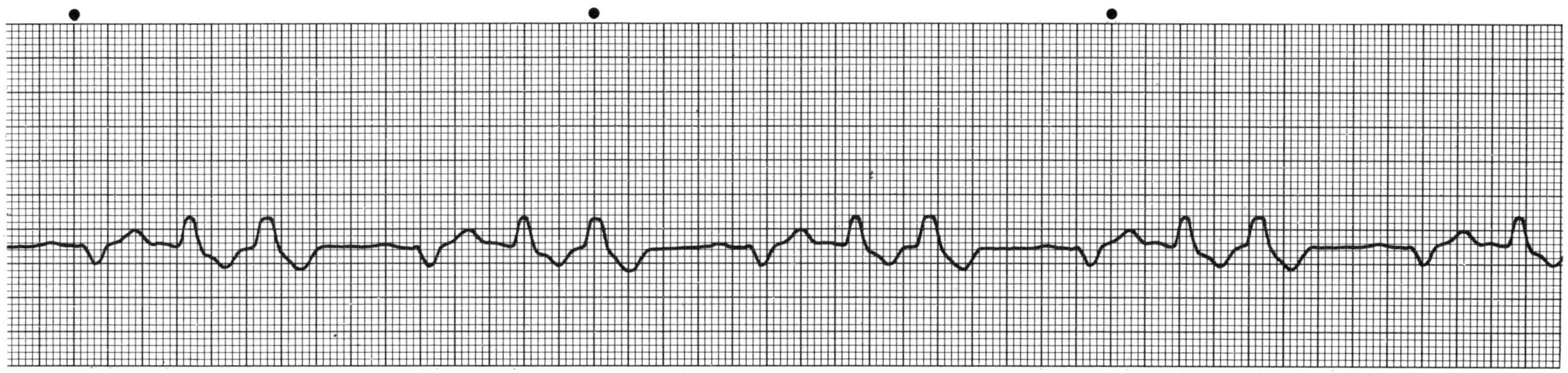

Question: This rhythm strip was recorded from a 14-year-old Siamese cat with a history of dyspnea and anorexia.

1. What is the rhythm diagnosis?
2. What are common causes of this arrhythmia?
3. What is the most likely underlying disorder?
4. What is the best therapeutic approach?

Case 166

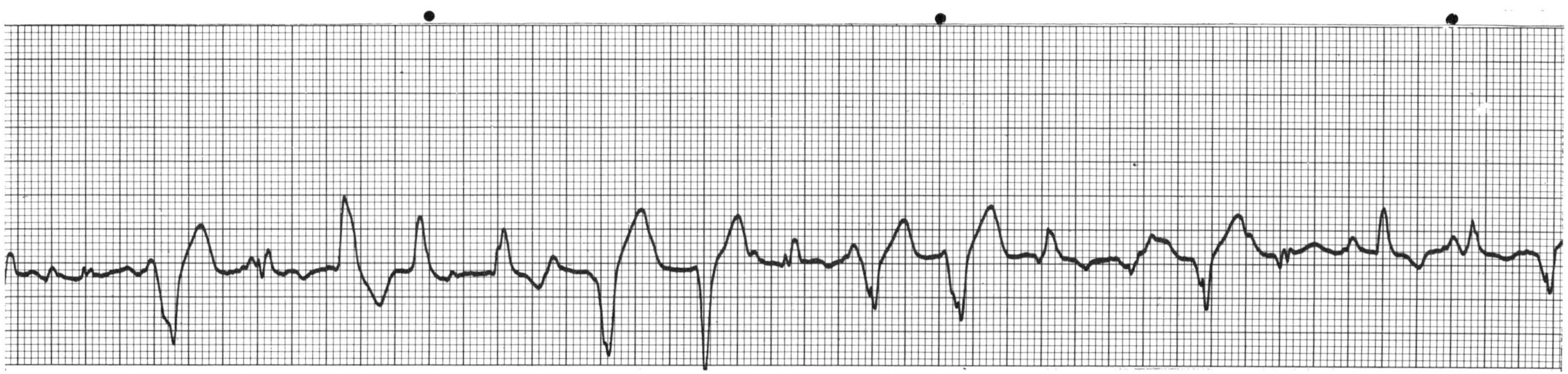

Question: This rhythm strip was recorded from a dog that had accidentally ingested digitalis tablets. Severe vomiting and diarrhea were present. A rapid heart rate and an abnormality in rhythm was auscultated on physical examination.

1. What is the rhythm diagnosis?
2. What is the best therapeutic approach?

Case 165

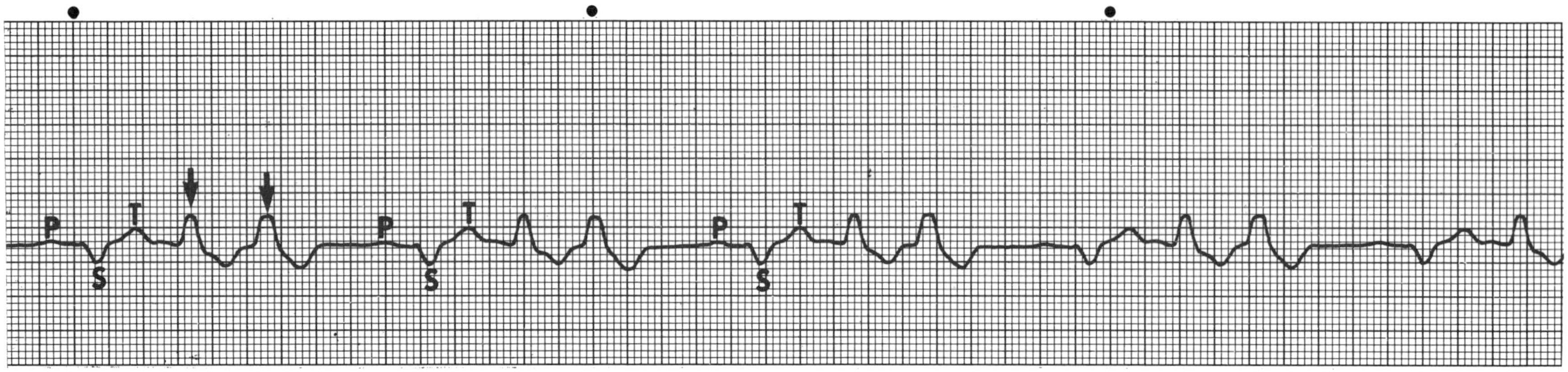

Answer: Sinus rhythm with frequent ventricular premature complexes (arrows). Heart rate is approximately 200 beats/min. The high normal P-R interval may be associated with cardiomyopathy, or it may reflect age-related degeneration or fibrosis of the AV node. The P-R interval tends to lengthen with age. The ventricular arrhythmia supports underlying myocardial disease. Sinus QRS complexes (labeled S) are wide and negative. Leads I and III were also negative. Right bundle-branch block and right ventricular enlargement should be considered. Radiographs revealed pleural effusion, and an echocardiogram confirmed hypertrophic cardiomyopathy. The arrhythmia should be treated with propranolol, but caution must be used because propranolol could worsen the conduction disturbance. A low dosage should be used initially, and the ECG should be monitored on a regular basis. Treating the congestive heart failure with furosemide and cage rest also helps to control the arrhythmia.

Case 166

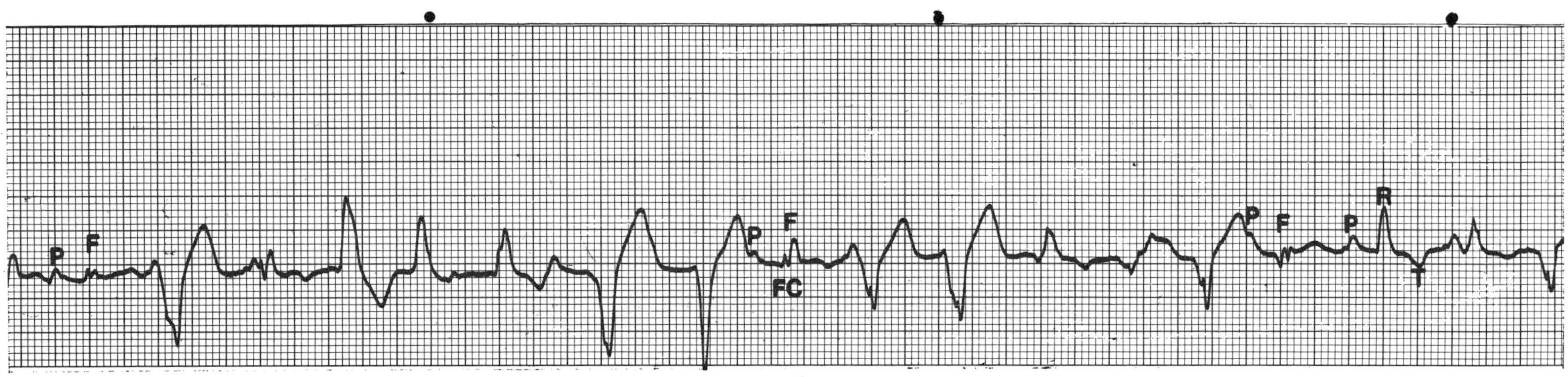

Answer: Multiform ventricular tachycardia. Heart rate is 220 beats/min. Digitalis acts directly on the myocardium, vagus nerve, and AV junction. The manifestations of digitalis toxicity are usually gastrointestinal, cardiac or neurologic. The lethal effects of digitalis toxicity are caused by its cardiac effects, i.e., the formation of arrhythmias. Digitalis can cause any cardiac arrhythmia. The P-R interval does not have to be lengthened to indicate digitalis toxicity. The rhythm is interrupted toward the end of the strip by a conducted sinus complex, which captures the ventricle. Numerous ventricular fusion complexes also are present (F). These complexes result from a simultaneous activation of the ventricle by a sinus impulse and a ventricular premature complex. Specific therapy for digitalis toxicity can include intravenous potassium, lidocaine, or phenytoin for ventricular arrhythmias, and phenytoin and a temporary transvenous pacemaker or atropine for symptomatic bradycardia. Digoxin immune Fab (Digibind) is the only available specific antidote for digitalis intoxication, but is very expensive.

Case 167

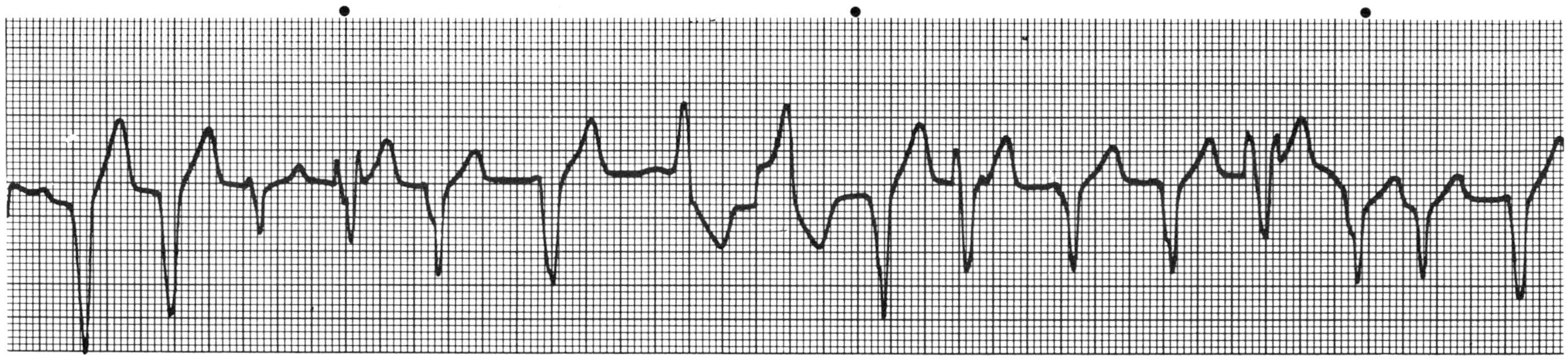

Question: This tracing was recorded from a dog with generalized weakness 2 days after having been hit by a car.

1. What is the rhythm diagnosis?
2. What is the best therapeutic approach?

Case 168

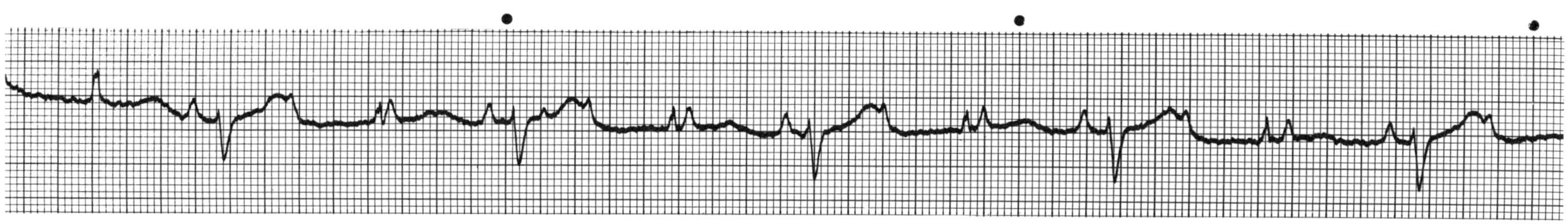

Question: This lead II tracing was recorded from a cat with a femoral pulse deficit. An echocardiographic examination revealed hypertrophic cardiomyopathy.

1. What is the rhythm diagnosis?
2. What abnormality in rhythm is likely to occur?
3. What is the best therapeutic approach?

Case 167

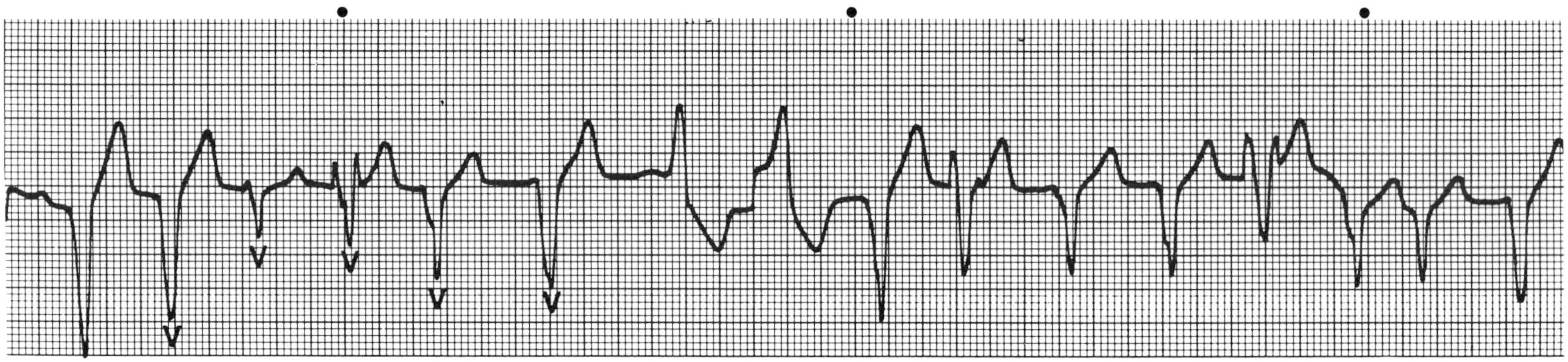

Answer: Ventricular tachycardia, a continuous series of ventricular premature complexes of variable shape (multiform) (V). Heart rate is approximately 210 beats/min. Ventricular tachycardia should be treated as soon as possible because ventricular fibrillation can easily follow. Animals with ventricular tachycardia must be continuously monitored. The drug of choice is lidocaine via continuous drip or intravenous bolus, or both. Electrical cardioversion is indicated if the animal is in a hemodynamic crisis and lidocaine fails. Any underlying acid-base and electrolyte abnormalities must be corrected. Oral antiarrhythmic therapy (quinidine or procainamide are the drugs of choice) is used to prevent recurrent ventricular tachycardia. Ventricular tachycardia is generally considered the most serious of all tachyarrhythmias. A marked fall in cardiac output, and consequently in cerebral as well as coronary and renal blood flow, usually occurs, especially when myocardial disease is present.

Case 168

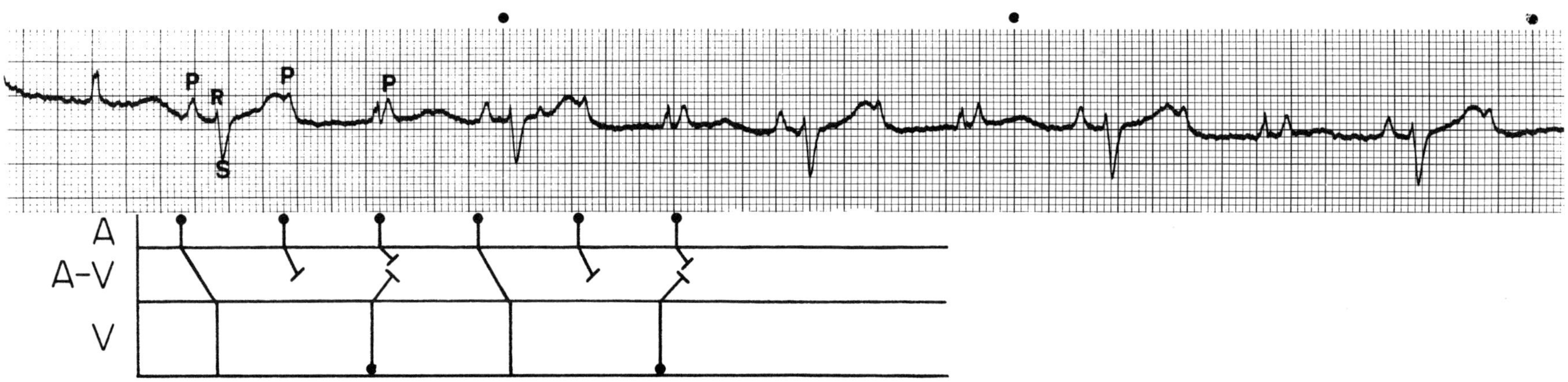

Answer: Escape—capture—bigeminy in the presence of second-degree AV block. Heart rate is variable. Two to one (2:1) AV block (two P waves for every conducted QRS complex) with ventricular escape complexes causing physiologic block of the third P wave in each series is present. The ladder diagram should help to explain this complex arrhythmia. Experience at this time indicates that the clinical cause and prognosis can be roughly estimated by studying the QRS duration. The conduction lesions in the cat are often quite variable and may be located in the AV node or His-bundle, or below the His bundle bifurcation. In this case, the abnormal QRS configuration indicates that complete AV block will probably result. Clinical signs, including fainting and weakness, will occur. Such animals are usually resistant to medical management, and thus, artificial pacing is the only treatment.

Case 169

A 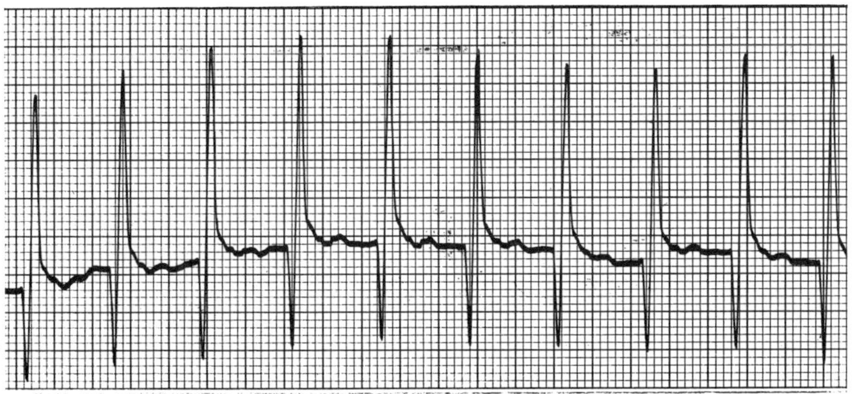

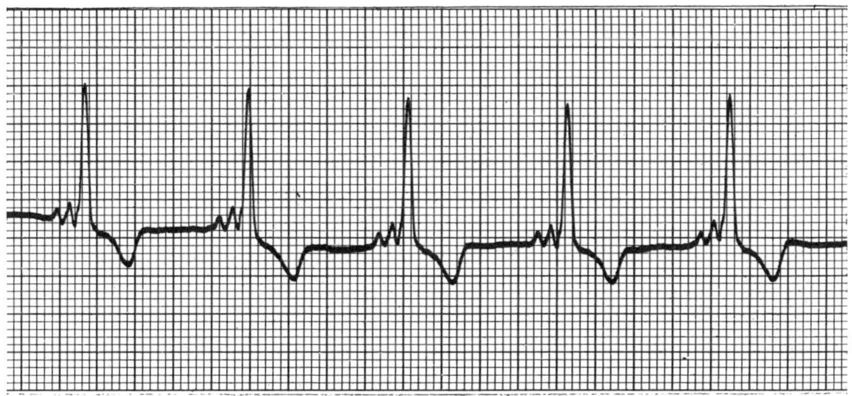 B

Question: These separate lead II rhythm strips were recorded from a dog with episodes of fainting. Strip B was recorded after ocular pressure.

1. What is the rhythm diagnosis in strip A, and what is the probable underlying cause based on strip B?
2. What is the best therapeutic approach?

Case 170

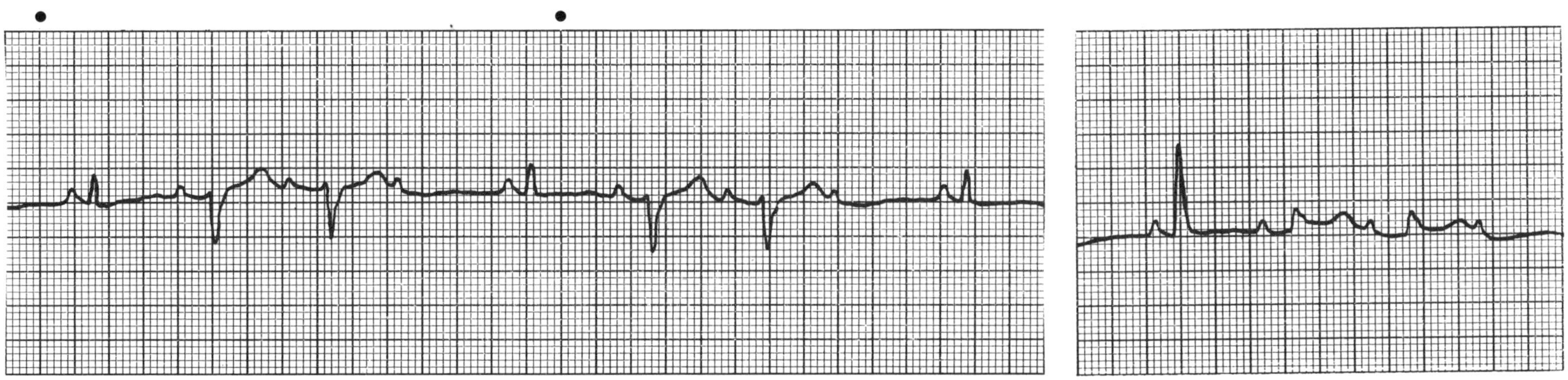

Question: This lead II ECG and lead CV_5RL tracing (right section) was obtained from a 10-year-old cat with a history of chronic bronchial asthma.

1. What is the rhythm diagnosis?
2. What is the best therapeutic approach?

Case 169

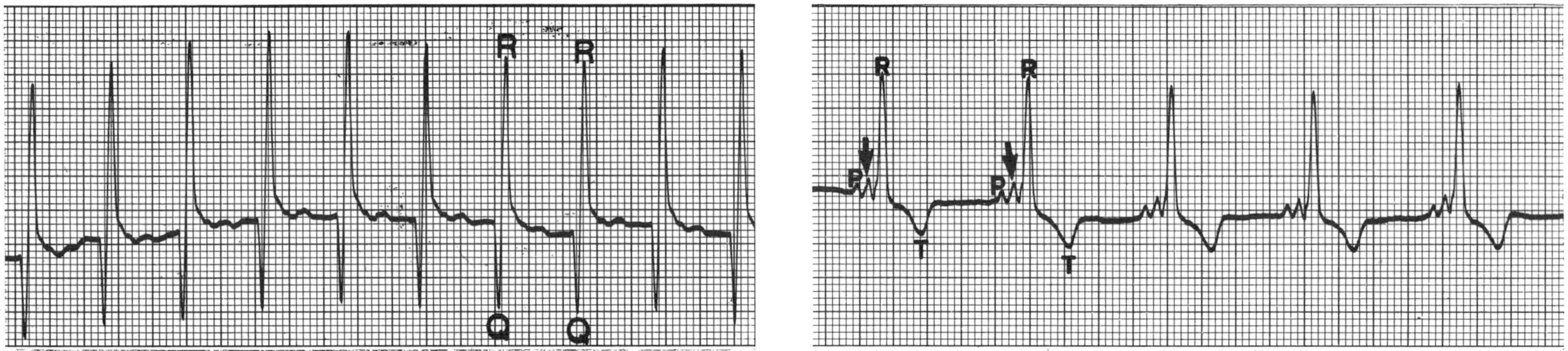

A

B

Answer: Wolff-Parkinson-White syndrome. A. Supraventricular tachycardia. Heart rate is approximately 260 beats/min. B. Ventricular pre-excitation. Heart rate is 140 beats/min. Wolff-Parkinson-White (WPW) syndrome consists of ventricular pre-excitation with episodes of paroxysmal supraventricular tachycardia. Ventricular pre-excitation occurs when impulses originating in the SA node or atrium activate a portion of the ventricles prematurely through an accessory pathway. Sinoatrial impulses are able to reach the ventricles early without going through the AV node. The paroxysmal tachycardia associated with ventricular pre-excitation (WPW syndrome) can be explained by the re-entry mechanism. An impulse traveling to the ventricles through the AV junction may turn around and re-enter the atria through the accessory pathway. A reciprocal rhythm or "electrical circuit" is thus established. Because the QRS complexes in strip A are wide and bizarre, the atrioventricular bypass tract is probably conducting impulses antegrade (atrioventricular) to the ventricles and retrograde (ventriculoatrial) to the AV node. Because ventricular activation is initiated at the site of the accessory AV pathway, the impulse does not travel through the normal intraventricular conduction system, thereby resulting in a wide and bizarre QRS complex. The QRS complexes in WPW syndrome can sometimes mimic those in ventricular tachycardia. The WPW syndrome in most cases requires conversion by (a) ocular or carotid sinus pressure, (b) use of cardiovascular drugs, or (c) direct-current shock. Considerations for drug therapy include procainamide, propranolol, and diltiazem.

Case 170

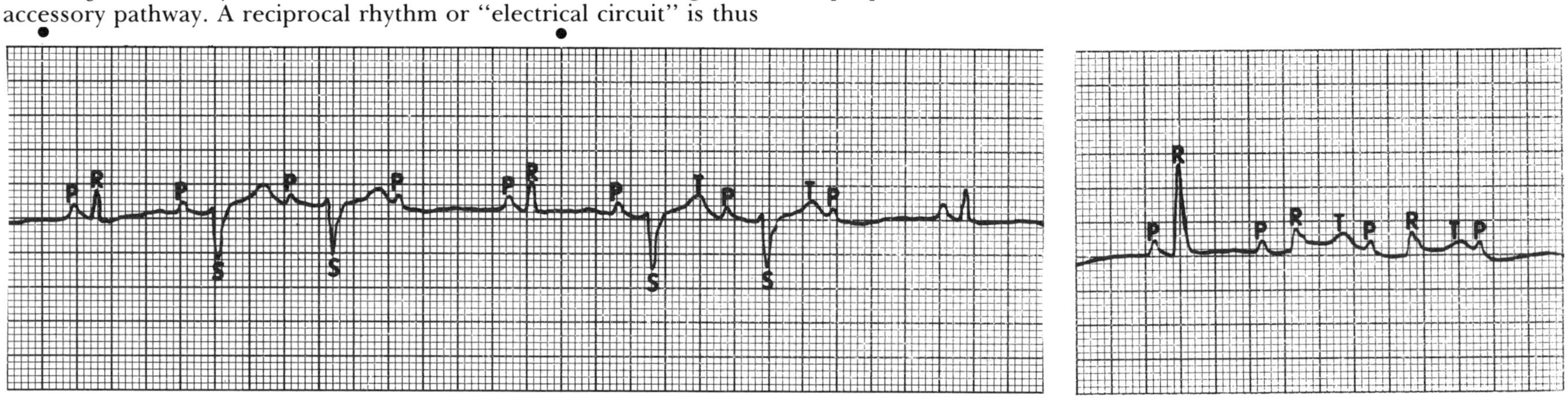

Answer: Sinus rhythm with Mobitz type I (Wenckebach) second-degree AV block and intermittent functional intraventricular conduction defect. Heart rate is approximately 170 beats/min. The best therapeutic approach is treatment of the asthma with bronchodilators and corticosteroids. Aminophylline or theophylline may enhance sympathetic tone, increase the sinus node discharge rate, and improve AV conduction. The P-R interval is prolonged with each successive cycle until a P wave fails to be conducted to the ventricles. The first P-R interval after the blocked P wave is the shortest. Although the P-R interval lengthens progressively, the incremental difference is greatest between the first and second P-R interval after the blocked P wave. The P-R interval lessens incrementally after the second P-R interval, thus resulting in a progressively shorter R-R interval. Type I AV block usually occurs in the AV node and is responsive to atropine. Rate-dependent right bundle-branch block (incomplete) occurs when, at a critical rate, the impulse finds the right bundle branch before it has fully repolarized. The QRS complexes in this intraventricular conduction defect can be misdiagnosed as ventricular premature complexes, thereby resulting in inappropriate treatment.

Case 171

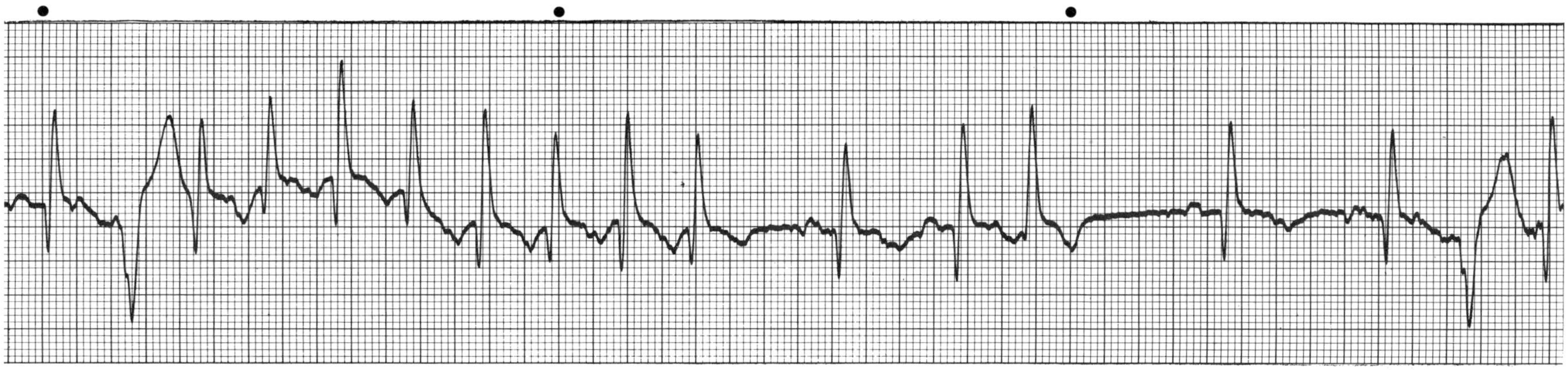

Question: This lead II ECG was obtained from a 6-year-old Doberman Pinscher with dyspnea and marked exercise intolerance.

1. What is the rhythm diagnosis?
2. What is the best therapeutic approach?

Case 172

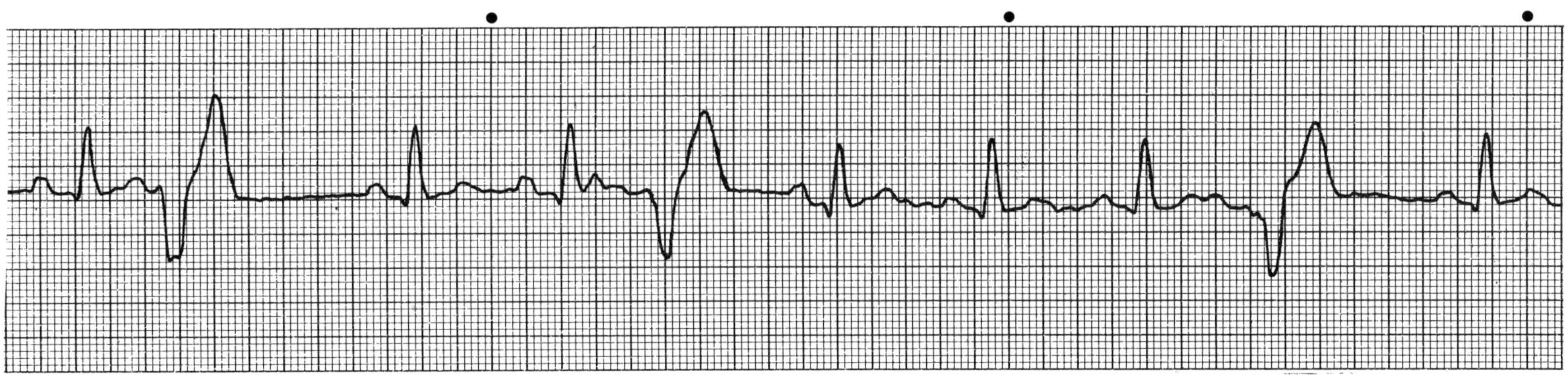

Question: This tracing was recorded from a geriatric dog with a grade III/VI holosystolic mitral murmur and no clinical signs.

1. What is the rhythm diagnosis?
2. What is the best therapeutic approach?

Case 171

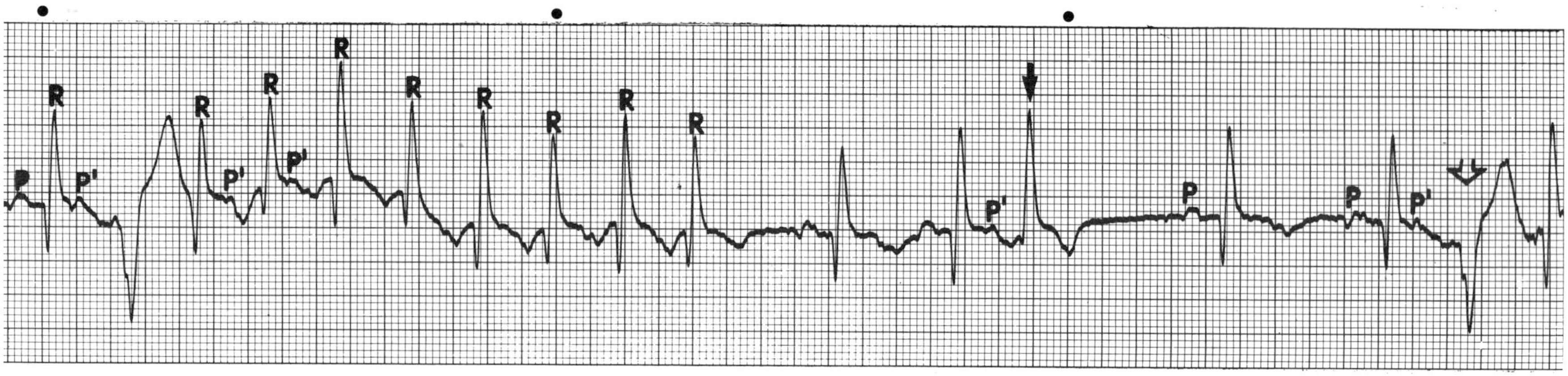

Answer: Sinus rhythm with atrial premature complexes with aberrant ventricular conduction and paroxysmal supraventricular tachycardia. Heart rate during tachycardia is 280 beats/min. Digoxin is the required drug for this arrhythmia in this patient. Thoracic radiographs confirm congestive heart failure. The first negative and wide QRS complex is preceded by a premature P′ wave. Therefore, the arrhythmia is an atrial premature complex with aberrant ventricular conduction rather than a ventricular premature complex. The atrial premature complexes persist for nine more complexes. Conduction normalizes after the first aberrantly conducted beat. The atrial premature complex (open arrow) with aberrant ventricular conduction demonstrates Ashman's phenomenon. The QRS-to-QRS complex (R-R) interval preceding the atrial premature complex (closed arrow) has a shorter cycle than the R-R interval preceding the second atrial premature complex (open arrow) with marked aberrant ventricular conduction (right bundle-branch block pattern). The longer cycle or slower rate of impulse transmission through the His-Purkinje system increases the refractory period of the bundle branches. Typically, the refractory period of the right bundle branch is longer than that of the left bundle branch. After a long interval, an atrial premature complex is more likely to find the right bundle in its refractory period, thereby resulting in aberrant conduction. Conduction usually normalizes during supraventricular tachycardia, because the bundle-branch refractory period resets to a shorter interval.

Case 172

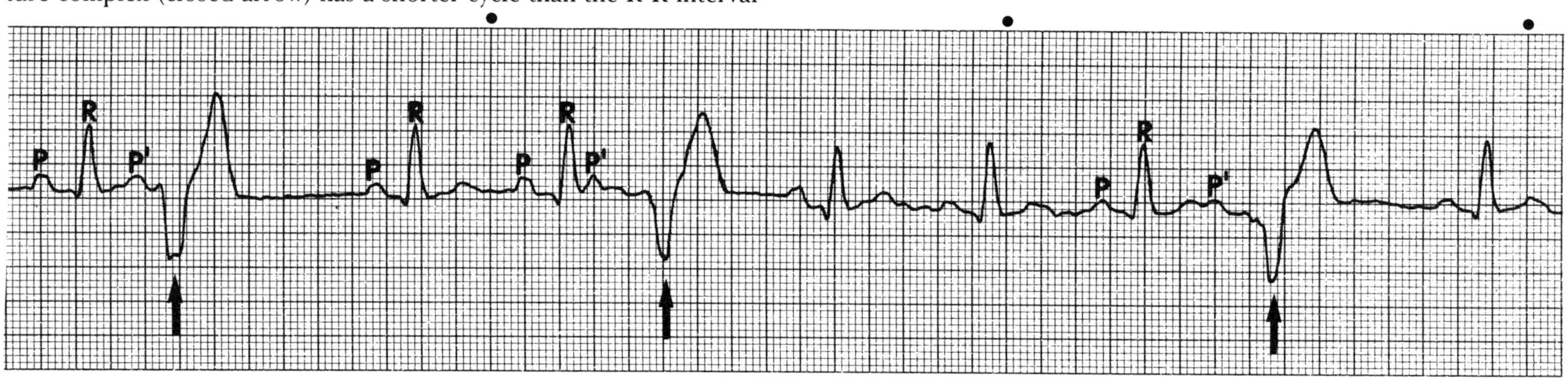

Answer: Sinus rhythm with atrial premature complexes that are conducted with aberrancy. Heart rate is approximately 130 beats/min. Premature complexes (arrows) are readily apparent. Morphologically, these complexes are quite different from the sinus complexes. On the surface, they could easily be mistaken for ventricular premature complexes. The presence of P′ waves in association with the premature complexes supports the diagnosis of atrial premature complexes. The P wave of the first premature complex is lost in the preceding QRS complex. The P-R interval of the premature complexes is prolonged, because the premature complex reaches the AV node during a relatively refractory period, thereby slowing conduction through the AV node. The QRS complexes reveal a right bundle-branch block appearance. The refractory period of the right bundle branch is longer than that of the left bundle branch. Consequently, premature complexes that are conducted aberrantly usually have a right bundle-branch block appearance. These atrial premature complexes are associated with aberrant conduction. The dog has no clinical signs and requires no treatment. If atrial tachycardia, weakness, or congestive heart failure develops, digoxin should be prescribed for the arrhythmia and an ECG should be re-evaluated in 3 to 7 days.

Case 173

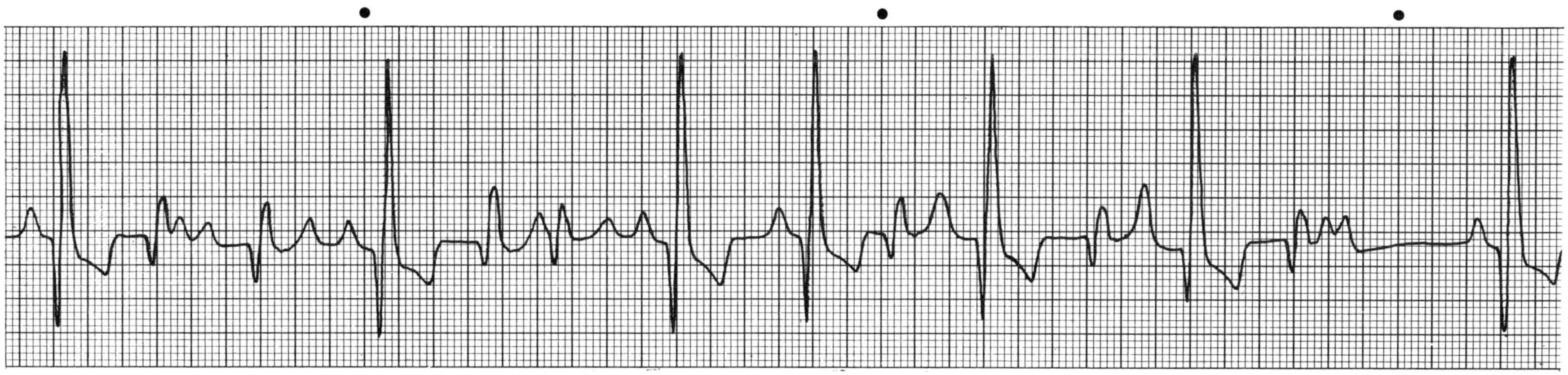

Question: This tracing was obtained from a 7-year-old Golden Retriever with a history of exercise intolerance and a mild cough.

1. What is the rhythm diagnosis?
2. What is the most likely underlying disorder?
3. What is the best therapeutic approach?

Case 174

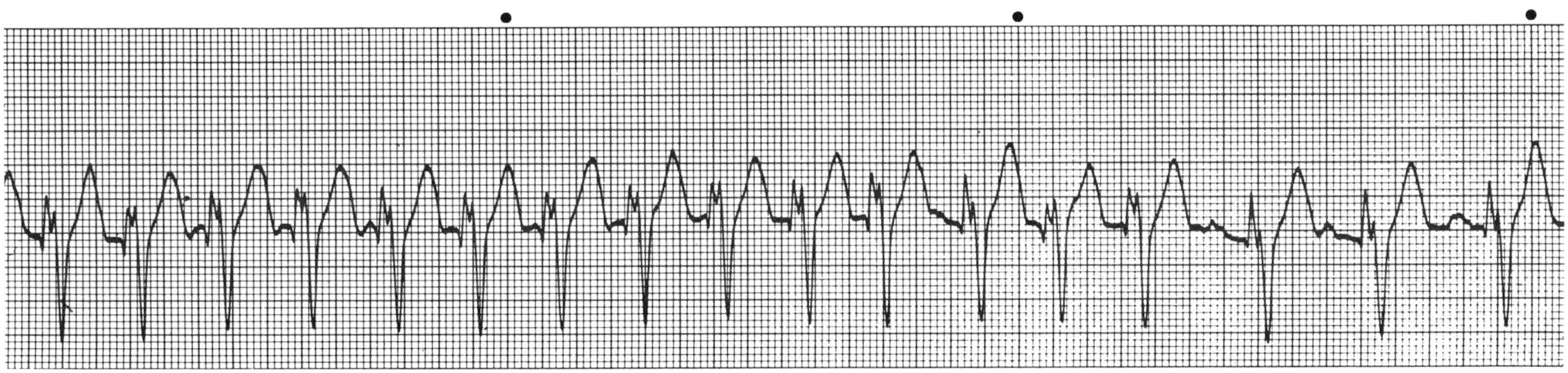

Question: This tracing was recorded from a 10-year-old dog with mitral valvular insufficiency and episodes of fainting. Ocular pressure was applied during the recording. Lead I was negative.

1. What is the rhythm diagnosis?
2. What is the best therapeutic approach?

Case 173

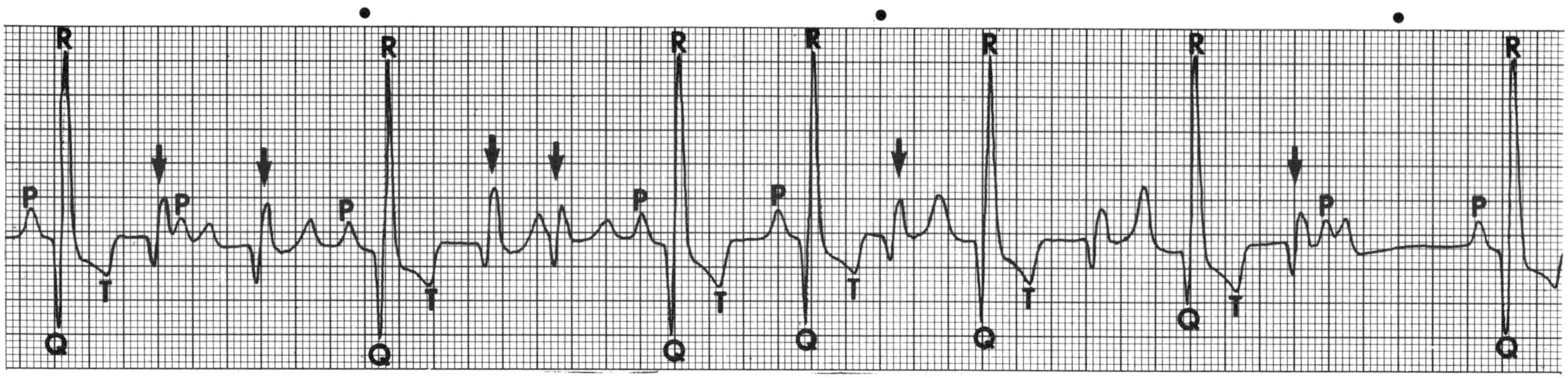

Answer: Sinus rhythm with frequent unifocal ventricular premature complexes occurring singly and in couplets. Heart rate is approximately 190 beats/min. Frequent ventricular premature complexes are present (arrows). Some P waves can be seen within the S-T segment of some ventricular premature complexes. These P waves are not conducted to the ventricles because of a physiologic block of the AV node caused by retrograde conduction of the ventricular premature complex into the AV node. The P waves and QRS complexes of the sinus complexes are wide, thus supporting a diagnosis of left ventricular enlargement. Slurring of the S-T segment also supports left ventricular enlargement. ECG evidence of left heart enlargement, coupled with the arrhythmia and history of coughing in this breed, suggests dilated cardiomyopathy. Antiarrhythmic therapy with procainamide, quinidine, or tocainide should be instituted, along with diuretics and vasodilators to treat cardiac failure. Digoxin is not recommended in this dog until the ventricular arrhythmia is controlled.

Case 174

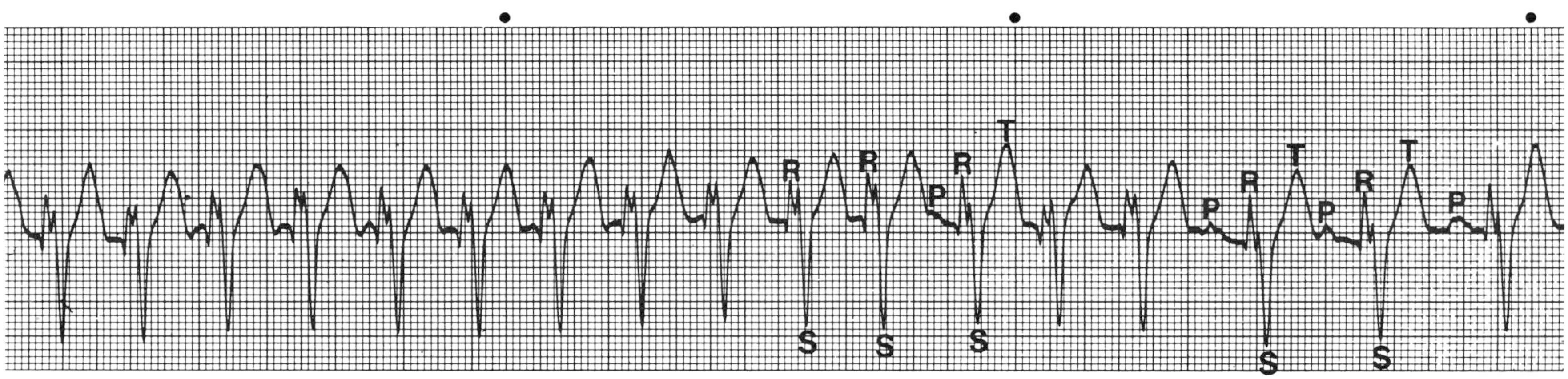

Answer: Supraventricular tachycardia with a pre-existing intraventricular block (right bundle-branch block). Heart rate is 250 beats/min. Whether the tachycardia in the tracing is ventricular cannot be determined until the end of the tracing. P waves are not visible. Vagal stimulation by ocular pressure eventually terminated the tachycardia. The last three complexes and the sixth complex from the end are sinus in origin, with QRS complexes identical to those present during the tachycardia. These sinus complexes are the result of atrial activity (P waves). Right bundle-branch block was confirmed by evaluating the other limb leads. The P waves are wide and notched, an indication of left atrial enlargement that may explain the source of the supraventricular tachycardia. Digoxin and/or propranolol or diltiazem can be used to prevent the attacks of tachycardia. This ECG can be confused easily with ventricular tachycardia.

Case 175

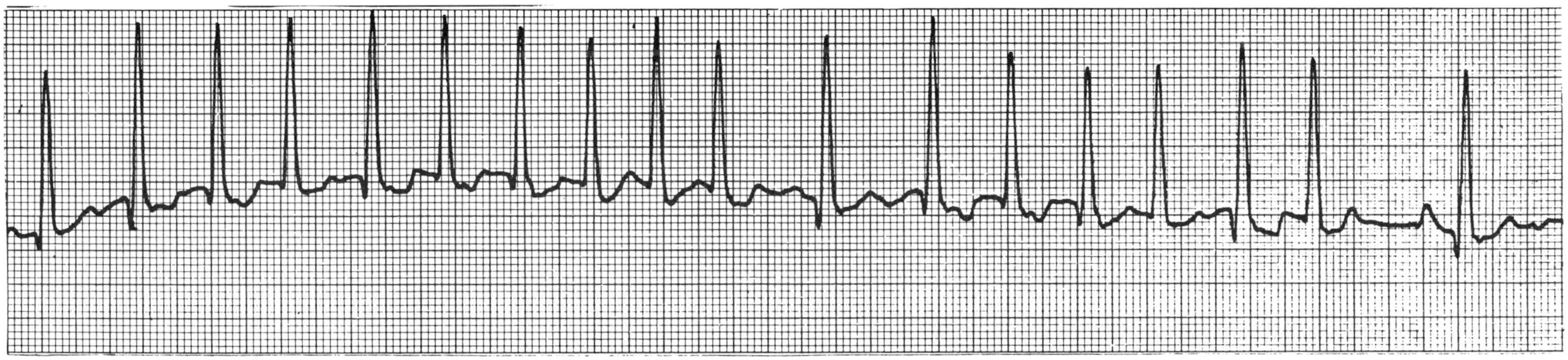

Question: This electrocardiogram was recorded from an Irish Wolfhound that had experienced episodes of collapse and weight loss during the last 2 weeks.

1. What is the rhythm diagnosis?
2. What is the most likely underlying disorder?
3. What is the best therapeutic approach?

Case 176

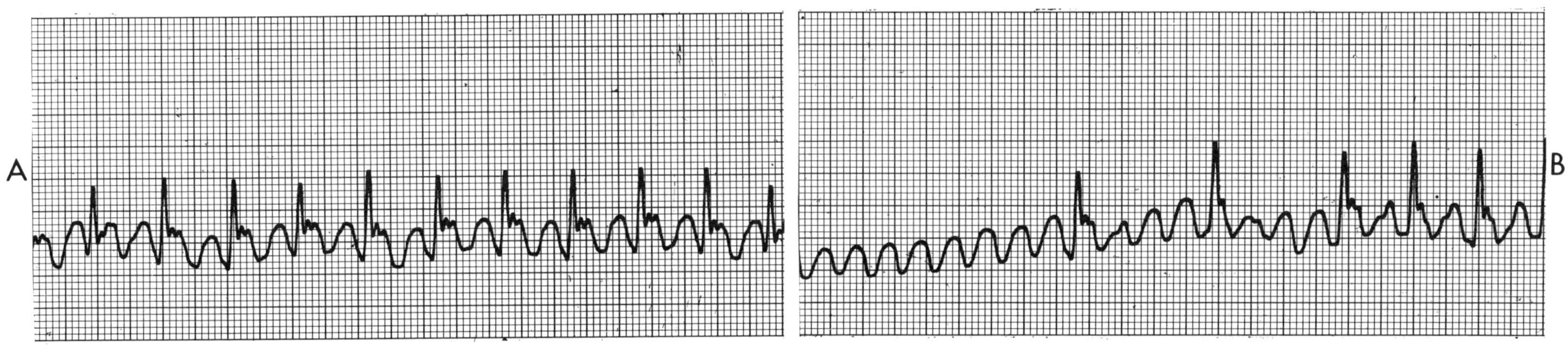

Question: These two ECG tracings were recorded from a dog with a rapid heart rate on auscultation.

1. What is the rhythm diagnosis?
2. What is the best therapeutic approach?

Case 175

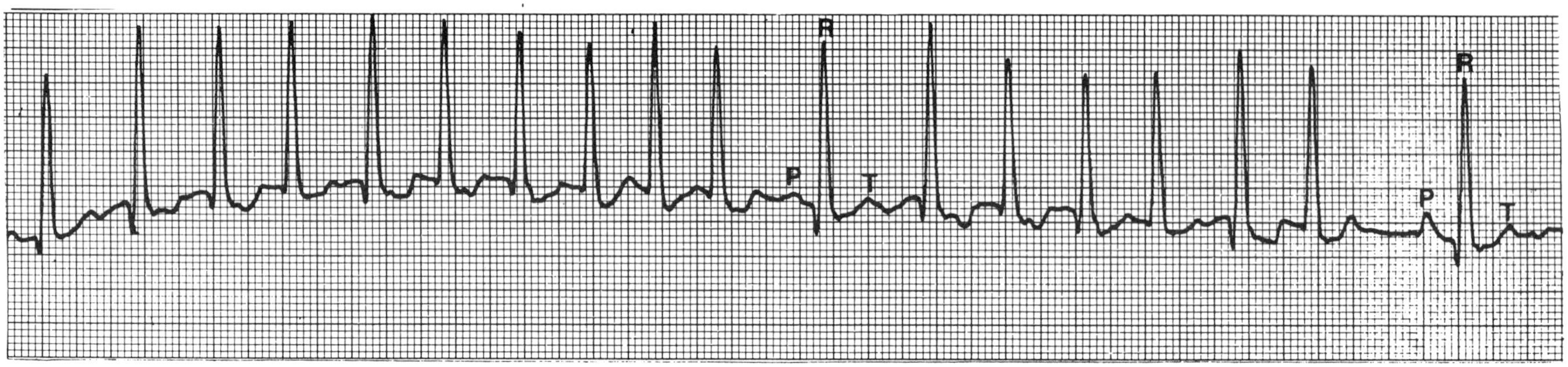

Answer: Paroxysmal atrial fibrillation. Heart rate is approximately 240 beats/min. Atrial fibrillation may resemble multifocal atrial tachycardia because of the rapid and irregular ventricular response. Well-defined P′ waves before each QRS complex are present in multifocal atrial tachycardia. Atrial flutter with varying ventricular response may also appear like atrial fibrillation. A careful search for flutter waves or P′ waves on other leads is essential. Note the two well-defined sinus complexes. The dilated form of cardiomyopathy should be considered first, with digoxin the drug of choice. This dog eventually had atrial fibrillation throughout the strip despite the use of digoxin. Blood flow in the coronary arteries and in the cerebral circulation is markedly reduced with rapid atrial fibrillation. Clinical signs can include heart failure, weakness, and syncope.

A

Case 176

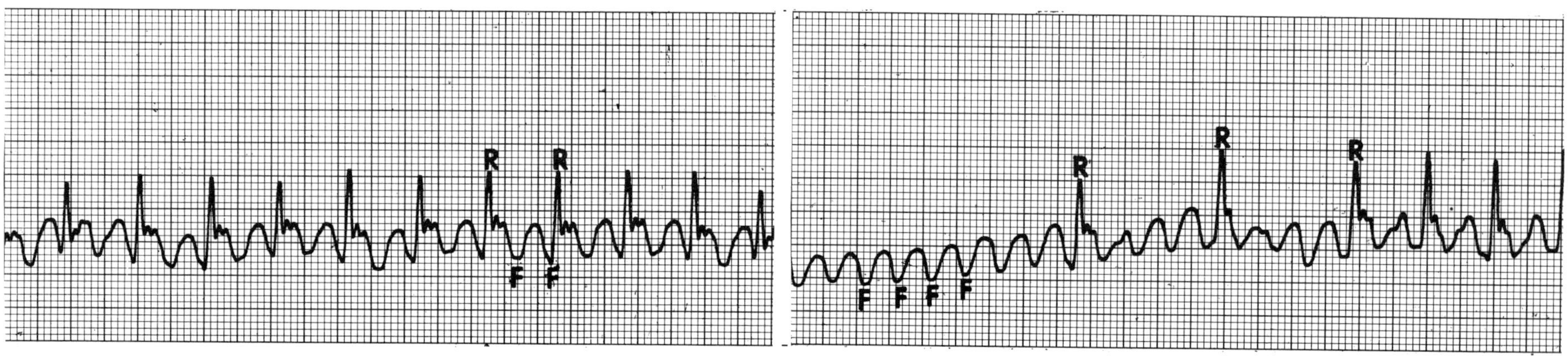

B

Answer: Atrial flutter. Heart rate is variable. Strip A reveals atrial flutter with a 2 : 1 response. The ventricular heart rate is 300 beats/min. In any rhythm in which the ventricular rate is 300 beats/min or above and is regular, the possibility of atrial flutter should be part of the differential diagnosis. The term "response" is sometimes used instead of "block" because the 2 : 1 AV conduction in atrial flutter is caused by a longer physiologic refractory period in the AV junction. With ocular pressure, the increased vagal activity in strip B increases the degree of response in the AV node, and the flutter waves (F) are more easily identified with their characteristic sawtooth pattern, as well as rate. The atrial rate is 600 beats/min. The therapeutic approach can be pharmacologic (e.g., digitalis, propranolol, and diltiazem) and/or electrical (e.g., cardioversion or right atrial pacing). Cardioversion is the treatment of choice if the condition of the animal is critical. Atrial flutter may reduce cerebral circulation, thereby producing clinical signs of weakness and syncope.

Case 177

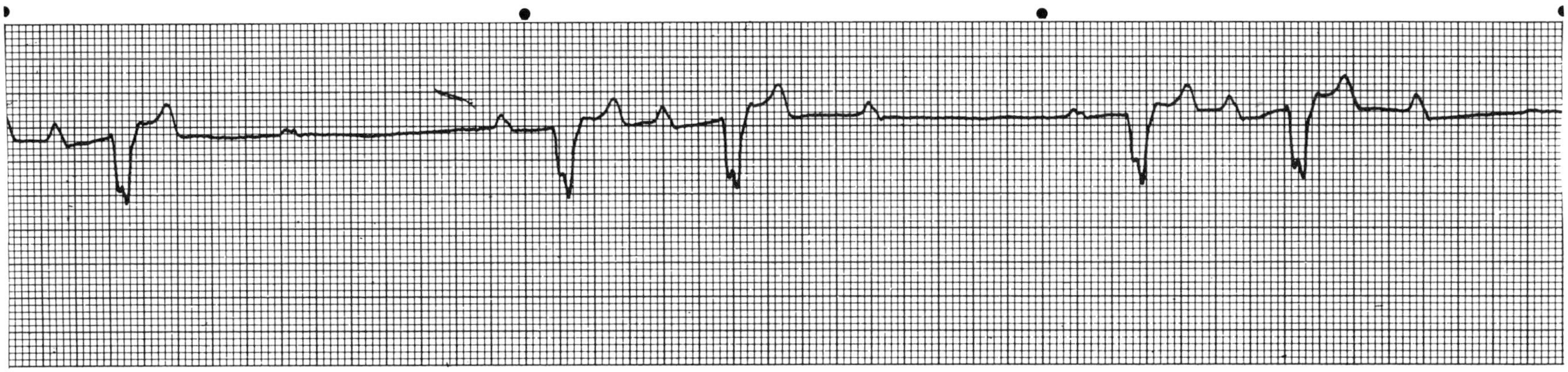

Question: This tracing was recorded from a dog with no clinical signs; however, an arrhythmia with varying intensity to the first heart sound was heard.

1. What is the rhythm diagnosis?
2. What is the best therapeutic approach?

Case 178

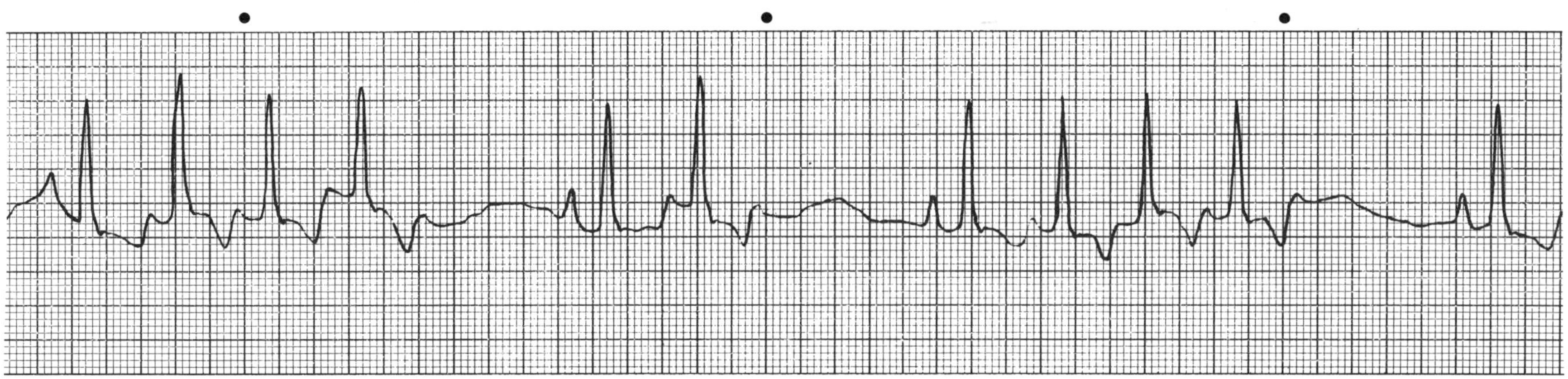

Question: This lead II ECG was obtained from a 12-year-old Miniature Poodle examined because of a worsening cough. A grade V/VI holosystolic murmur was auscultated equally in the left and right hemithorax.

1. What is the rhythm diagnosis?
2. What is the most likely underlying disorder?
3. What is the best therapeutic approach?

Case 177

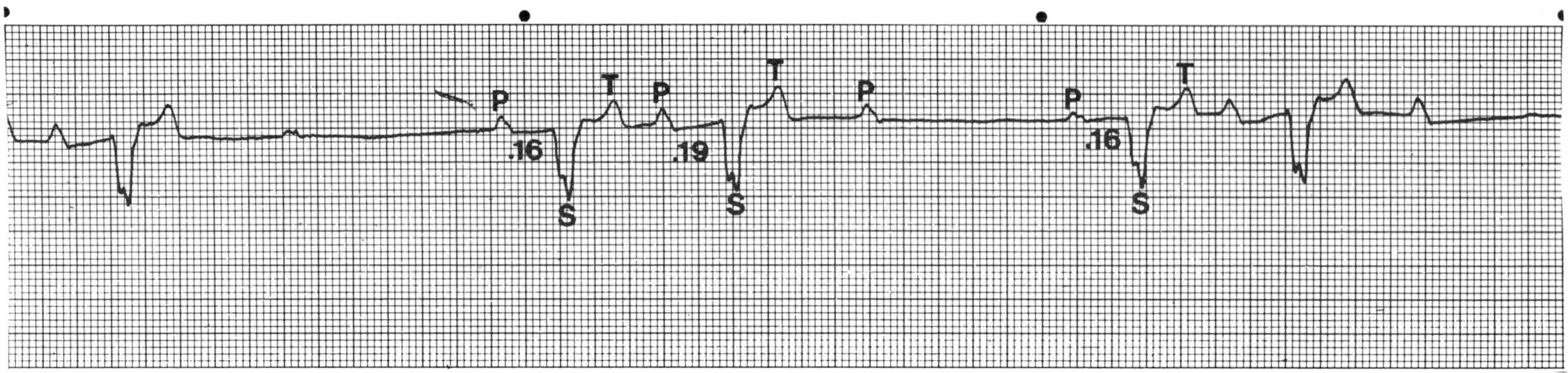

Answer: Mobitz type I AV block (Wenckebach type) with a 3 : 2 ventricular response. Ventricular rate is approximately 70 beats/min. This type of AV block is characterized by progressive lengthening of the P-R interval until a point is reached at which no ventricular complex follows the P wave. Following the blocked atrial impulse, the P-R interval shortens to its original value (0.16 sec or 8 boxes), and the sequence is repeated. First-degree AV block is also present as the P-R interval is prolonged. The changing configuration of the P wave represents a wandering pacemaker. The wide and negative QRS complex (right bundle branch block) may indicate that the conduction defect is below the AV node. An artificial pacemaker may be indicated if clinical signs (syncope, lethargy) occur or if the rhythm progresses to complete AV block.

Case 178

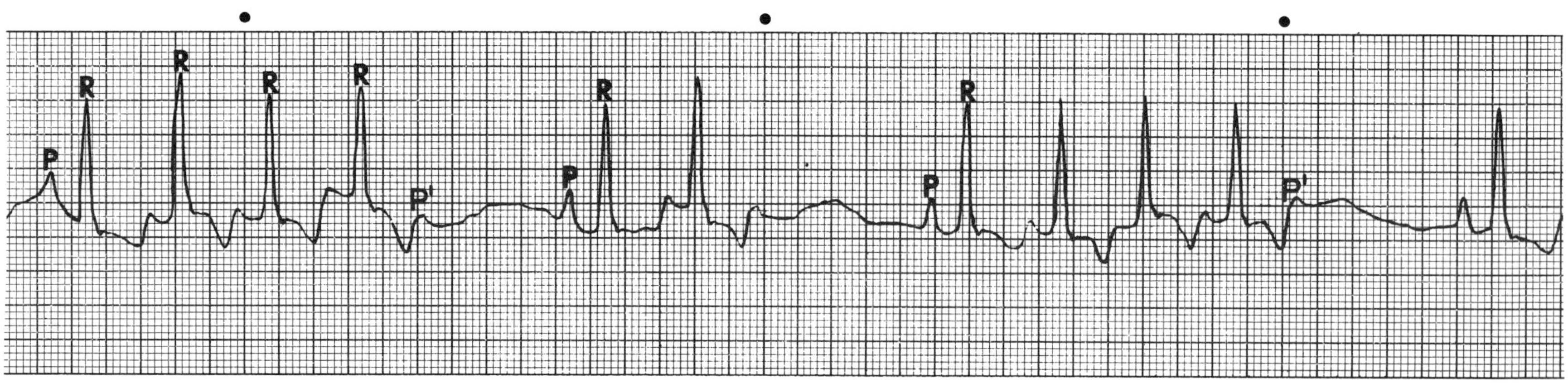

Answer: Sinus rhythm with paroxysmal runs of multifocal atrial premature complexes. Heart rate is variable. Mitral and tricuspid valvular insufficiency are the most likely disorders. Chronic pulmonary disease is reportedly the most common cause of multifocal atrial premature complexes in humans. Notice the irregular R-R intervals during the third run of atrial premature complexes. Also notice that the last premature P′ wave in each run is not followed by a QRS complex (nonconducted atrial premature complexes). This physiologic block is responsible for pauses that are longer than expected between the runs of atrial premature complexes. Thoracic radiographs should be obtained and the underlying disorder should be treated. Diuretics and vasodilators are advised for congestive heart failure and bronchodilators for pulmonary disease. Digoxin is recommended to control atrial tachycardia, especially if the dog has congestive heart failure.

Case 179

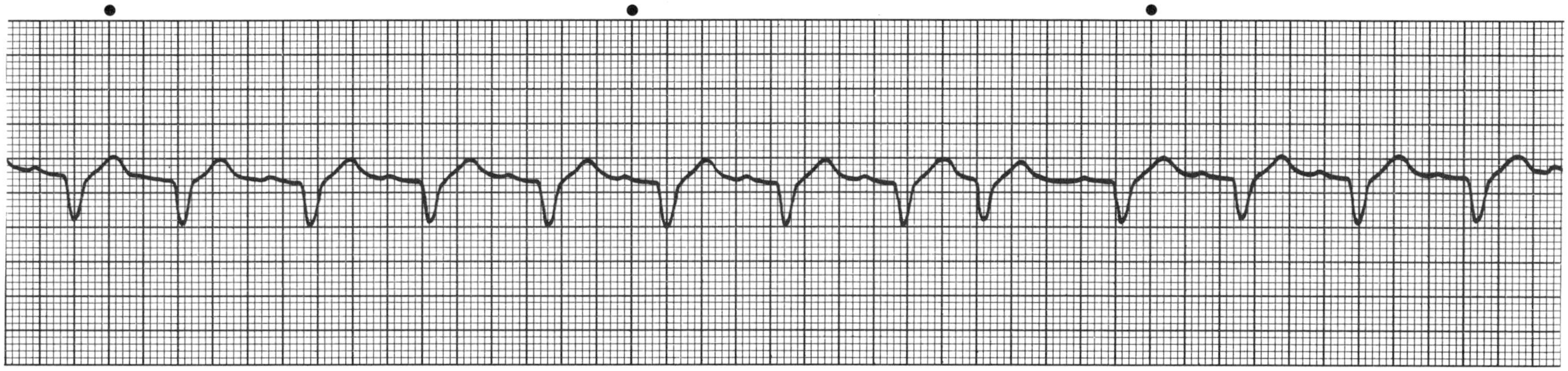

Question: This rhythm strip was obtained from a 15-year-old domestic shorthair cat as part of a geriatric profile.

1. What is the rhythm diagnosis?
2. What is the common cause of this arrhythmia?
3. What is the most likely underlying disorder?
4. What is the best therapeutic approach?

Case 180

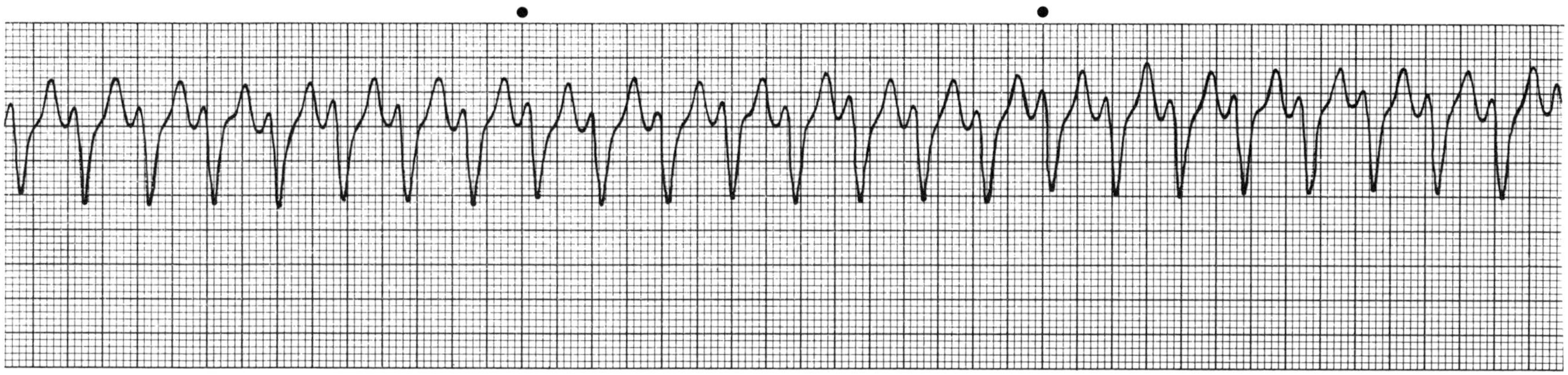

Question: This lead II ECG was obtained from a 6-month-old Standard Poodle puppy examined because of a recent episode of collapse.

1. What is the rhythm diagnosis?
2. What is the most likely underlying disorder?
3. What is the best therapeutic approach?

Case 179

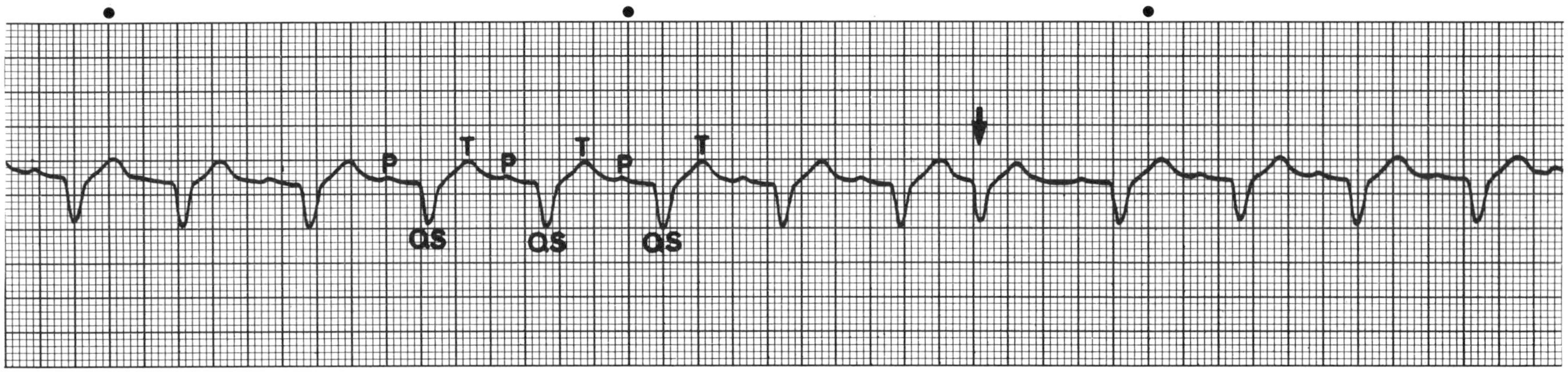

Answer: Sinus rhythm with one atrial premature complex (arrow), first-degree AV block, and right bundle-branch block. Heart rate is 170 beats/min. The P-R interval is prolonged at 0.10 sec (first-degree AV block). The QRS complexes (QS) are wide and negative in lead II, thus suggesting a conduction disturbance. Ventricular tachycardia is not present because the P-R interval is constant. Leads I and III were also negative, thus resulting in a right-axis deviation. The right axis and wide complexes support a diagnosis of right bundle-branch block. The right bundle-branch block coupled with first-degree AV block could indicate diffuse conduction disease. Conduction system disease in geriatric cats can result from degeneration or fibrosis or from cardiac changes associated with cardiomyopathy. The atrial premature complex (arrow) may be an incidental finding or could be associated with atrial distention. First-degree AV block and bundle-branch blocks do not adversely affect cardiac output. They require no treatment. An occasional atrial premature complex also does not warrant antiarrhythmic therapy.

Case 180

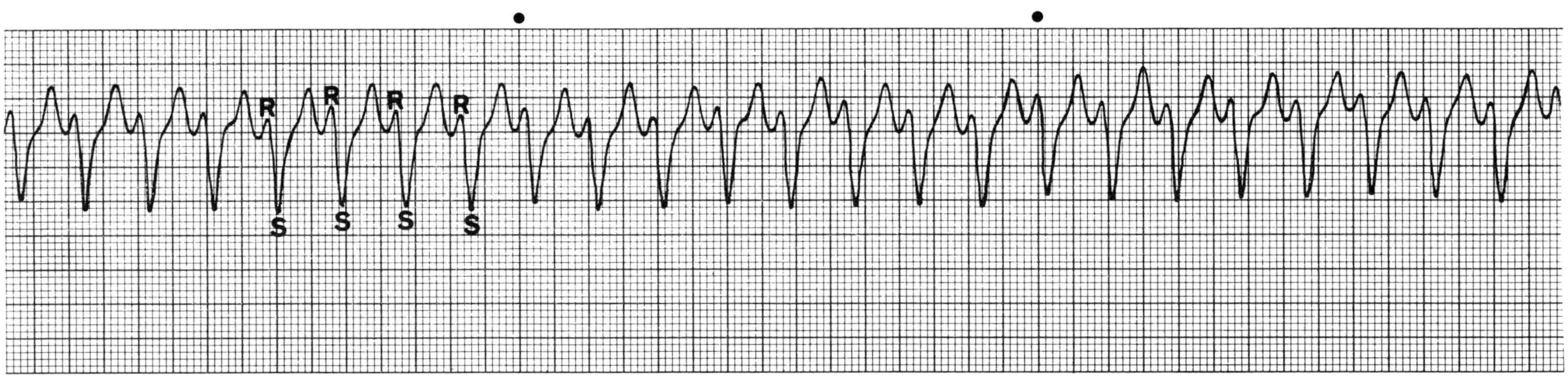

Answer: Supraventricular tachycardia with right bundle-branch block or ventricular tachycardia. Heart rate is 320 beats/min. A congenital heart defect and viral myocarditis are common causes of this arrhythmia. A vagal maneuver (carotid sinus stimulation or ocular pressure) and, if that is unsuccessful, a lidocaine bolus are the best diagnostic as well as therapeutic approaches to this wide complex tachycardia. Abrupt termination of the tachycardia, with visible sinus beats with a QRS complex resembling complexes during tachycardia, supports a diagnosis of supraventricular arrhythmia. Appropriate treatment with administration of digoxin, diltiazem, or propranolol can then be initiated. If a lidocaine bolus terminates this tachyarrhythmia with the emergence of sinus beats with QRS complexes of different morphology, the diagnosis is ventricular tachycardia. A lidocaine infusion should be instituted and either procainamide or quinidine should be administered orally, with or without propranolol. Additional treatment may be indicated on the basis of radiographic and echocardiographic findings. Control of heart failure with a diuretic and vasodilator may also be required.

Case 181

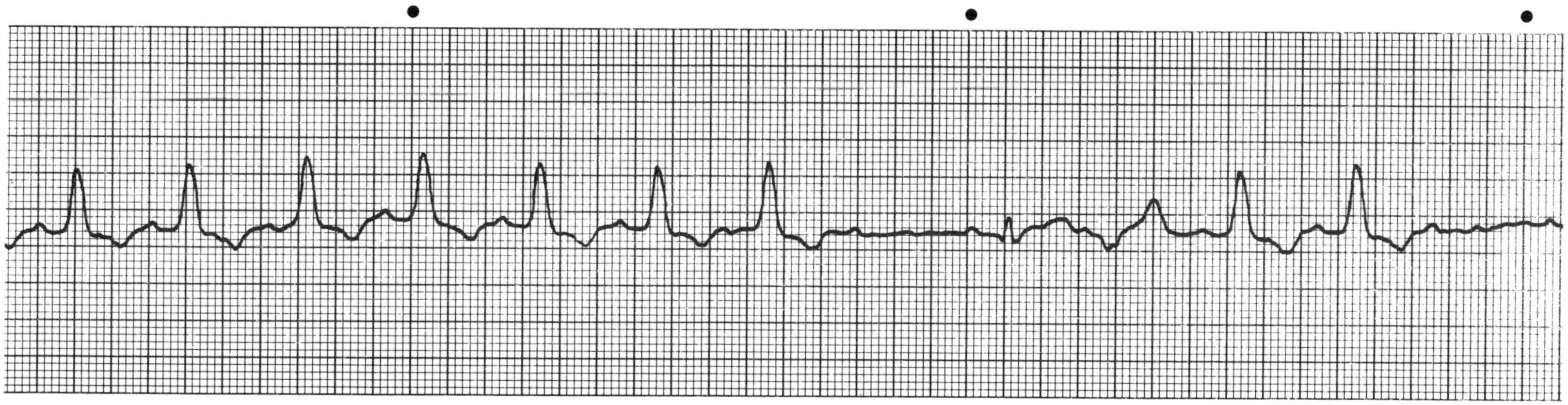

Question: This complex lead II rhythm strip was recorded from a cat with a history of seizures.

1. What is the rhythm diagnosis? This lead II rhythm strip represents a complex abnormality.

Case 182

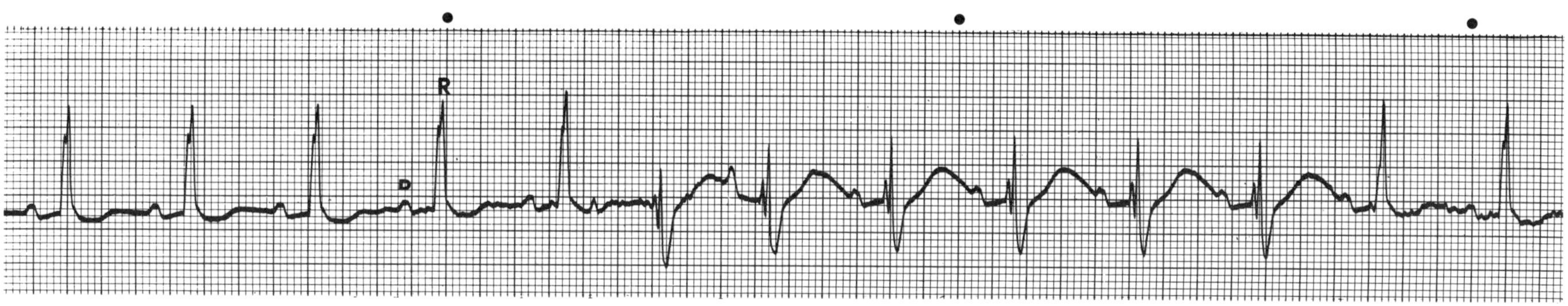

Question: This tracing was recorded from a dog with no clinical signs, but an arrhythmia was heard on auscultation.

1. What is the rhythm diagnosis? This lead II rhythm strip represents a complex abnormality.

Case 181

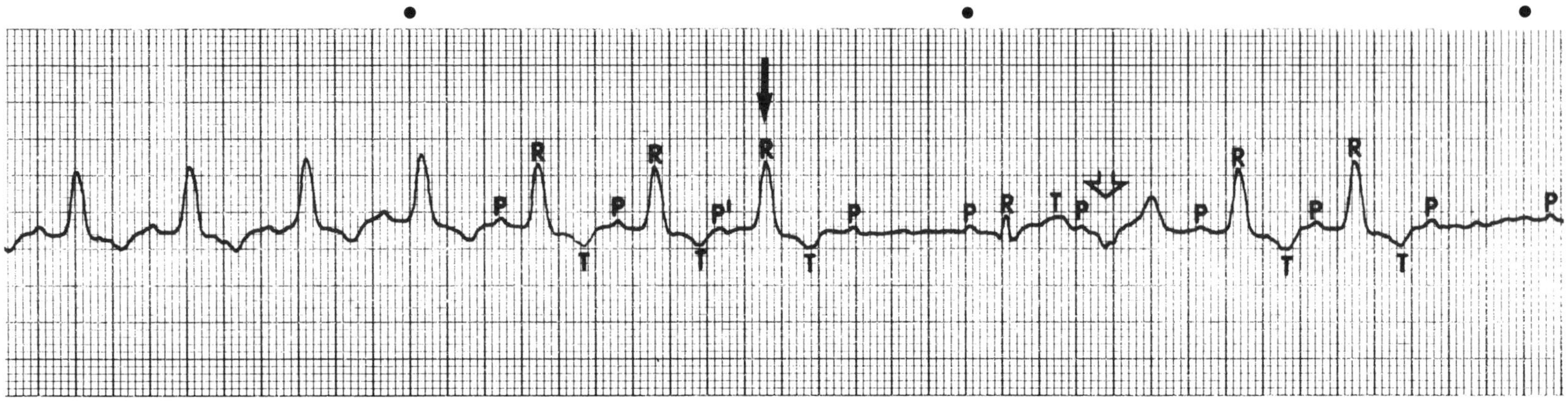

Answer: Sinus rhythm with rate-dependent bundle-branch block, intermittent second-degree AV block, and one ventricular premature complex. Heart rate is variable. The positive wide QRS complexes indicate a left bundle-branch block pattern (also seen in leads I, III, and aVF). For a diagnosis of bundle-branch block, the QRS complex must be 0.06 sec or more in duration. The absence of left ventricular enlargement on thoracic radiographs lends support to a diagnosis of left bundle-branch block. The development of intermittent bundle-branch block or aberrant ventricular conduction during a series of consecutive complexes depends on the heart rate. Above a critical heart rate, impulses reach the bundle branch during a prolonged refractory period, thereby causing a conduction block. Typically, the right bundle Purkinje cells have a refractory period longer than that of the left bundle Purkinje cells. In diseased hearts, a crossover of refractoriness may occur, with the refractory period of the left bundle becoming longer than that of the right bundle. Below a critical rate, conduction becomes normal, because impulses now reach the affected bundle after recovery is completed. The rate was changed after the occurrence of one probable atrial premature complex (closed arrow) followed by second-degree AV block. One normally conducted sinus QRS complex then occurs after the pause. A ventricular premature complex (open arrow) then occurs. The left bundle-branch block pattern returns for two more consecutive complexes, and then is followed by more blocked P waves.

Case 182

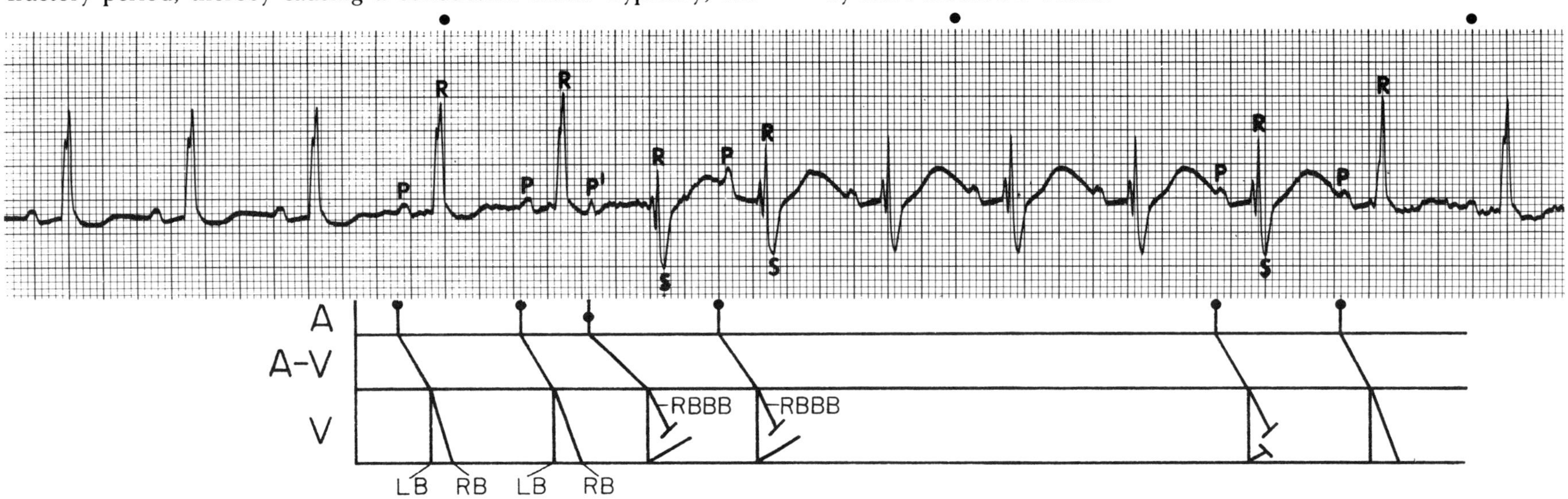

Answer: Aberrant ventricular conduction (incomplete right bundle-branch block) after an atrial premature complex (P′) (sixth complex). Heart rate is approximately 165 beats/min. The ladder diagram technique should help to clarify the underlying mechanism for this complex arrhythmia. The aberrant ventricular conduction is caused by concealed transseptal activation of the right bundle branch after an initial atrial premature complex with aberrancy. The premature complex finds the right bundle in its refractory period. The refractory period of the right bundle branch is usually longer than that of the left bundle branch. The right bundle-branch block pattern persists for six complexes, and then the retrograde conduction finally blocks for some reason. When an atrial premature complex activates the His-Purkinje system while a bundle branch is refractory, the QRS complex shows a bundle-branch block pattern, thus reflecting the delay in or failure of impulse transmission down that bundle branch. An atrial premature complex with aberrant intraventricular conduction is distinguished from a premature junctional or ventricular abnormality in rhythm by the presence of a premature ectopic P wave preceding the complex. LB = left bundle; RB = right bundle; RBBB = right bundle-branch block.

Case 183

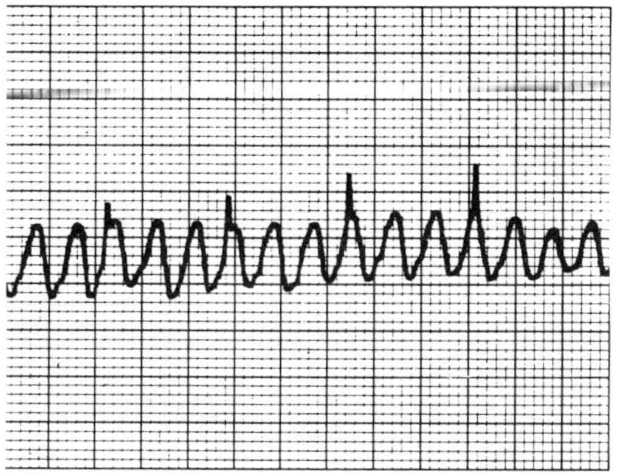

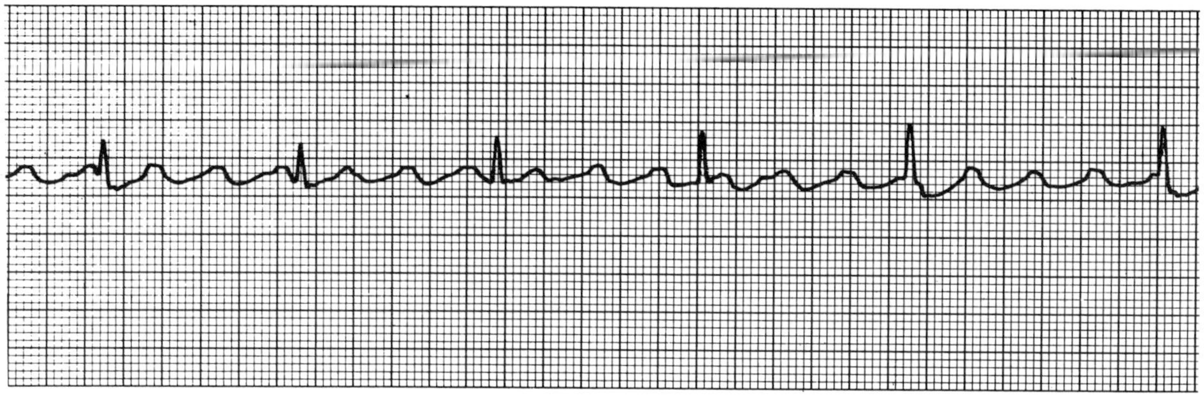

Question: Strip A and strip B were recorded from a dog with a history of six fainting episodes. These tracings were recorded after ocular pressure. Strip A paper speed: 25 mm/sec.

1. What is the rhythm diagnosis?
2. What is the best therapeutic approach?

Case 184

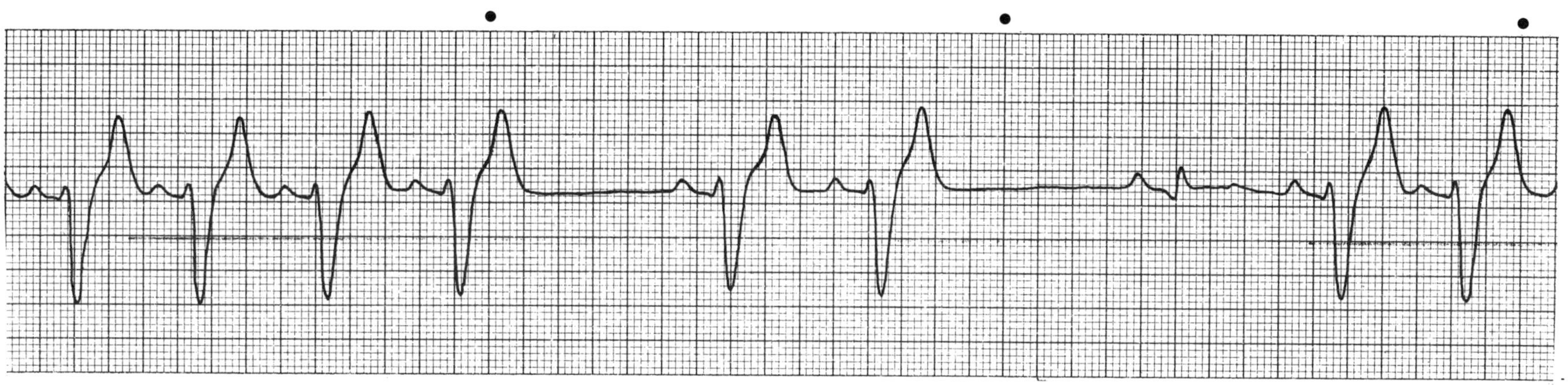

Question: This lead II ECG was obtained from a 10-year-old Irish Setter that was undergoing a geriatric screen.

1. What is the rhythm diagnosis?
2. What is the best therapeutic approach?

Case 183

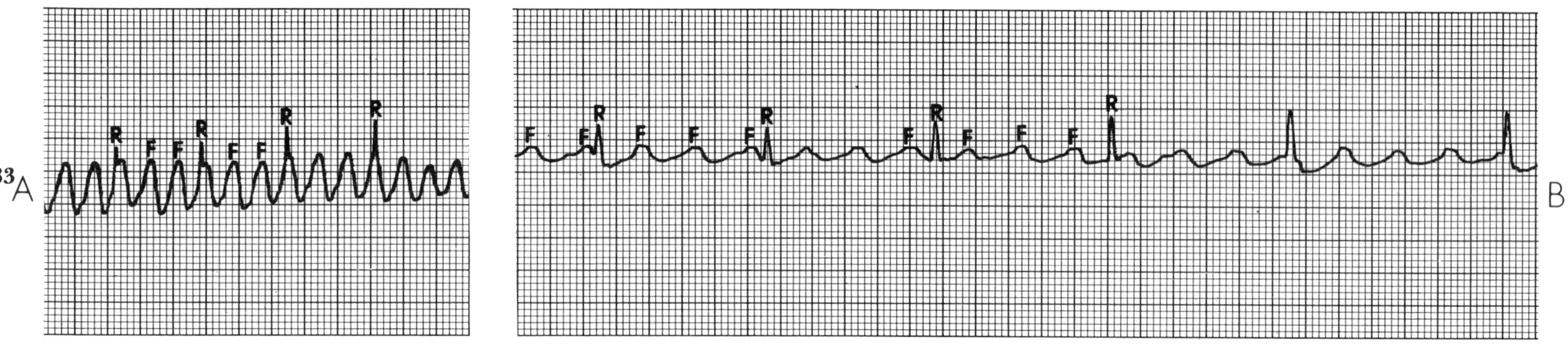

Answer: Atrial flutter at atrial rates of over 375 beats/min with varying degrees of conduction to the ventricles. Strip A at a paper speed of 25 mm/sec accentuates the sawtooth appearance of the flutter wave. Varying degrees of AV conduction are usually present. The atrial rhythm (F waves) is regular, with a rate usually greater than 300 beats/min. The ventricular rhythm and rate depend on the atrial rate and the state of AV conduction (same as atrial rate, 1 : 1 conduction; half the atrial rate, 2 : 1; 3 : 1; 4 : 1; etc.). By increasing vagal tone, AV nodal conduction slows. By slowing the ventricular rate, identification of flutter waves, ectopic P waves, or atrial fibrillatory waves may be made. The urgency of therapy depends on the ventricular rate, because fast ventricular rates usually cause heart failure, hypotension, or electrical instability. Digoxin is usually the drug of choice for atrial flutter. Low-energy precordial shock (cardioversion) usually converts atrial flutter. If the condition of the animal is critical, propranolol, verapamil, or adenosine may also be effective.

Case 184

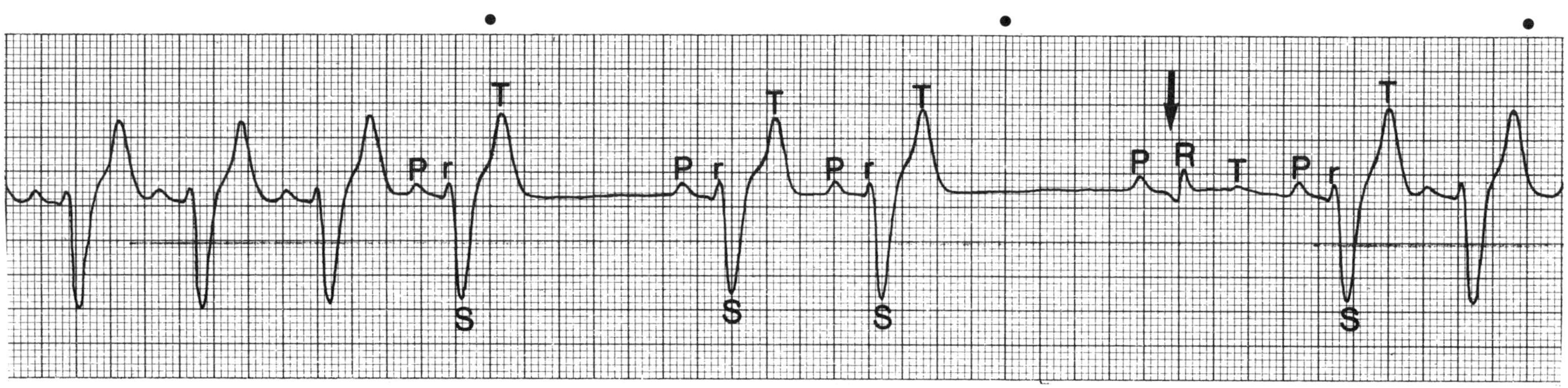

Answer: Sinus rhythm with intermittent right bundle-branch block. Heart rate is approximately 100 beats/min. No specific treatment exists for intermittent or sustained right bundle-branch block. Right bundle-branch block is typified by a prolonged duration of the QRS complex, a consistent P-R interval, deep and wide S waves in leads I, II, III, aVF, and left precordial chest leads, and a right-axis deviation pattern. Intermittent bundle-branch block that occurs with an increase in heart rate is also called acceleration or tachycardia-dependent aberrancy. The exact mechanism for this type of aberrancy is not known. The right bundle branch is able to function normally when the heart rate is slow and results in a sinus beat with normal conduction (arrow). Intermittent bundle-branch block is insignificant clinically but may cause confusion in the interpretation. The term "aberrancy" is applied to intraventricular conduction abnormalities of supraventricular impulses (premature or after a pause) that result in a widened, bizarre QRS complex. It is clinically important to distinguish aberrantly conducted beats from ventricular arrhythmias.

Case 185

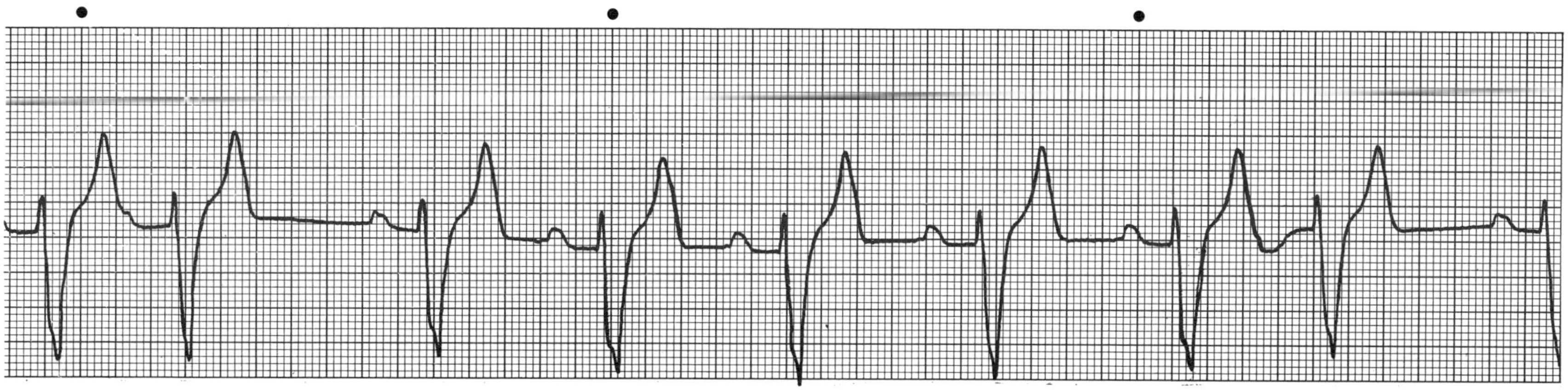

Question: This lead II ECG was obtained from a 9-year-old Beagle examined because of progressive coughing and exercise intolerance of 2 weeks' duration. A grade IV/VI holosystolic murmur was heard in the left fifth intercostal space, and pulmonary crackles (rales) were evident. Large, wide S waves were present in leads I, III, and aVF.

1. What is the rhythm diagnosis?
2. What is the best therapeutic approach?

Case 186

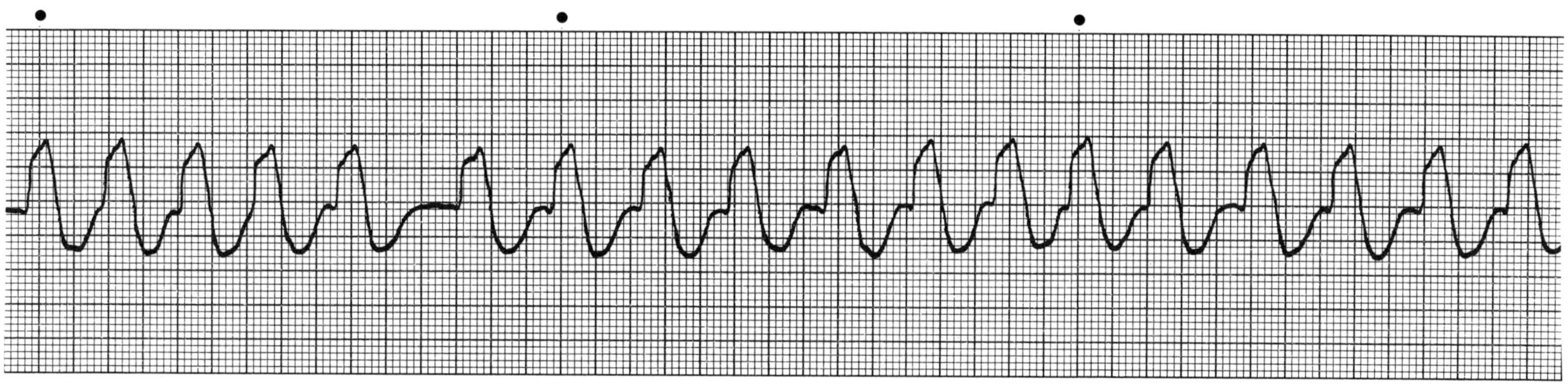

Question: This lead II ECG was obtained from a 5-year-old male Boxer with acute signs of dyspnea and syncope.

1. What is the rhythm diagnosis?
2. What is the most likely underlying disorder?
3. What is the best therapeutic approach?

Case 185

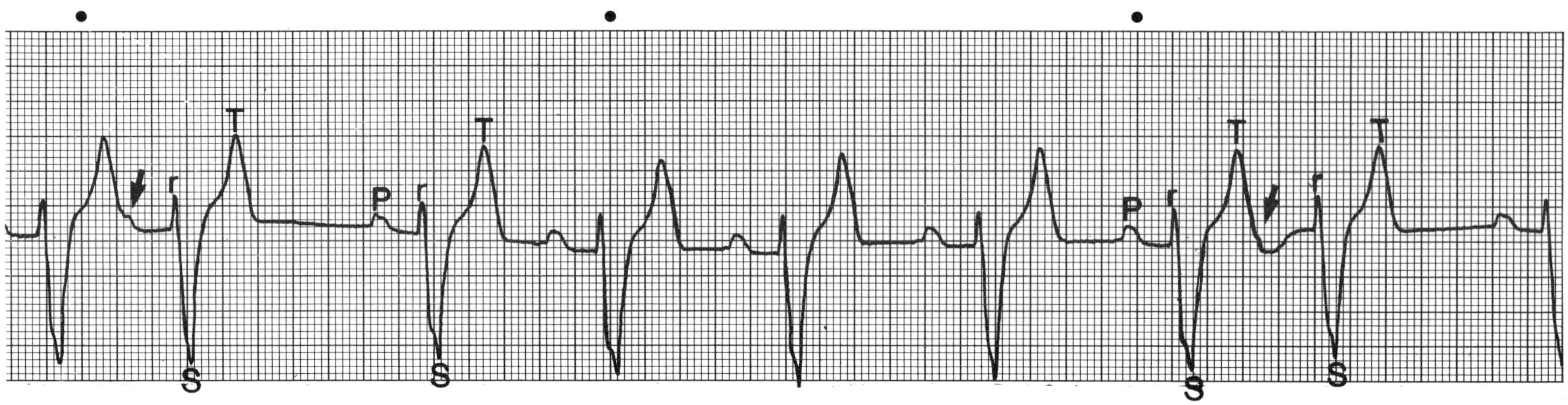

Answer: Sinus rhythm with atrial premature complexes and right bundle-branch block. Heart rate is approximately 120 beats/min. Digoxin can be administered to treat the atrial arrhythmia. A diuretic and vasodilator can be added if the radiographs reveal congestive heart failure. The criteria for right bundle-branch block include prolongation of the QRS complex (> 0.07 sec); consistent P-R interval; deep and wide S wave in leads I, II, III, aVF, and left precordial chest leads; and, usually, right-axis deviation pattern. Although the QRS complexes resemble ventricular premature complexes, the consistent P-R interval rules out ventricular arrhythmia. The atrial premature complexes are characterized by premature P waves (arrows) that are barely visible on the downslope of the T waves and by QRS complexes that resemble QRS complexes of the sinus beats in animals with right bundle-branch block.

Case 186

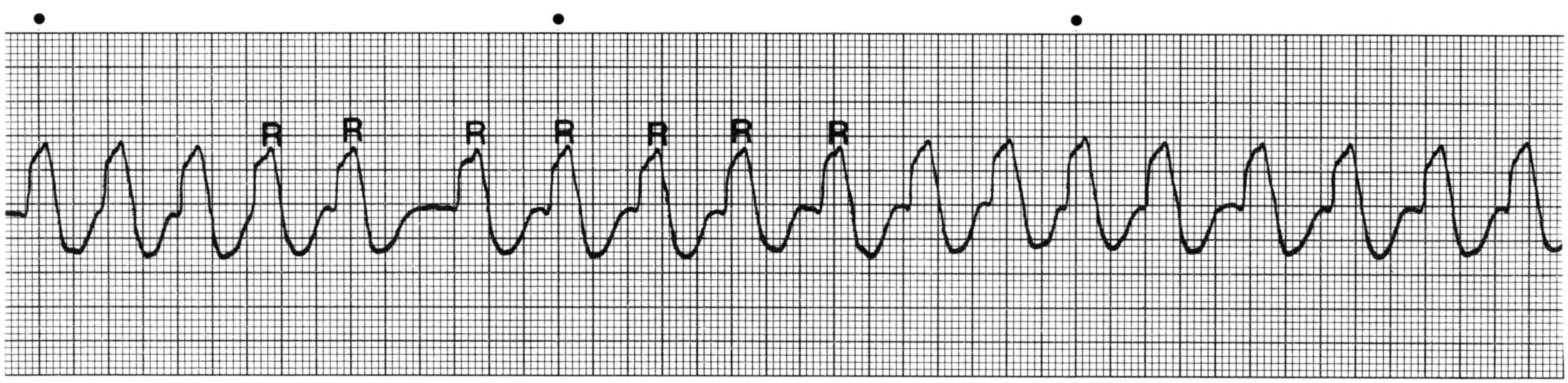

Answer: Atrial fibrillation with left bundle-branch block. Heart rate is 240 beats/min. Cardiomyopathy is the most likely underlying disorder. Digoxin is the recommended drug, especially if clinical signs of congestive heart failure are present. Without such evidence, diltiazem or propranolol is an alternative drug for treating atrial fibrillation. The rapid heart rate, lack of visible P waves, and irregularly irregular cardiac rhythm support the diagnosis of atrial fibrillation as the underlying rhythm. The prolonged duration of the QRS complexes (> 0.07 sec) and normal mean electrical axis are characteristics of left bundle-branch block. Left bundle-branch block must be differentiated from left ventricular enlargement. This wide complex tachyarrhythmia can easily be confused with ventricular tachycardia.

Case 187

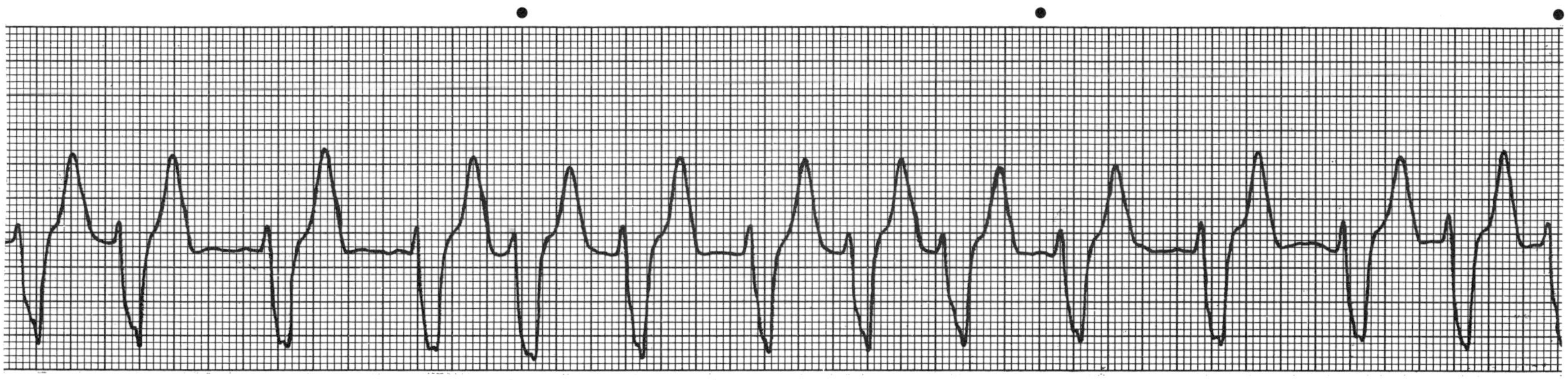

Question: A 3-year-old male Boxer with a history of difficult breathing and collapse was examined. An irregular heart rhythm was auscultated.

1. What is the rhythm diagnosis?
2. What is the most likely underlying disorder?
3. What is the best therapeutic approach?
4. What serious arrhythmia can be confused with this rhythm diagnosis?

Case 188

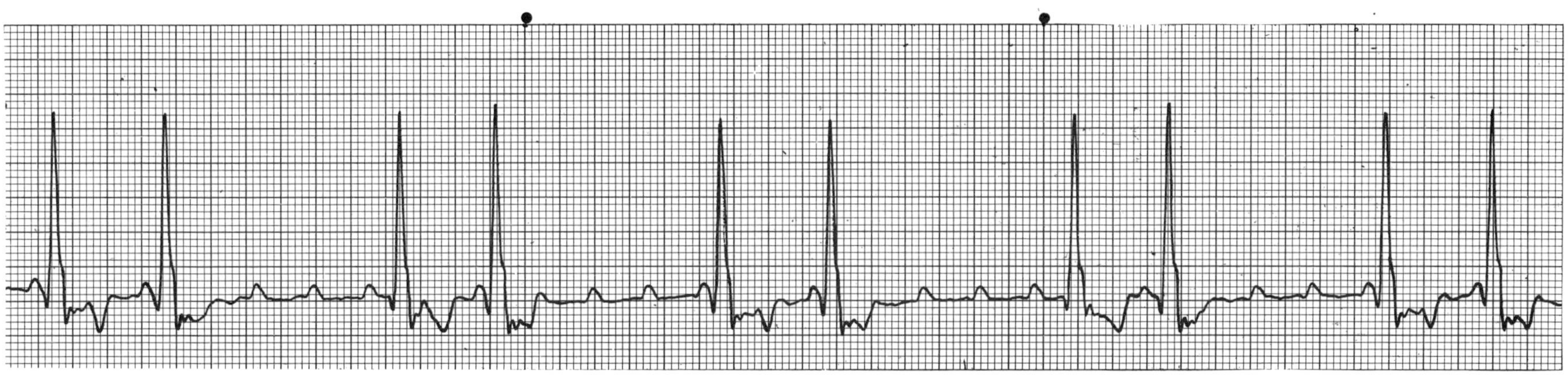

Question: This complex rhythm strip recorded from a dog could be explained by multiple interpretations, and many cardiologists would disagree as to which interpretation was correct. The diagnosis of complex arrhythmias and an understanding of the mechanisms are added stimulations, as well as frustrations, to clinicians with expertise in electrocardiography.

1. What is the rhythm diagnosis?
2. What are the possible mechanisms for this regular grouping of complexes?

Case 187

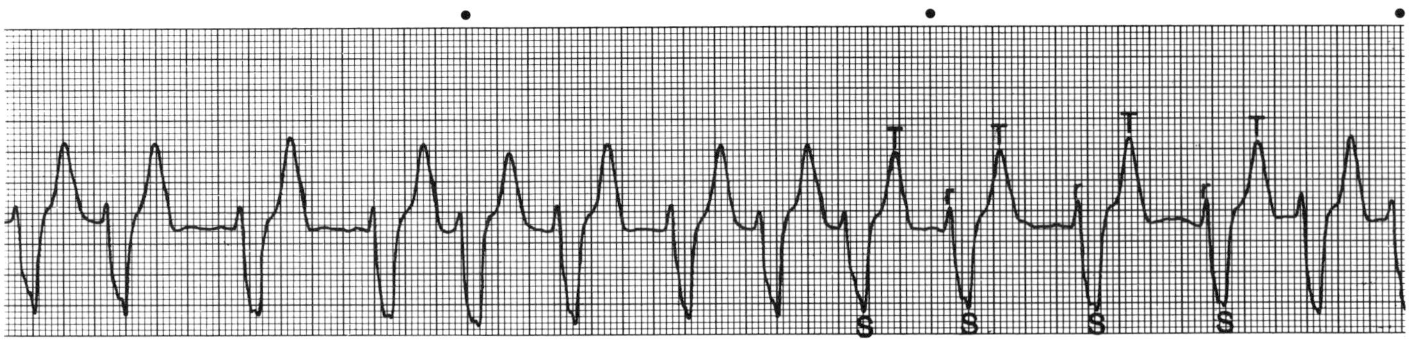

Answer: Atrial fibrillation with right bundle-branch block. Heart rate is 180 beats/min. Dilated cardiomyopathy is often associated with atrial fibrillation. Digoxin is the drug of choice for atrial fibrillation when the animal is in heart failure. Ventricular tachycardia is always on the differential diagnosis for wide complex tachycardia. In this instance, ventricular tachycardia was considered, but the rapid, irregularly irregular rhythm with no visible P waves supported a diagnosis of atrial fibrillation. Right bundle-branch block was suspected, because large, wide S waves were also present in leads I, III, and aVF. A lidocaine bolus can be administered to animals with suspected ventricular tachycardia. Lidocaine may increase the rate of AV conduction and adversely raise the ventricular rate in animals with atrial fibrillation. The differential diagnosis for wide complex tachycardia includes ventricular tachycardia, atrial tachycardia with pre-existent bundle-branch block or aberrant ventricular conduction, and ventricular pre-excitation. A His bundle electrogram and measurement of the H-V interval may be needed to differentiate some atrial from some ventricular wide complex tachycardias.

Case 188

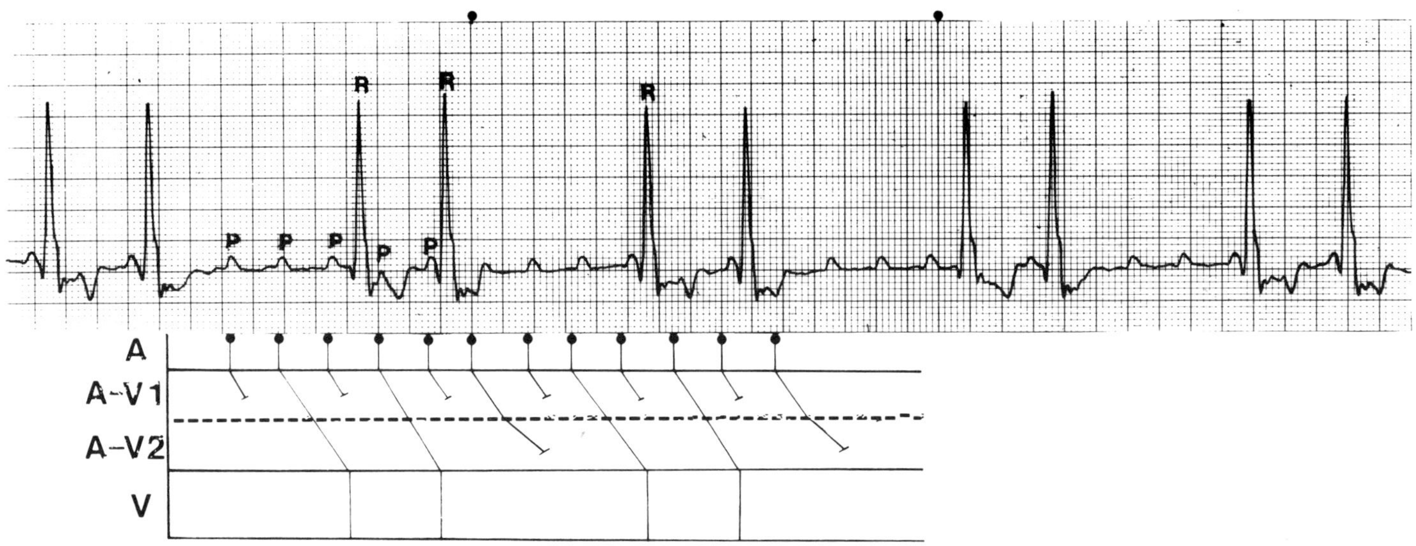

Answer: Atrial tachycardia with alternating 2 : 1 block at level 1 (upper portion) in the AV junction and 3:2 block at level 2 (lower portion) in the AV junction. Heart rate is variable. The ladder diagram technique for this strip should help to understand this complex arrhythmia. The grouping of complexes results from these two levels of block. Because the refractory period of the AV junction is longer than that of the atria, all the atrial impulses cannot be conducted to the ventricles. The usual 2 : 1 AV conduction is not caused by block, but by physiologic interference in the AV junction. AV conduction ratios greater than 2 : 1 are indicative of AV block. Two regions of block are most likely present with conduction ratios greater than 2 : 1. All impulses penetrate for the same distance into the upper portion of the AV junction, but only alternate impulses are transmitted to the lower portion. In the lower portion, another region of block may cause some of the arriving impulses to be dropped in a sequence. This block usually occurs with the Wenckebach phenomenon. Even-numbered conduction ratios, such as 2 : 1, are most common with atrial flutter or tachycardia, whereas odd-numbered conduction ratios are rare and suggest the presence of a pathologic conduction disturbance in the AV junction. Electrophysiologic studies are indicated to confirm these two regions of AV block. Paroxysmal atrial tachycardia with varying block at one level should also be considered.

Case 189

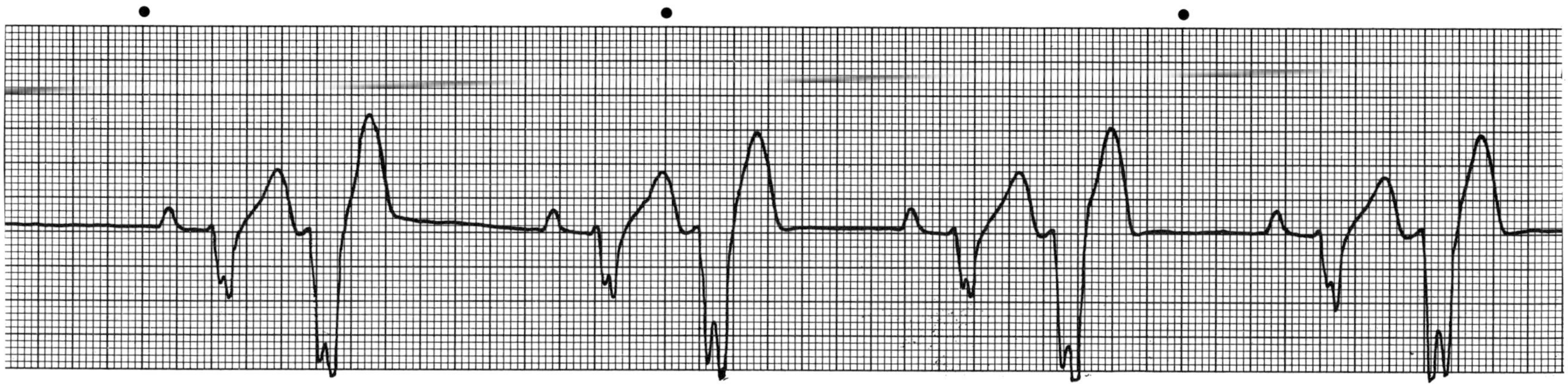

Question: This rhythm strip was obtained from a 7-year-old Beagle.

1. What is the rhythm diagnosis?
2. What is the best therapeutic approach?

Case 190

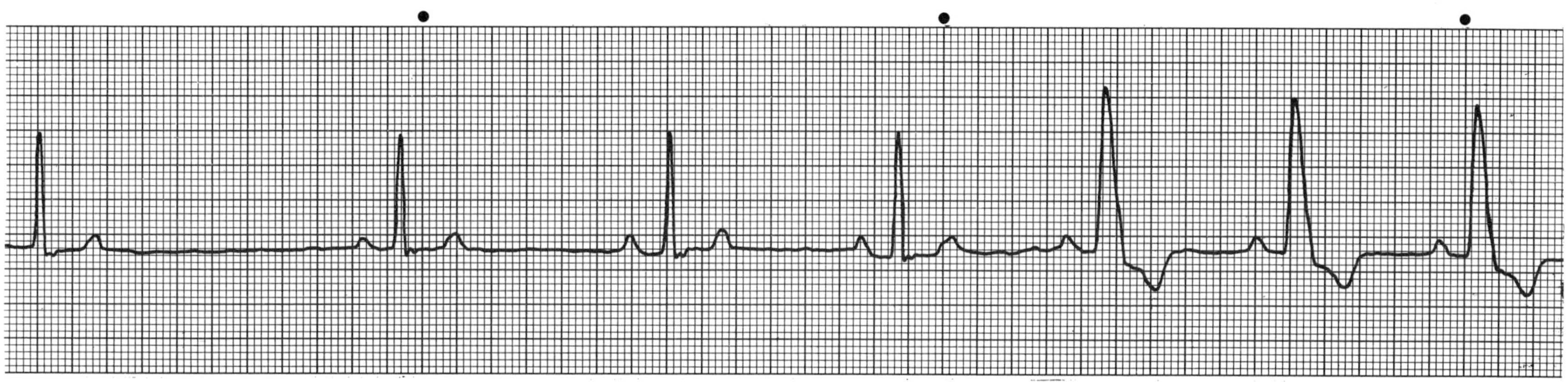

Question: This lead II ECG was obtained from a 10-year-old Irish Setter with no clinical signs that was examined because of low exercise intolerance.

1. What is the rhythm diagnosis?
2. What is the best therapeutic approach?

Case 189

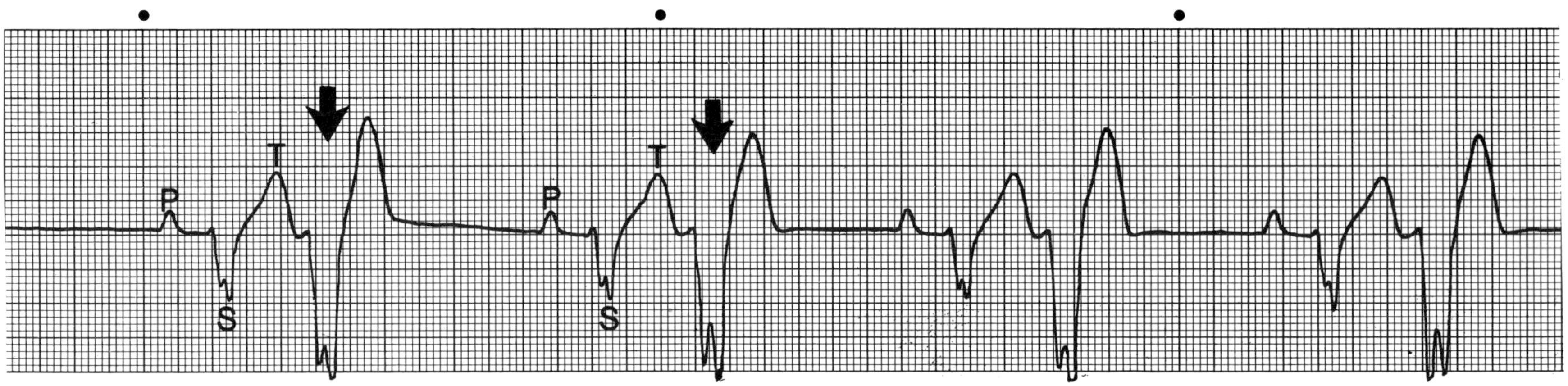

Answer: Sinus rhythm with ventricular bigeminy. Heart rate is approximately 120 beats/min. The sinus complexes are conducted with a right bundle-branch block pattern (leads I and III negative). A bigeminy pattern is present. The premature complexes (arrows) are similar to the sinus complexes, but are larger and wider. Atrial bigeminy with ventricular aberrancy should be considered as a possible diagnosis. The smaller, negative, wide QRS complexes can also be confused with ventricular premature complexes, but the consistent P-R interval supports sinus complexes with right bundle-branch block. The sinus complexes also are not premature. In this dog, lidocaine converted the rhythm to a sinus rhythm. This response supports the diagnosis of ventricular bigeminy. The arrhythmia was controlled with procainamide.

Case 190

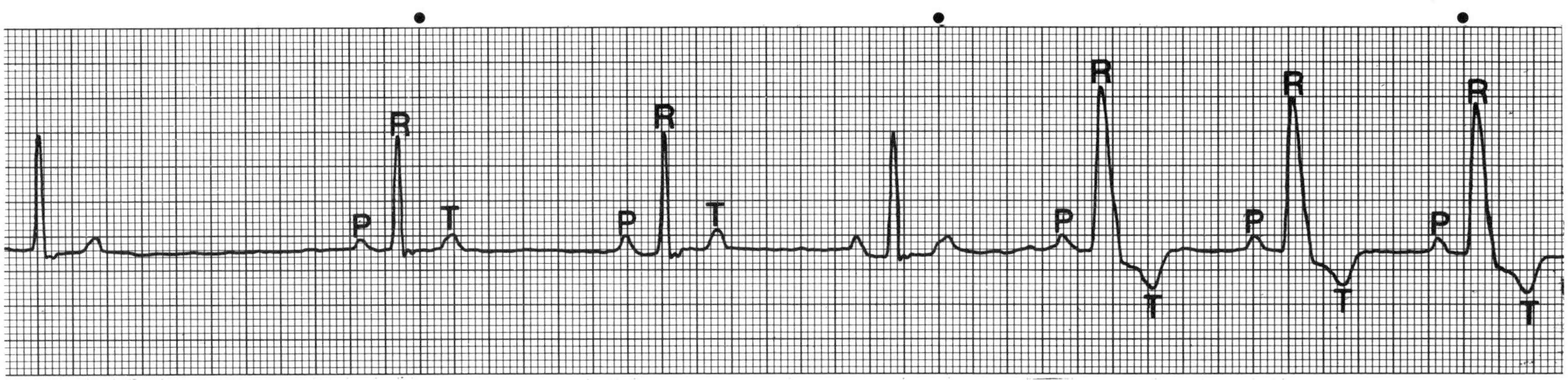

Answer: Sinus arrhythmia with intermittent, rate-dependent left bundle-branch block. Heart rate is approximately 80 to 100 beats/min. No treatment is required. As the rate of impulse transmission through the His-Purkinje system increases, the refractory period of the bundle branch normally decreases. Above a critical rate, impulses may find either the right or the left bundle branches incompletely repolarized, thus blocking the impulse conduction to the ventricular myocardium. Typically, the right bundle branch has a refractory period longer than that of the left bundle branch. Conversely, as in this dog, pathologic changes in the heart may cause a crossover of bundle-branch refractoriness, with the left bundle having a refractory period longer than that of the right bundle. The left bundle-branch block pattern occurred suddenly at a heart rate of 100 beats/min. The 3 wide and bizarre QRS complexes (last 3 complexes) can be confused with a run of ventricular premature complexes, but the consistent P-R interval supports conducted P-QRS-T complexes. The criteria for left bundle-branch block include QRS complexes of prolonged duration (> 0.07 sec) and absence of left ventricular enlargement on thoracic radiographs.

Case 191

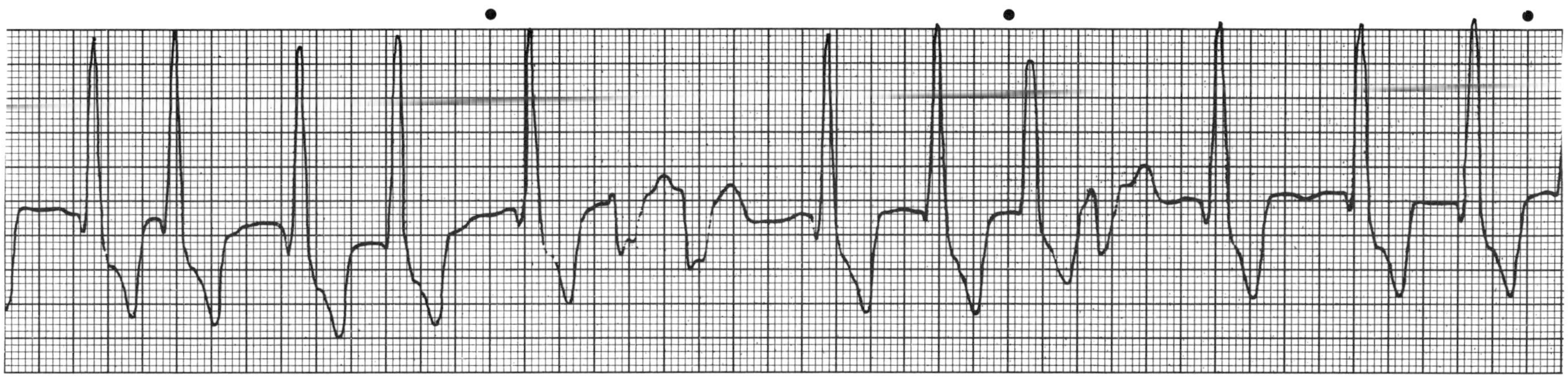

Question: This lead II rhythm strip was recorded from a 5-year-old female Doberman Pinscher that had a history of coughing.

1. What is the rhythm diagnosis?
2. What is the most likely underlying disorder?
3. What is the best therapeutic approach?
4. What is the prognosis?

Case 192

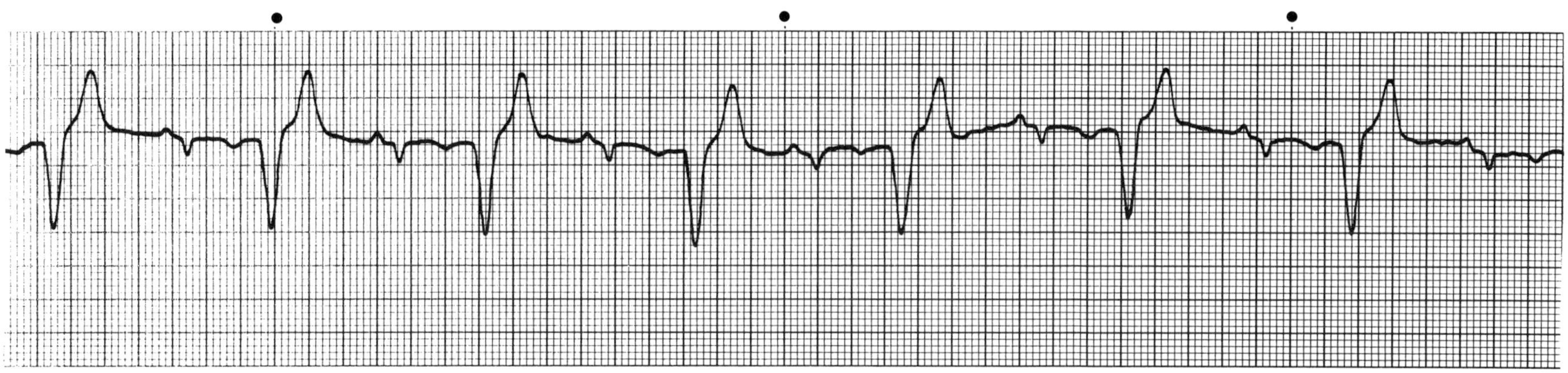

Question: This ECG was recorded from a cat that had been hit by a car.

1. What is the rhythm diagnosis?
2. What is the best therapeutic approach?

Case 191

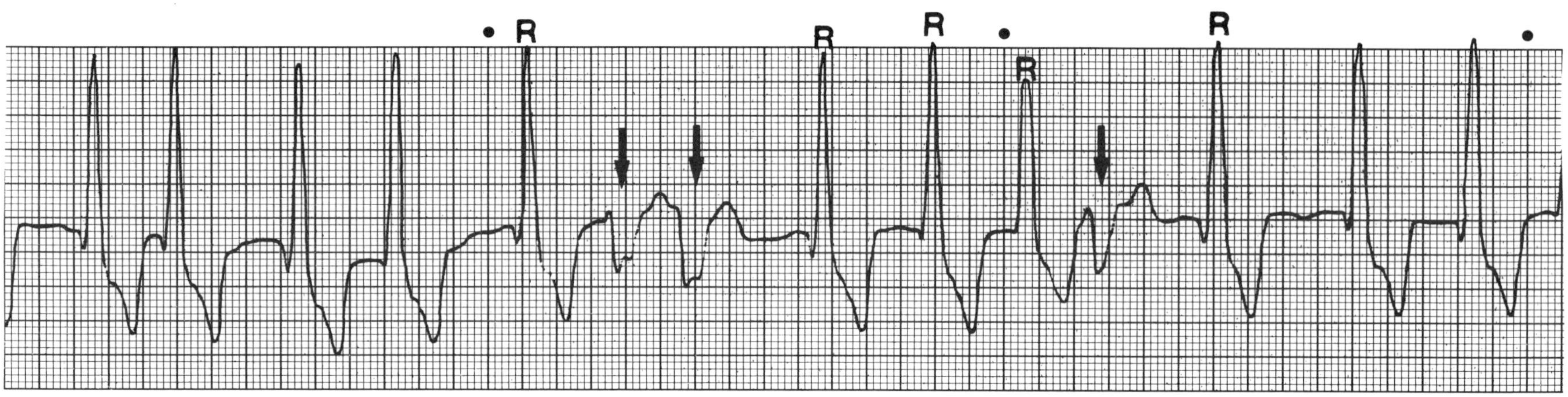

Answer: Atrial fibrillation with ventricular premature complexes. Heart rate is approximately 200 beats/min. Atrial fibrillation is characterized by a rapid, irregularly irregular rhythm without P waves. Ventricular premature complexes are also present (arrows). Differential diagnosis for these negative complexes should include aberrantly conducted supraventricular beats. The cycle preceding the two negative complexes is longer than the previous R-R interval and resets the Purkinje system with a longer refractory period. The right bundle branch has a refractory period longer than that of the left bundle. A long cycle followed by a short cycle may result in a supraventricular impulse that is conducted aberrantly in a right bundle-branch block pattern (often termed Ashman's phenomenon). A His bundle ECG would be required to differentiate between ventricular premature complexes and aberrant ventricular conduction. Dilated cardiomyopathy is the most likely diagnosis on the basis of ECG, history, and signalment. Atrial fibrillation in this dog should be treated with digoxin. If radiographs confirm congestive heart failure, furosemide and a vasodilator should be prescribed. The ECG should be repeated in 5 to 7 days. If the heart rate is greater than 160 beats/min, either propranolol or diltiazem should be added to the treatment regimen. If the ventricular arrhythmia worsens, procainamide, tocainide, or mexiletine should be added. Quinidine is not recommended because it may cause digoxin toxicity. The prognosis is poor. The owners should be alerted to the possibility of sudden death.

Case 192

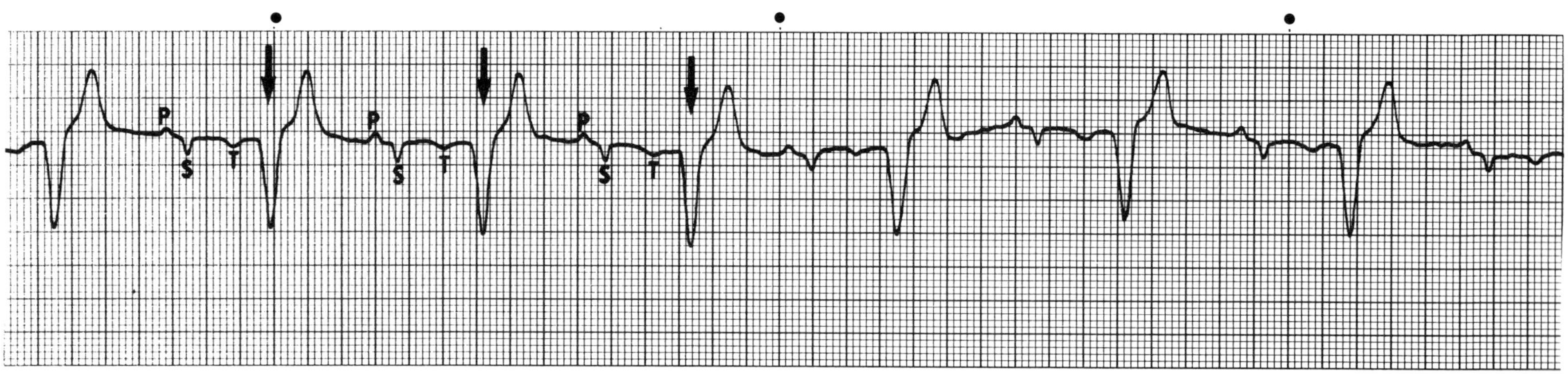

Answer: Ventricular bigeminy. Heart rate is approximately 190 beats/min. Ventricular premature complexes (arrows every other beat in this case) are impulses that arise from an ectopic focus in the ventricles. They spread through both ventricles with delay, thereby causing a bizarre widened QRS complex. The repetitive coupling of a ventricular premature complex to consecutive sinus beats is known as ventricular bigeminy. If every third complex is a ventricular premature complex, the rhythm is called ventricular trigeminy. The presumed mechanism for these rhythms is re-entry of the impulse through a portion of ventricular tissue. The compensatory pause following the ventricular premature complex tends to favor the occurrence of another ventricular premature complex, and thus, once initiated, ventricular bigeminy tends to be self sustained (the rule of bigeminy). Ventricular premature complexes rarely require aggressive treatment in the cat because they tend to decrease and often disappear spontaneously. Supportive measures are important. Shock therapy in this cat resulted in a normal sinus rhythm within 3 hours.

Case 193

A 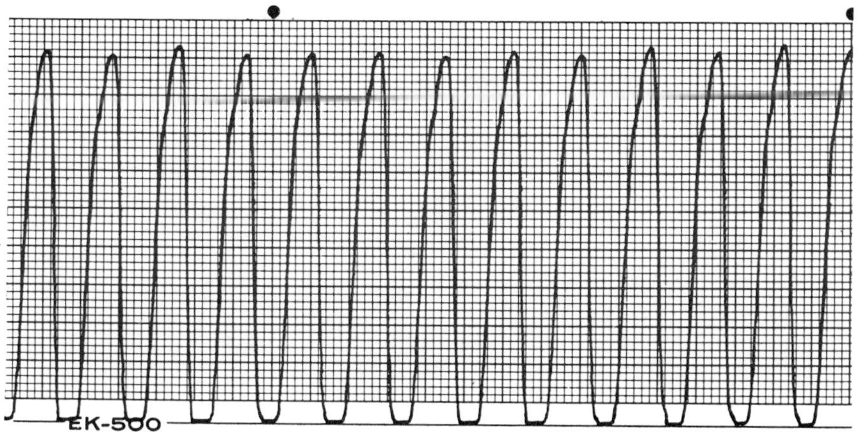

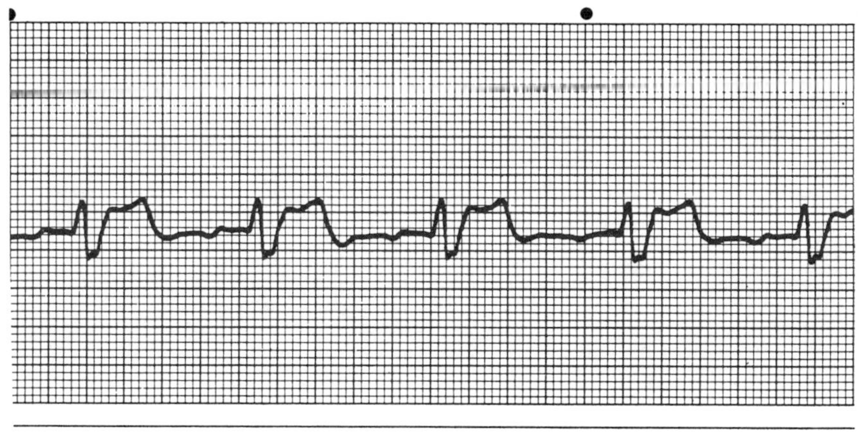 B

Question: Strip A was recorded from a dog with an acute onset of collapse preceded by 2 days of vomiting and diarrhea. Strip B was recorded after an intravenous cardiac drug was given.

1. What are the differential diagnoses for the tachycardia in strip A?
2. What drug was given?
3. What are the abnormalities in strip B?

Case 194

A 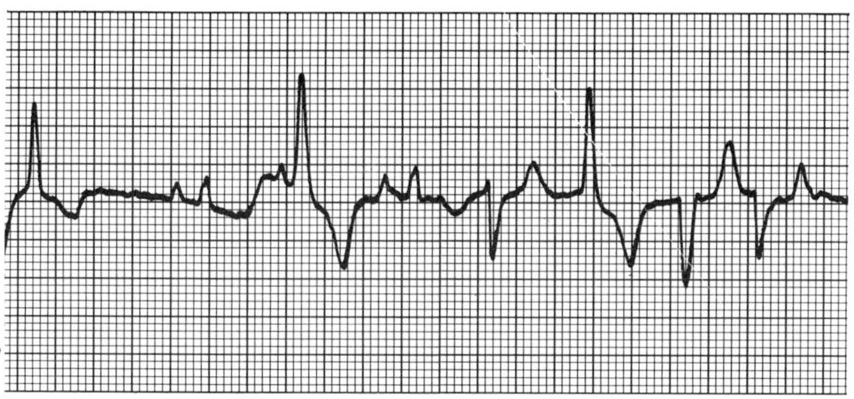

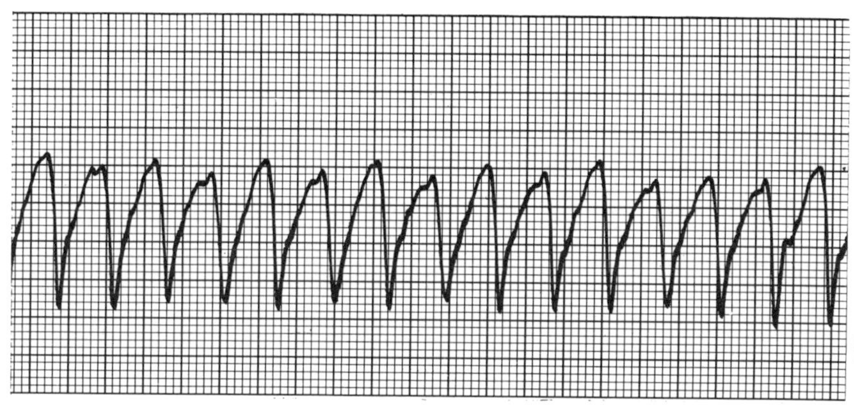 B

Question: This series of ECG rhythm strips was recorded from a cat with episodes of fainting.

1. What is the rhythm diagnosis?
2. What are the hemodynamic effects of this cardiac abnormality in rhythm?

Case 193

A

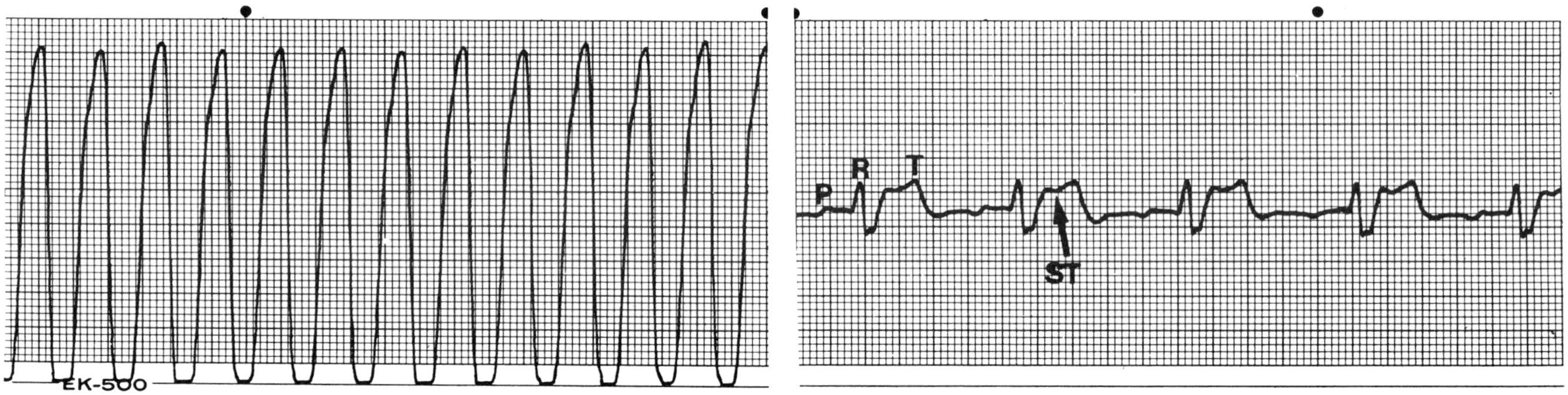

B

Answer: A. Ventricular flutter. B. Normal sinus rhythm (after lidocaine injection). The rhythm is regular and rapid with extremely bizarre QRS complexes. No P waves can be seen. The boundary between the QRS complexes, S-T segment, and T wave is unclear so that each entire complex appears to be a continuous loop. Differential diagnoses should also include supraventricular tachycardia (e.g., atrial tachycardia) with bundle-branch block, aberrant QRS complex, Wolff-Parkinson-White syndrome, or nonspecific QRS widening (hyperkalemia/acidosis, or severe left heart enlargement). The clinical significance of ventricular flutter is almost the same as that of ventricular fibrillation. The first treatment of choice for ventricular flutter is the intravenous infusion of lidocaine. Direct current shock may be required. The small P waves and S-T segment elevation after injection of lidocaine probably represent electrolyte abnormalities and/or hypoxia. The increased duration of the QRS complex may represent an intraventricular conduction defect. An intravenous drip of lidocaine should be continued, and a biochemistry blood profile should be carefully evaluated. Procainamide or quinidine also can be started when the dog is stable.

Case 194

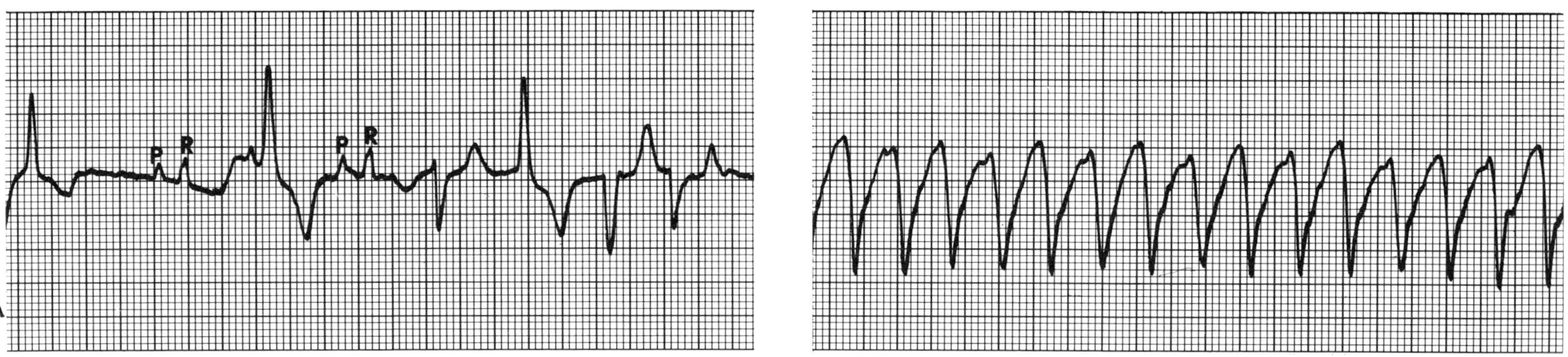

A

B

Answer: A and B. Ventricular tachycardia. Heart rate is variable. Strip A reveals a multiform (varying configuration of ventricular premature complexes) paroxysmal ventricular tachycardia. The second and fourth complexes (P-R) are capture complexes. Strip B, recorded at a different time, reveals a ventricular tachycardia that is now an "active" rhythm resulting from the repetitive firing of one ectopic ventricular focus at a rapid rate. A supraventricular tachycardia with abnormal QRS complexes should be considered, but the contour of the capture complexes in strip A is different from that of the ectopic complexes in strip B. Ventricular tachycardia in the cat is considered the most serious of all tachyarrhythmias. Severe underlying disease is usually present. Physical examination reveals weak pulses as the cardiac output is decreased. A reduction in cardiac output is of great significance when the cat has pre-existing heart disease.

Case 195

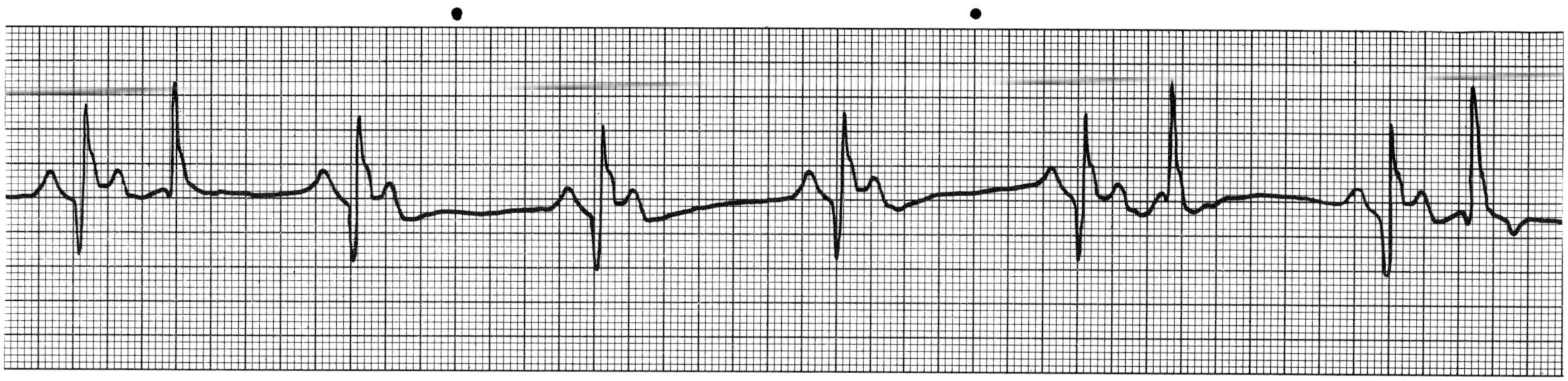

Question: This complex lead II rhythm strip was recorded from a Golden Retriever with aortic stenosis.

1. What is the rhythm diagnosis?
2. What is the best therapeutic approach?

Case 196

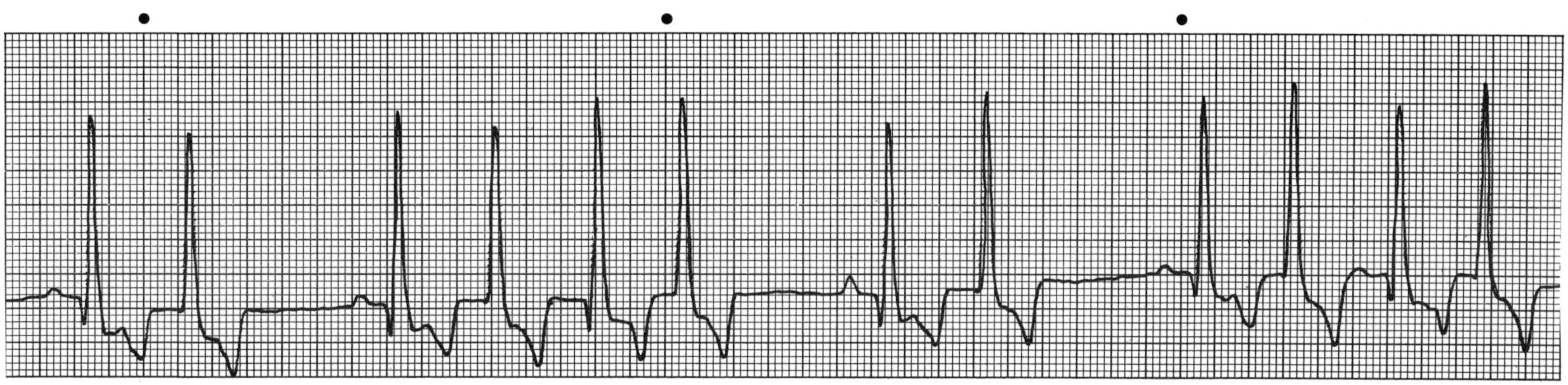

Question: This lead II ECG was obtained from an 11-year-old Miniature Poodle with progressive mitral valvular insufficiency and a chief complaint of coughing.

1. What is the rhythm diagnosis?
2. What is the best therapeutic approach?

Case 195

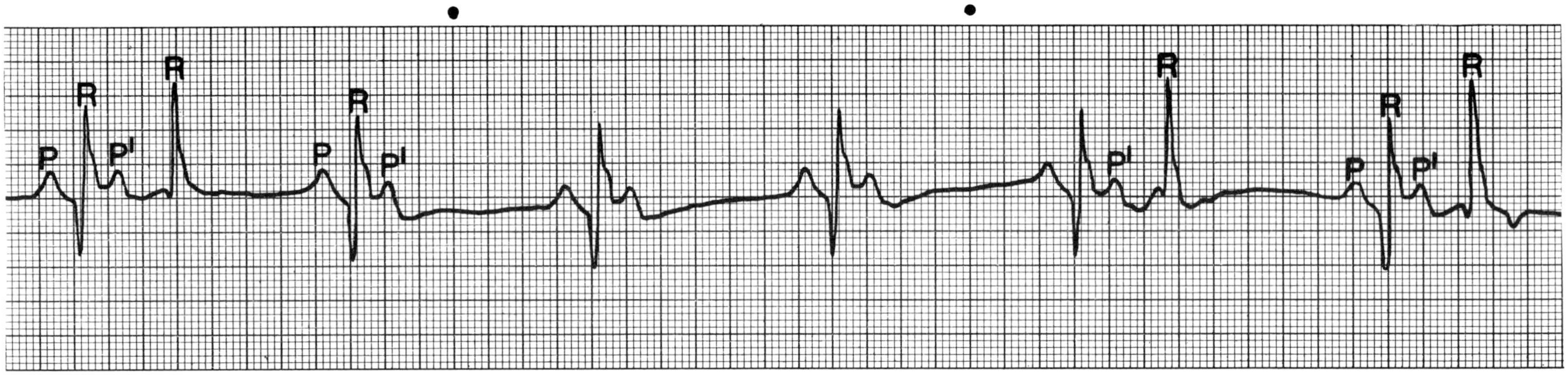

Answer: Blocked atrial premature complexes. Atrial premature complexes with aberrant intraventricular conduction. Heart rate is variable. Blocked atrial premature complexes coupled to sinus QRS complexes occur when the coupling interval is sufficiently short so that the AV node–His-Purkinje system is refractory to conduction of premature impulses. Ectopic P′ waves distort the S-T segment or T wave of each sinus QRS complex. Aberrant ventricular conduction results when an atrial premature complex (beats 2, 7, 9) conducts to the ventricle with the QRS complex morphology that is different from that of the normal sinus QRS. The atrial premature complex conducts normally down the AV node and His bundle, but because of the prematurity, a portion of the bundle-branch system has not recovered its ability to conduct. Conduction therefore is blocked in the unrecovered (refractory) area. Conduction does proceed through the remaining recovered tissue to the ventricle. Aberrant conduction can thus be thought of as a functional bundle-branch block or conduction delay. Treatment is the same for atrial premature complexes. Aberrant complexes must be differentiated from ventricular ectopic complexes because each condition is usually treated differently and may have a different prognosis.

Case 196

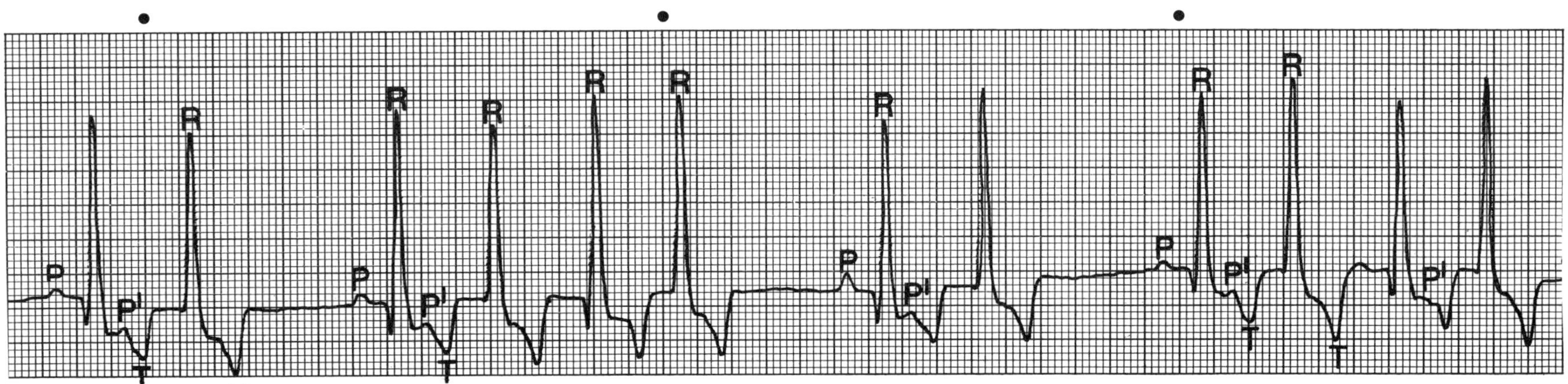

Answer: Sinus rhythm with intermittent runs of multifocal atrial premature complexes. Heart rate is approximately 140 beats/min. Digoxin is the drug of choice for this atrial arrhythmia, along with a diuretic and vasodilator for treatment of probable congestive heart failure. Thoracic radiographs should be taken. The premature QRS complexes of differing intervals that resemble the QRS complexes of the sinus beats support the diagnosis of multifocal atrial premature complexes. The premature P′ waves are fused and obscured in the preceding T waves. Arrhythmias can cause or aggravate congestive heart failure.

Case 197

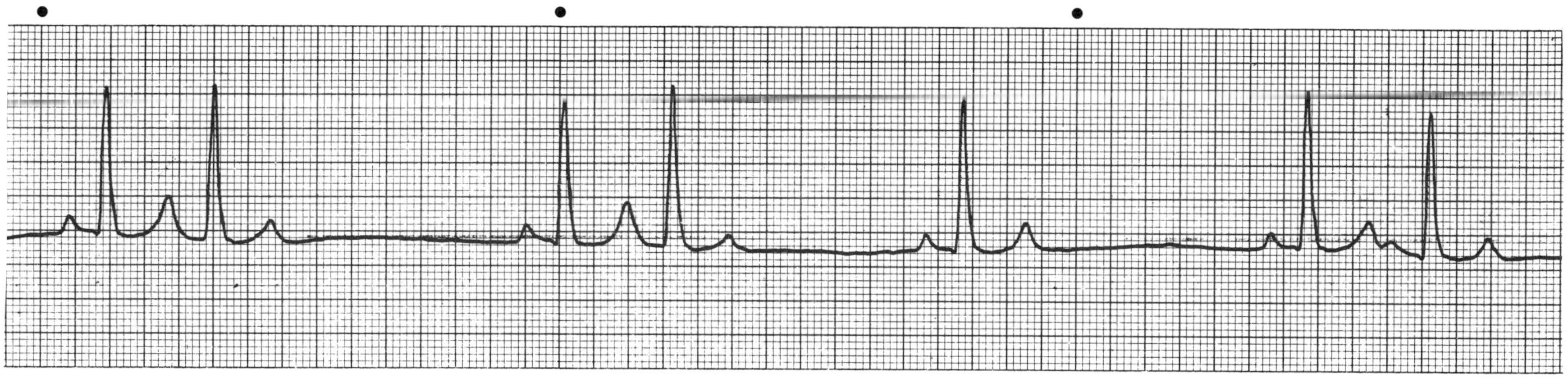

Question: This ECG was obtained from a 5-year-old female Cocker Spaniel during routine physical examination.

1. What is the rhythm diagnosis?
2. What are the common causes of this arrhythmia?
3. What is the best therapeutic approach?

Case 198

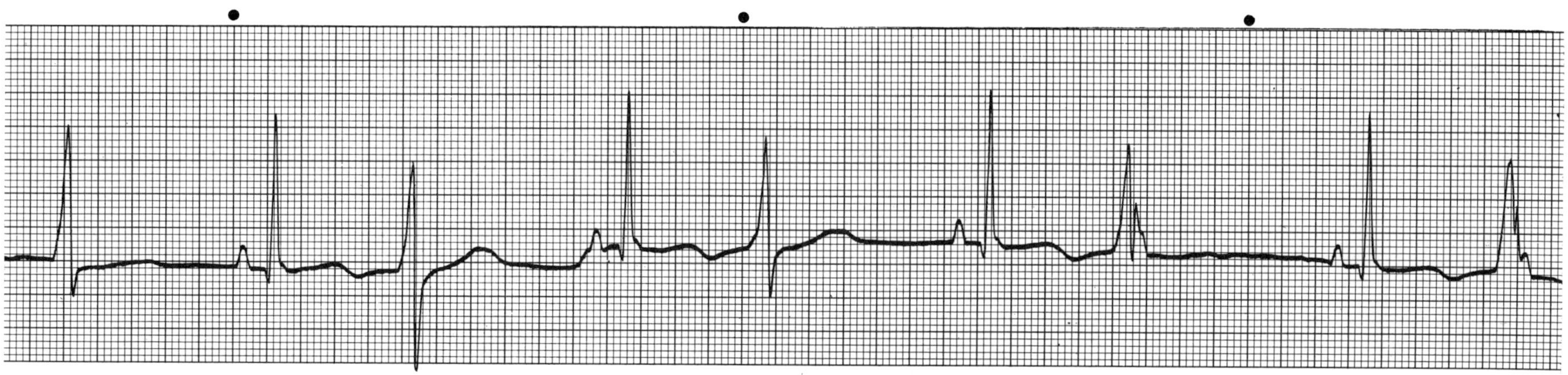

Question: This rhythm strip was recorded from a 7-year-old Poodle with no clinical signs. An arrhythmia was noticed on routine physical examination. A murmur does not exist, and the lungs sound clear.

1. What is the rhythm diagnosis?
2. What is the best therapeutic approach?

Case 197

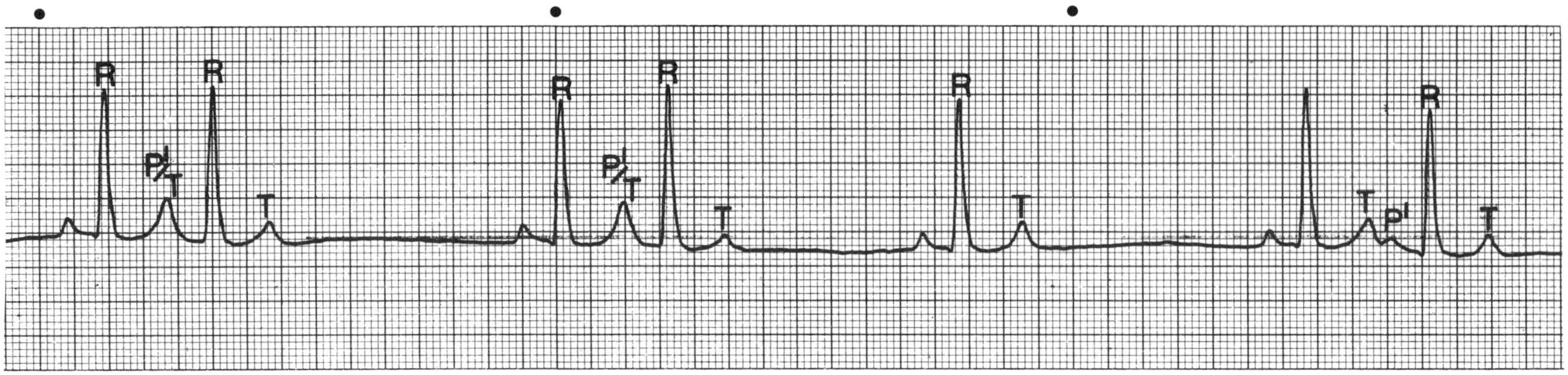

Answer: Sinus rhythm with frequent atrial premature complexes. Heart rate is approximately 100 beats/min. The T waves preceding the first two atrial premature complexes are longer than the T wave of the one isolated sinus complex. The T waves are longer because of the superimposed premature P′ waves. The premature P′ wave of the last atrial premature complex comes slightly later, so the preceding T wave can be clearly distinguished from the P′ wave. Atrial premature complexes frequently accompany atrial distention and disease. The history does not reveal underlying problems. Thoracic radiographs would be indicated to assess heart size. Although the atrial premature complexes occur frequently, the overall heart rate is normal and the dog has no clinical signs. Therefore, treatment is not recommended at this time.

Case 198

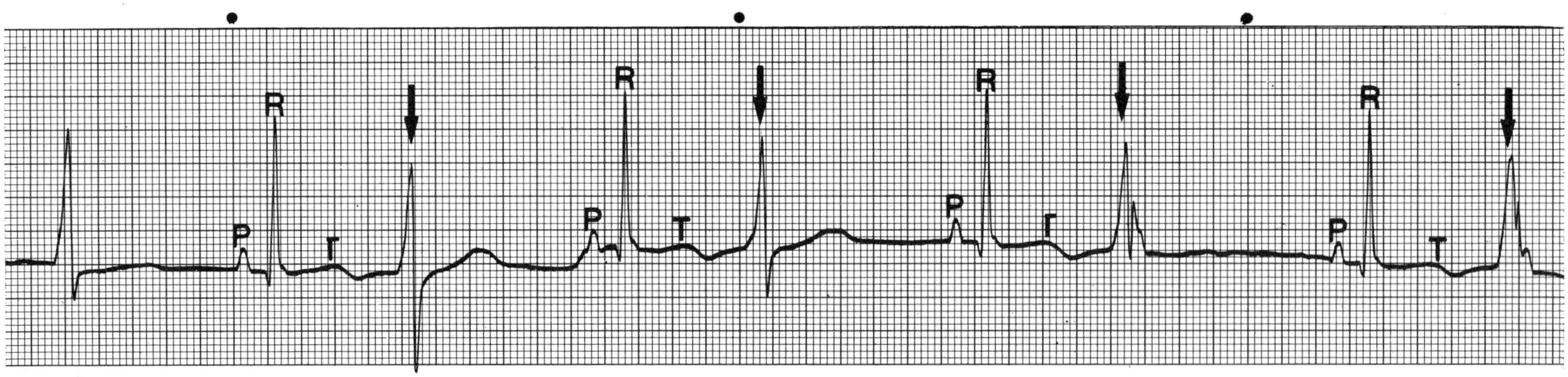

Answer: Sinus rhythm with periods of ventricular bigeminy. Heart rate is 120 beats/min. Ventricular premature complexes (arrows) occur every other complex (ventricular bigeminy). Differential diagnoses for the arrhythmia include myocarditis, neoplastic infiltration, and scarring of the myocardium. Thoracic radiography is recommended, and echocardiography should be performed if the heart is enlarged or the arrhythmia persists. A biochemical blood profile should be done. The best therapeutic approach for this dog is controversial. Although the ventricular premature complexes are frequent, the dog has no clinical signs, and ventricular tachycardia is not evident. All class I antiarrhythmic agents (e.g., procainamide and quinidine) have been shown to have proarrhythmic potential, and in some human studies, certain class I drugs (e.g., flecainide and encainide) have been shown to increase mortality. Therefore, treatment of the arrhythmia in this dog is not recommended. The owner should watch for exercise intolerance, weakness, and collapse. If signs develop, treatment then should be initiated, especially if radiographic or echocardiographic evidence reveals underlying cardiac disease.

Case 199

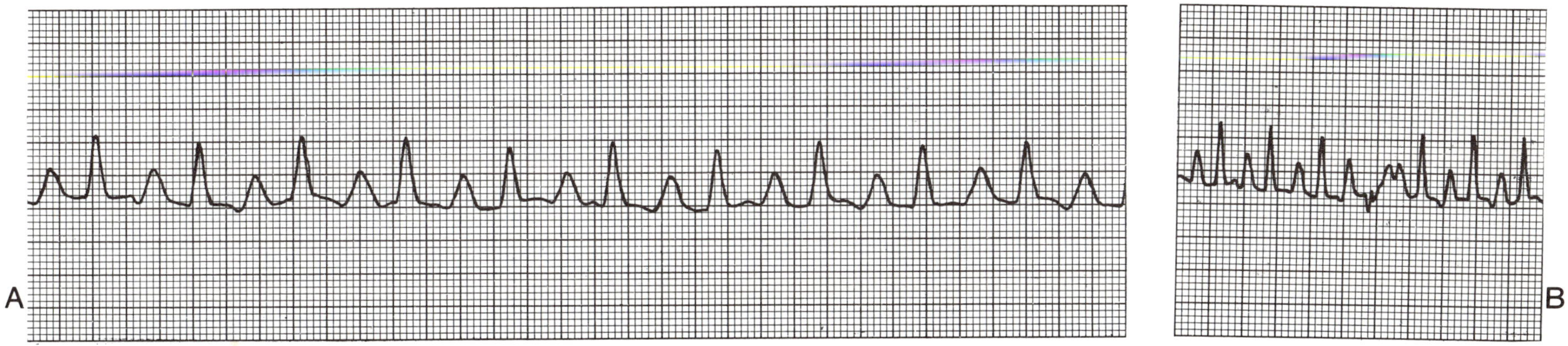

Question: This lead II ECG was obtained from a 2-year-old male Great Dane that was examined because of a history of dyspnea and severe exercise intolerance. Strip A and strip B were recorded sequentially. Strip A paper speed: 50 mm/sec; strip B paper speed: 25 mm/sec.

1. What is the rhythm diagnosis in strip A and strip B?
2. What is the most likely underlying disorder?
3. What is the best therapeutic approach?

Case 200

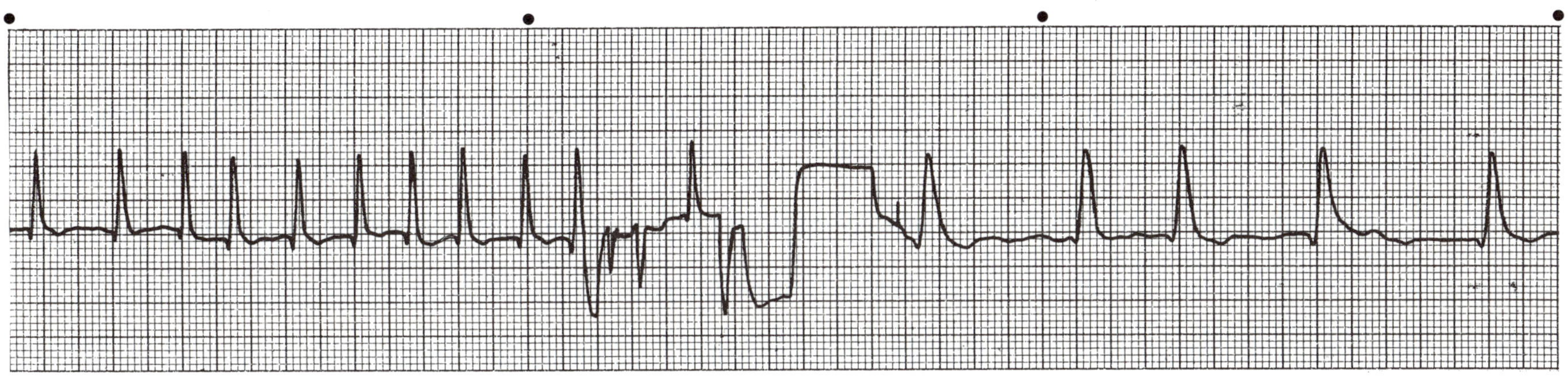

Question: This tracing was obtained from a lethargic 4-year-old Irish Wolfhound.

1. What is the rhythm diagnosis?
2. What is the most likely underlying disorder?
3. What is the best therapeutic approach?
4. What cautions should be given to the owners?

Case 199

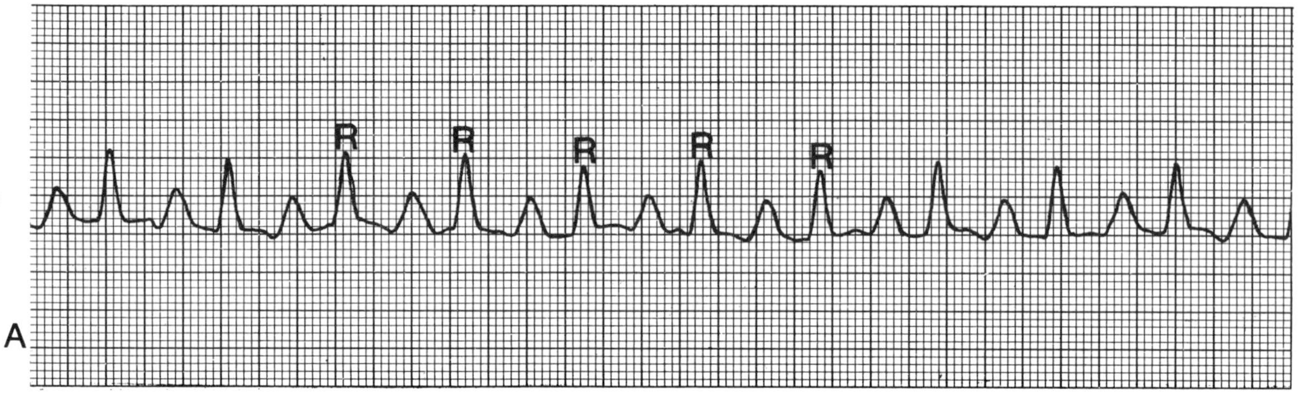

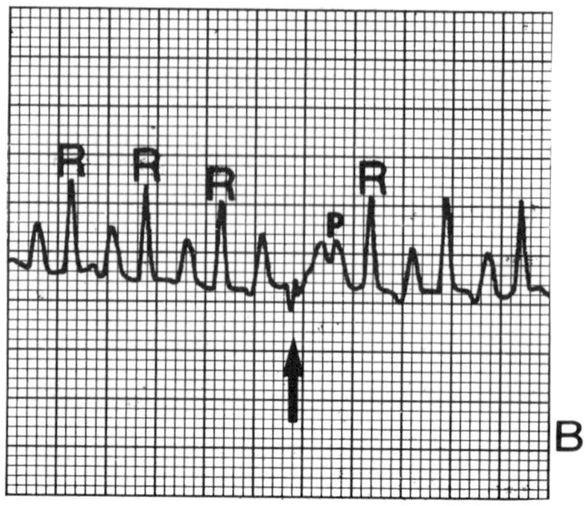

Answer: A. Supraventricular tachycardia. B. Supraventricular tachycardia with one ventricular premature complex (arrow). Heart rate is approximately 190 beats/min. Dilated cardiomyopathy is the most likely underlying disorder. Administration of digoxin, a diuretic, and of an angiotensin converting enzyme inhibitor is the best therapeutic approach. The QRS complexes seen in strip A appear wide, and the P waves are not discernible. Accordingly, the rhythm can be confused with ventricular tachycardia. In strip B, the negative ventricular premature complex interrupts the tachycardia. The T wave following the ventricular premature complex (arrow) is slightly separated from the following P wave, which precedes the next positive QRS complex. This finding indicates that the rhythm is supraventricular rather than ventricular in origin. Supraventricular tachycardia must be differentiated from ventricular tachycardia because of the differences in therapy and prognosis for each condition.

Case 200

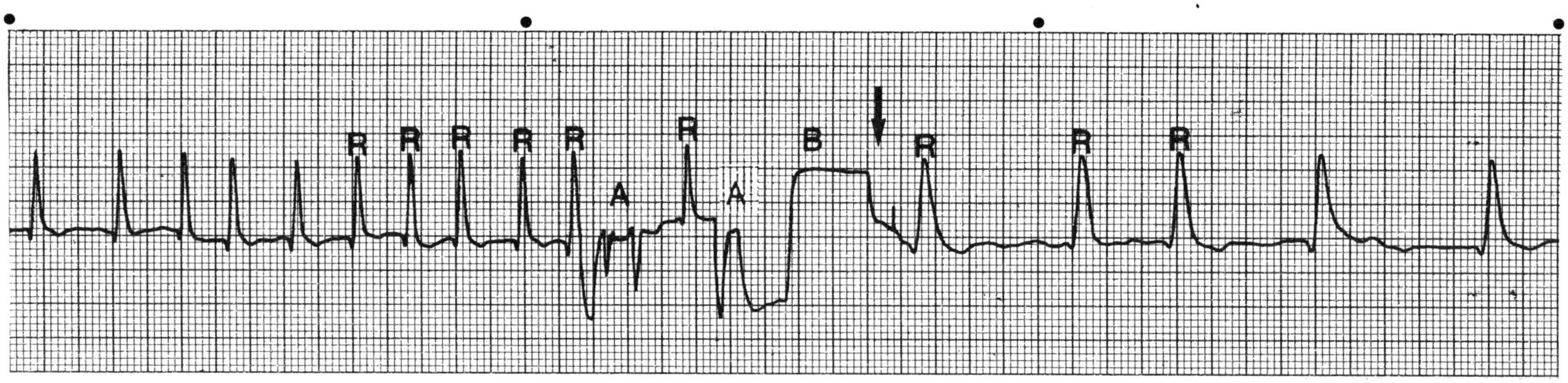

Answer: Atrial fibrillation. Heart rate is approximately 170 beats/min. Atrial fibrillation is characterized by a rapid, irregularly irregular rhythm and the absence of P waves. Movement artifact is present (A). The standardization button was depressed in the middle of the strip (B). The paper speed was changed from 25 mm/sec to 50 mm/sec at the arrow. The slower paper speed accounts for the narrower complexes in the first half of the strip. The history of lethargy and atrial fibrillation in this breed strongly suggests dilated cardiomyopathy. Digoxin should be used to slow the rate of atrial fibrillation. A return to sinus rhythm in this dog is unlikely. Congestive heart failure may eventually develop. In this breed, atrial fibrillation can also be a relatively benign arrhythmia not associated with cardiomyopathy or clinical signs. Digoxin is used in this dog because the heart rate is > 160 beats/min.